MICROCIRCULATION REVISITED - FROM MOLECULES TO CLINICAL PRACTICE

Edited by **Helena Lenasi**

Microcirculation Revisited - From Molecules to Clinical Practice
http://dx.doi.org/10.5772/61893
Edited by Helena Lenasi

Contributors

Cathryn Kolka, Radu Badea, Attila Tama Szora, Alexandru Florin Badea, Iulian Opincariu, Mihai A. Socaciu, Robert Schier, Matija Zupan, Diogo André Fonseca, Pedro Antunes, Maria Dulce Cotrim, Ian Wright, Rebecca Dyson, Darinca Carmen Todea, Mariana Miron, Silvana Cânjău, Bogdan Vitez, Gheorghe Nodiţi, Leoné Malan, Gavin W Lambert, Roland Von Kaenel, Nicolaas T Malan, Wayne Smith, Walthard Vilser, Nina Eikelis, Manja Reimann, Claudio Aguayo, Estefania Nova-Lamperti, Felipe Zuñiga, Valeska Ormazabal, Carlos Escudero, Ines Drenjančević, Helena Lenasi

Published by InTech

Janeza Trdine 9, 51000 Rijeka, Croatia

Publishing Process Manager Andrea Koric

Technical Editor SPi Global

Cover InTech Design team

First published November, 2016

Printed in Croatia

Additional hard copies can be obtained from orders@intechopen.com

Microcirculation Revisited - From Molecules to Clinical Practice, Edited by Helena Lenasi

p. cm.

Print ISBN 978-953-51-2730-7
Online ISBN 978-953-51-2731-4

For EU product safety concerns:
IN TECH d.o.o., Prolaz Marije Krucifikse Kozulić 3, 51000 Rijeka, Croatia,
info@intechopen.com or visit our website at intechopen.com.

Meet the editor

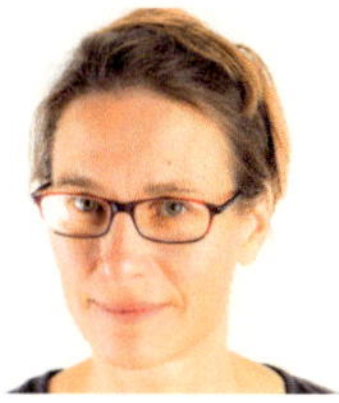

Helena Lenasi is currently an assistant professor of physiology at the Institute of Physiology, Faculty of Medicine, University of Ljubljana, Slovenia. She obtained her MD title in 1996 and her PhD title in 2003 at the University of Ljubljana, after working as a researcher at the Institute of Cardiovascular Physiology, JWG University in Frankfurt/Main in Germany. Her working activities are education and research. She teaches physiology for pre- and post-graduate students at the Faculty of Medicine and Faculty of Sport at the University of Ljubljana, Slovenia. Her main fields of interest are cardiovascular and exercise physiology. Her research is mainly focused on studying human microcirculation in health and disease in collaboration with clinics. She is an editor of Slovenian Medical Journal.

Contents

Preface

Microcirculation has long attracted scientists; first attempts to investigate microcirculation reach as far as the seventeenth century and are connected with the discovery of light microscopy. Many researchers have since tried to unravel the mystery of mechanisms governing the supply of tissues with nutrients and the removal of waste products.

Over the past decades, the knowledge on the physiology and pathophysiology of microcirculation has expanded also due to evolvement of modern techniques, which enable in vivo assessment of microcirculatory dynamics. Yet, the existing knowledge is far from optimal as the microvascular network is very complex regarding its structure and functional organization.

Adequate tissue perfusion is a prerequisite for normal organ functioning. On the other hand, tissue perfusion primarily depends on intact microcirculation and preserved vascular tone regulation. It is well known that microvascular dysfunction in terms of deranged endothelial or smooth muscle function is one of the earliest events in the pathogenesis of many cardiovascular and metabolic diseases, leading to an impairment of the corresponding organ. Compromised microcirculation could finally be detrimental for the whole organism. Thus, understanding the normal organization and function and early detection of dysfunctional microcirculation are of crucial clinical importance. An early diagnosis and proper clinical interventions may thus considerably postpone the development of the disease.

However, microcirculation should not be regarded as independent entity but rather as a circuit strongly coupled to events occurring at the cellular level in tissues on one side and to systemic factors such as blood pressure and fluid balance on the other, which in turn encompass cardiovascular system as a whole. Thus, it must always be considered in a broader context taking into account an interdisciplinary approach. In this respect, the chapters in the book usually refer to the system as a whole, stressing some important characteristics at the cellular and molecular level up to clinical settings reflecting normal and pathological conditions.

Although a lot of studies are investigating the mechanisms of microvascular dynamics at the molecular level, which could mainly be performed on animal models and isolated organs, the situation in situ is far more complicated and could hardly be simulated on appropriate models. In this respect, in vivo studies on humans are encouraged as they in fact reflect the real situation and could strongly support the clinical work with patients. As such, newer accomplished techniques are urgently needed that in conjunction with the clinical picture would enable an early recognition of microvascular pathology and improvement in some treatment strategies as well as assessing the outcomes.

Obviously, microcirculation is a complex and heterogenous network that includes many elements interacting with each other. Concerning the complexity and a vast number of studies that at the time are being conducted all over the world, it is obvious that the book cannot cover all aspects of microcirculation but rather a small part of the spectrum. In this respect, the book addresses some important facts and recent findings on the physiology and pathophysiology of microcirculation, each chapter focusing on a particular issue. The chapters in the book are organized systematically, the first ones presenting some characteristics of coronary microcirculation, the skeletal muscles, and the newborn's microcirculation, respectively. In addition, some molecular mechanisms of vascular tone regulation are presented, followed by chapters, describing pathological conditions caused by dysfunctional microcirculation. Finally, some clinical aspects are presented and potential therapeutic interventions to treat microcirculatory dysfunction briefly outlined.

Scientists and researchers all over the globe contributed their interesting findings and speculations on the microcirculation and helped to unravel some puzzles in the complex microcirculatory mosaic. I would like to express my many thanks to the authors for their invaluable contribution and comprehensive overviews. Last but not least, I would also like to thank the publishers for inviting me to be part of their team as an editor. My special gratitude goes to the publishing process manager Ms. Andrea Korić who was always there to answer my questions.

I hope that the book will be of help to medical and other public health providers in expanding their knowledge or finding some interesting references in the field of microcirculation as it looks today.

Assistant Professor Helena Lenasi, MD, PhD,
University of Ljubljana,
Faculty of Medicine, Institute of Physiology,
Ljubljana, Slovenia

Chapter 1

Introductory Chapter: Microcirculation in Health and Disease

Helena Lenasi

Additional information is available at the end of the chapter

http://dx.doi.org/10.5772/64680

Microcirculation is the terminal vascular network where the exchange of substances between the blood and the tissues occurs. Usually, the term refers to functional unit comprising vessels with a diameter of less than 100 μm, including arterioles, capillaries, and venules. Appropriate vascularization of tissues and an intact microcirculatory bed are prerequisites for adequate tissue perfusion and thus normal organ functioning. The unique feature of microcirculation is its large area which in conjunction with low velocity of blood flow enables appropriate conditions for the exchange of substances between the blood and the tissues. Another important issue is its adaptability either to acute changes of organ demands or to chronic changes in its environment. These tasks are primarily accomplished by arterioles as the main targets and effectors of vascular tone regulation including the vascular endothelium and smooth muscle cells, as well as adjacent cells and humoral and nervous factors all playing in a fine orchestrated concert. The principal characteristics of fluid and substances trafficking across the capillary wall according to classical Fick and Starling principles and depending on the concentration gradients of substances transported, on capillary permeability, and on hydrostatic and oncotic pressures are described elsewhere.

1. Structural and functional organization: some general and special features

The structural organization of the microcirculation is tightly coupled to its physiologic function. As organs serve different functions and have different metabolic demands, the microcirculatory networks differ among organs. The complexity and heterogeneity in blood flow and metabolism in respect to one tissue as well as in different tissues have been confirmed in animal experiments and in patients due to advanced imaging techniques.

The book starts with a comprehensive overview of the coronary microcirculation written by Fonseca et al., thoroughly describing the characteristics of coronary microcirculation, from anatomical and histological aspects to physiology with emphasis on the regulatory mechanisms, and finally elucidating some pathophysiologic mechanisms in relation to systemic cardiovascular diseases. Of interest is the impact of perycites to the regulation of microcirculation as pointed out in the chapter, as well as a rather neglected field of venous part of the microcirculation [1]. The chapter specially focuses on the regulation of coronary microvasculature with the presentation of all known mechanisms that might be applied also to other vascular beds, i.e., the myogenic control, the endothelial component, and the metabolic regulation [2]. The latter presumably plays the most important role in the coronary microcirculation due to constantly changing demands of the working heart muscle [3]. Additionally, systemic factors such as the autonomic nervous system and humoral mediators are elucidated. As diseases of the cardiovascular system nowadays represent the leading cause of morbidity and mortality all over the world, the most frequent pathologies of the coronary vessels are presented [4]. The heart vessels are very prone to structural remodeling, vascular rarefaction, and perivascular fibrosis finally culminating in luminal obstruction what might be detrimental for the patient; apart from macrocirculation, it is the microcirculation that is suggested to play a key role in the coronary pathophysiology [5]. The impact of risk factors, oxidative stress and inflammation, and the interplay between various regulatory mechanisms, all predisposing to heart disease development are comprehensively exposed with a brief link to some metabolic diseases.

The dependence of the cellular metabolism on tissue blood flow and vice versa is more extensively described in the following chapter written by Kolka, which focuses on the microcirculation of skeletal muscle and also proposes some therapeutic interventions in targeting the skeletal muscle microcirculation to treat both vascular and metabolic diseases. The skeletal muscle microcirculation is subjected to the greatest variations of blood flow and nutrients breakdown during strenuous exercise as compared to resting conditions. During resting conditions, only about 20% of capillaries are perfused: the blood flow is estimated to amount 5–10 mL/min/100 g, compared up to 80–100 mL/min/100 g during exercise [6], pointing to complex mechanisms of blood flow regulation. Worth to mention is the difficulty to estimate these changes and microvascular dynamics at the capillary level with the available techniques. In the chapter, an interesting scientific approach for the evaluation of substrate exchange in the microenvironment of skeletal muscle is presented, namely, the lymph sampling [7, 8]. Taking into account great variations in the metabolic rate as well as the type and rate of substrates metabolized regarding intensity and mode of exercise, it is compelling to speculate that changes in blood flow will affect metabolism. In this respect, vasoactive compounds affecting vascular tone and perfusion could also indirectly affect the metabolism. Insufficient perfusion might in turn lead to deranged metabolic pathways making one more susceptible to metabolic diseases, such as diabetes and obesity [9]. Interestingly, nitric oxide (NO) as a key endothelial vasodilator also directly affects metabolism by competing with mitochondria for oxygen and consequently inhibiting the oxidative phosphorylation and potentially switching the metabolism to some other (anaerobic) pathways [10]. Apart from classical vasoactive substances mainly released from the endothelium, many hormones are themselves vasoactive; glucagon-like peptide has been shown to increase capillary perfusion on acute basis and angiogenesis on longer term, and considering this, might represent a potential therapeutic target [11, 12]. In addition, some important interactions among vasoactive compounds and hormones have been elucidated in the chapter, such as the interference of angiotensin II (Ang) and NO systems [8], and the prevention of endothelin-induced vasoconstriction by insulin and adiponectin [13, 14]. Insulin also directly affects capillary recruitment and at supraphysiologic concentrations, it has been shown to increase blood flow in human skeletal muscles and skin [15]. Capillary density has been directly correlated with insulin sensitivity thus strengthening the hypothesis that capillary recruitment importantly contributes to insulin-mediated glucose uptake [16]. As exposed in the chapter of Kolka, an important question to be resolved is the process of insulin trafficking across the endothelial barrier. At this place, a word should be devoted to endothelial glycocalix, which presents an additional structural and functional endothelial barrier that in turn affects the composition of the muscle interstitium and consequently the supply of nutrients to the cells. Glycocalix has thoroughly been investigated as a potential therapeutic target [17].

2. The central role of endothelium in the regulation of vascular tone

Although endothelium also plays an important role in the processes of inflammation, hemostasis, and tissue repair, its prominent role in the physiological regulation of vascular tone along with a vast number of endothelial vasoactive substances and their interactions are most extensively exposed in the book. Accordingly, all endothelial mediators might represent a potential therapeutic target as briefly pointed out in some chapters.

The importance of functionally intact endothelium is already obvious in the newborn as exposed in the chapter of Wright and Dyson. Apart from the involvement of the autonomic nervous system and the sympathoadrenal activation at birth, substances released from endothelium importantly contribute to the delicate balance between vasodilators and vasoconstrictors which is a prerequisite for normal circulatory function. To list just a few, isoprostanes and prostaglandins released in response to increased partial oxygen pressure at birth play a major role in the closure of ductus arteriosus, thus enabling the transition to the adult-type circulation taking place at birth [18]. In preterm infants, this delicate balance is disturbed in terms of enhanced vasodilation and diminished vasoconstriction rendering them more susceptible to hypotension resulting in organ hypoperfusion and potentially irreversible end-organ damage [19]. An interesting feature pointed out in the chapter is greater susceptibility of male preterm newborns to developing potentially fatal hypotension, which has been speculated to be due to increased levels of gaseous neurotransmitter hydrogen sulfide (H_2S) in males [20]. Accordingly, the assessment of urinary concentrations of thiosulfate, a metabolite of H_2S [20, 21] and normetanephrine, a measure of total body sympathoadrenal activity [22], respectively, might predict the outcome. The impact of other gaseous compounds is additionally described in the chapter, with the leading role of NO, presumably involved in the regulation of basal vascular tone, and carbon monoxide (CO), apparently playing a crucial regulatory role in the cerebral circulation during the transition period [23, 24]. While most observations were deduced from animal studies or isolated models, far more complex interplay takes part in humans *in vivo*. A lot of potential crosstalks and the influence of one mediator on the other one could merely be speculated, as exposed in the chapter [23]. Their potential adaptive role and their impact in the neonatal period are emphasized. Of interest, the interplay of NO, CO, and H_2S differ in neonates and in the adults, which in addition to the chapter of Wright and Dyson is also exposed in the chapter of Fonseca et al. [25].

The role of NO as a key endothelial vasodilator has briefly been corroborated in the chapters of Fonseca et al., Zupan, and Schier et al. Yet, other vasodilators presumably are even more important at the level of microcirculation, the central role being played by the metabolites of arachidonic acid (AA), extensively exposed in the chapter of Drenjančević et al. Three important pathways of AA metabolism are presented, including: the cyclooxygenase (COX) pathway, the lipopxygenase (LOX) pathway, and the cytochrome (CYP) pathway. In the chapter, the mostly investigated products of these metabolic pathways and their potential interactions at the level of the vascular smooth muscle are thoroughly presented. Worth to emphasize is the dual role of the above-mentioned enzymes, namely, they catalyze the production of vasoconstrictors as well as vasodilators and it is their delicate balance that finally determines the proper vascular tone. In many diseases, this fine balance is disturbed, such as in obesity, diabetes, hypertension, and other metabolic and cardiovascular diseases. Of the CYP metabolites of AA, epoxyeicosatrienoic acids (EETs) have been implicated as endothelium-derived hyperpolarizing factors (EDHF), contributing to proper vasodilation in the settings with reduced bioavailability of NO [26], such as in increased production of reactive oxygen species (ROS), which uncouple the endothelial nitric oxide synthase (eNOS), and consequently augment additional release of ROS from eNOS itself.

An interesting aspect is the nonenzymatic metabolism of AA, mainly mediated by ROS which nowadays are widely recognized as mediators of cellular immunity, inflammation, and tissue repair, and also indirectly affect vascular tone [27]. The impact of ROS as potential (noxious) vascular messengers is also dealt with in some other chapters.

Additional interesting suggestion presented in the chapter of Drenjančević et al is potentially positive contribution of Ang, which has usually been presented as a foe in the vascular homeostasis. Contrary to the common accepted knowledge, they propose that sufficient levels of Ang actually are essential for normal vascular function, as confirmed in the studies which have demonstrated that a decrease in the circulating levels of Ang lead to impaired microvascular endothelial function [28]. As for Ang, Kolka additionally exposes its effect on blood vessel permeability which indirectly also affects the tissue metabolism [29].

Yet, the effects of endothelial vasoactive compounds are not that straightforward, as there are many interactions depending also on the vascular bed studied and being also tissue and species specific.

The deranged interplay of endothelial mediators in the pathogenesis of various diseases of modern era has long been implicated. As stated in the subsequent subheading, some chapters address the question of endothelial dysfunction as a hallmark of many diseases. Moreover, the dysfunction of endothelium often precedes the clinical manifestation of the disease.

3. Dysfunctional microcirculation is a hallmark of many diseases

The importance of intact and functional microcirculation with preserved adaptability to meet organ metabolic demands has long been appreciated. It has been confirmed in many independent studies that deranged microcirculation compromises normal organ function and finally the organism as a whole. Either deranged vascular control in terms of deranged autonomic nervous system as pointed out in the research chapter of Malan et al. as well as in terms of endothelial dysfunction have been implicated. Increased sympathetic tone or disturbed responsivity to adrenergic challenges might induce increased vasoconstrictor tone finally leading to hypertension and inappropriate structural remodeling of the vessel wall. Endothelial vasoconstrictors and increased oxidative stress also augment the vasoconstrictor component causing ischemia and tissue failure on a larger time scale. Microvascular dysfunction has been shown to be the primary event in the pathogenesis of many metabolic and cardiovascular pathologies which is shortly mentioned in other chapters. On the other hand, injury and inflammation subsequently trigger angiogenesis and structural adaptation that have the potential of restitution, which takes part after say surgical procedures as pointed out in the chapter of Schier et al. The potential to restitute *ad integrum* strongly depends on the preoperative state of the microcirculation and on other known vascular risk factors such as hypertension, smoking, diabetes, obesity, etc. [30]. Potential risk factors can partly be overcome by changes in lifestyle and some interventions such as exercise. Moreover, the letter may strongly affect the outcome of a therapeutic procedure as stressed in the chapter of Schier et al. [31].

A good model of microvascular dysfunction potentially leading to impairment of the central nervous system and causing high mortality and morbidity is leukoaraiosis. The term, potentially unfamiliar to broader medical public, denotes diffuse confluent changes in the cerebral white matter often accidentally detected on neuroradiological imaging. Its prevalence in the population aged between 50 and 75 years has been estimated to comprise up to 25% and, as such, undoubtedly must be regarded as highly clinical significant in terms of predisposing to various degrees of cognitive impairment, ischemic events, and stroke [32]. In his chapter, Zupan thoroughly describes the pathogenesis of leukoaraiosis, which includes a spectrum of factors, often apparently discordant, ranging from endothelial dysfunction to leaky blood-brain barrier on one side [33], to ischemia on the other [34], yet all causing chronic perfusion impairment. Similar factors and causes could actually be applied also to other microcirculatory networks. In his chapter, Zupan reports that the prevalence of leukoaraiosis is higher in the Blacks than in the Whites. This might be connected to increased prevalence of hypertension in the Blacks which has extensively been discussed also in the chapter of Malan et al. [35]. Interestingly, Malan et al. also showed a close link between depressive disorders and vascular dysfunction of the retinal artery in terms of sympathoadrenal disbalance. The correlation was significantly more pronounced in the Blacks compared to the Whites pointing out an important role of ethical predisposition and genetic susceptibility on one side, but also risk factors on the other side [36]. Interestingly, chronic depression has been related to attenuated cortisol levels which would impact the synthesis of epinephrine [37], as proposed in the chapter of Malan et al. All these facts must be taken into account when designing the therapeutic strategies and a proper follow-up of patients.

Another interesting aspect of endothelial dysfunction addressed in the chapter of Drenjančecić et al. is the impact of high salt diet on vascular function [38]; vascular pathologies linked to increased salt intake undoubtedly represent a great burden of the civilized world. As already stated, other aspects of endothelial dysfunction are extensively presented also in the chapters of Fonseca et al. with emphasis on the involvement of coronary microcirculation in the pathogenesis of cardiovascular events, and in the chapter of Kolka on skeletal muscle microcirculation and its involvement in metabolic (obesity, diabetes) and cardiovascular diseases (hypertension).

While those chapters mainly deal with mechanisms of endothelial dysfunction, more clinical aspects in terms of the determination of microvascular and endothelial dysfunction are illustrated in the chapters of Tamas-Szora et al. and Todea et al. They present some potential diagnostic tools for an early detection of microvascular dysfunction as well as for tracing the outcome and the evaluation of the effectiveness of treatment.

4. *In vivo* applicability of some methods for clinical evaluation of microcirculation

Modern techniques with relatively high spatial resolution have enabled a timely detection of the disease, which is a prerequisite for an adequate treatment. Within the noninvasive imaging, sound- and light-based imaging techniques are able to provide high resolution and clinically relevant information in assessing microcirculation.

Mostly applied optical imaging techniques for clinical evaluation of the microcirculation today include (dynamic) capillaroscopy, confocal microscopy, two photon imaging, and stimulated emission depletion microscopy for tracing superficial structures; optical coherence tomography, hyperspectral imaging, side stream dark field imaging, and incident dark field imaging for assessing subsuperficial microvascular beds; and diffusion correlation spectroscopy, functional near infrared spectroscopy, and photoacoustic tomography to assess deeper structures [39]. Obviously, each technique is designed for determination of special microcirculation network and its position regarding the depth of a tissue.

In spite of many methods available, in the book, only two noninvasive techniques are extensively presented, namely, the contrast enhanced ultra-sonography (CEUS) and the laser Doppler (LD) fluxmetry (LDF) in the chapters of Tamas-Szora et al. and Todea et al., respectively. Their applicability in the assessment of vascular dearrangement in tumor evolvement, angiogenesis, inflammation, and some other pathologies and in the assessment of dental pathologies, respectively, is presented along with some advantages and disadvantage of both. Both methods are based on optical and acoustic penetration of a tissue and exploit the Doppler effect causing the frequency shift of illuminated light and sound, respectively, due to reflections from moving particles, i.e., predominantly erythrocytes. Both chapters give insight into potential clinical applicability of CEUS and LDF for tracing microcirculation and emphasize the need and importance of performing *in vivo* studies on humans.

In their chapter, Tamas-Szora et al. comprehensively describe the principles governing CEUS as well as some modifications and their various applicability, substantiated with representing illustrative figures that accompany the text and enable a better perception of the method for unfamiliar readers. CEUS has rendered itself a valuable clinical tool for assessing vascularization in various tissues, specially parenchymal organs, such as liver [40], testicles, kidney [41], and mammary glands [42]. Yet, the limitation inherent to all sonographic methods described so far is that CEUS enables the discrimination of the vessels of size of around 100 μm and, in this respect, does not accurately evaluate the proper "microcirculation" [43]. Nevertheless, it is highly applicable in the clinical settings as it enables the detection of blood flow down to velocities less than 2 cm/s, and the discrimination between inflammatory and degenerative pathology as in musculoskeletal diseases [44]. In this regard, capillary perfusion could be indirectly estimated, i.e., either increased perfusion in say inflammation or cessation of blood flow in ischemic tissues.

To improve the CEUS technique, different contrasting agents that augment the signals under observation might be applied; yet, they increase the diagnostic costs. The advantages of CEUS over some other methods include repeatability, lack of harmful effects as in computer tomography (CT) caused by ionizing radiation, and high spatial and temporal resolution to list just a few. Target-specific structures might additionally be detected by combining the contrast agent with specific antibodies.

LDF and its update, LD imaging [45] with its varieties remain the gold standard for clinical evaluation of microcirculation as described in the chapter of Todea et al. In the chapter, some results of authors' own experiments evaluating the outcome of therapy in terms of microvascular function are exposed. LDF has proven to be an effective tool of choice to evaluate microcirculation in the oral cavity, preferentially of the gingiva and dental pulp, respectively [46, 47]. LD techniques enable assessment of tooth vitality after various procedures including bleaching, tooth implants and prepared teeth, surgical intervention after trauma, as well as tracing microcirculation following treatment of gingival disease, such as inflammation, and gingival blood flow resolution after surgical procedures. Supposedly, LDF also enables to evaluate the redistribution of blood flow through arteriovenous anastomoses that are a unique feature of the cutaneous and mucous microcirculation.

5. Therapeutic interventions at the level of microcirculation: potential role of endothelial progenitor cells (EPCs)

Interventional studies have focused on various aspects of microvascular function, as already outlined in the chapters of Fonseca et al., Kolka, Drenjančević et al., and Zupan. Many vasoactive compounds might represent therapeutic targets, either by targeting their endothelial receptors or interfering with their synthesis by acting on the corresponding intracellular enzymes. In addition, interfering with the renin-angiotensin-aldosterone [48] system seems a promising therapeutical intervention to treat vascular and associated metabolic diseases as pointed out in the chapter of Kolka. The effects of phosphodiesterase inhibitors (Sildenafil and Tadalafil), and thiazolidinediones on vascular function, capillary recruitment, and consequently metabolism have also been investigated, as exposed by Kolka. The potential intervention on the level of glycocalyx has already been mentioned [17]. An interesting target affecting the metabolism of fat and increasing energy expenditure and angiogenesis might be brown adipose tissue, as briefly exposed in the chapter of Kolka [49]. Moreover, the supplementation of L-arginine might ameliorate vascular complications in patients suffering from neurodegenerative and vascular diseases as mentioned in the chapter of Zupan [50].

Apart from the above-mentioned targets, endothelial progenitor cells have evolved over the last few years as a promising new strategy for targeting microvascular and subsequently organ dysfunction. Nowadays, many studies are being conducted on how the injection of EPCs on the site of injury or damaged organ affects potential improvement of organ function. Apart from acute adjustments, chronic adjustments in terms of increased angiogenesis are crucial for tissue regeneration. Angiogenesis and vasculogenesis are key events in directing proper organ function, not only during fetal life, but also later in adulthood. EPCs also play an important role in vascularization in pregnancy [51]. They are important component in tissue regeneration and, in this respect, might represent a potential therapeutic niche. Thus, improvements of techniques to obtain sufficient number of EPCs from the peripheral circulation, or from the bone marrow, proper harvesting and breeding are prerequisites for efficient therapy. Some important aspects of EPCs are presented in the chapter of Nova-Lamperti et al., where the crucial technical steps in obtaining and manipulating the cells are presented as well as the results of some studies investigating the effects of therapy with EPCs. Furthermore, the stimuli for migration, recruitment, and differentiation of stem cells affecting angiogenesis *in vivo* are corroborated. Unfortunately, the potential of EPCs for proper angiogenesis strongly depends on the clinical condition and risk factors of the individuum. Namely, it has been shown that the number of EPCs conversely correlated with cardiovascular risk factors, such as hypercholesterolemia, hypertension, smoking, diabetes mellitus, and dyslipidemia. Moreover, lower numbers of EPCs as compared to healthy ones have been shown in patients suffering from unstable angina, myocardial infarction, as well as atherosclerosis, and erectile dysfunction, as described in the chapters of Schier et al. and Nova-Lamperti et al. On the other hand, some cytokines, hormones, drugs, and physical activity increase the number and function of EPCs. In this respect, the importance of physical activity could not be overemphasized. Some good and positive examples are presented in the chapter of Schier et al. who have shown that even short lasting submaximal exercise performed preoperatively to assess the cardiopulmonary status of a patient might significantly improve the outcome after major surgery in patients [31, 52]. In this respect, regular exercise should be strongly encouraged in all groups of patients, let alone in healthy populations in general practice. Clinical applicability of EPCs has already been confirmed in many clinical trials, when *ex vivo* expanded EPCs were injected into the damaged area of tissue, such as in the treatment of acute myocardial infarction [53], in the recovery from deep venous thrombosis, in the recanalization of organized venous thrombi

[54], in pulmonary arterial hypertension [55], in attenuation of peripheral artery disease [56], and in liver regeneration [57]. Yet, the disadvantage of such therapy is a very low number of EPCs in peripheral blood and relatively high costs of mobilization. Nevertheless, EPCs seem to represent a promising future therapeutic approach for the treatment of "modern era" diseases.

6. Conclusion

In the introductory chapter, I intended to briefly sum up the content of the book, exposing some interesting features of separate chapters. Basic principles of the microvascular blood flow and vascular tone regulation are briefly presented with endothelium playing a central role. Today, researchers are focused on complex interactions of vasoactive compounds trying to elucidate their potential interplays in health and disease, which would accomplish therapeutic strategies. Prototypes of alternative therapeutic approach presented in the book might be exercise as a type of self-governed therapy on one side, and EPCs as a kind of complex hospital-based therapy. As diseases of the cardiovascular system are the leading cause of morbidity and mortality in modern world, additional efforts in establishing new diagnostic tools and efficient therapies are urgently needed. The authors have provided comprehensive overviews and opened up new challenging questions that I hope would be useful to scientists involved in the microcirculation which remains an unlimited field of inspiration. A lot has already been unrevealed, and the rest is yet to be discovered.

Author details

Helena Lenasi*

Address all correspondence to: helena.lenasi.ml@mf.uni-lj.si

Institute of Physiology, Faculty of Medicine, University of Ljubljana, Ljubljana, Slovenia

References

[1] O'Farrell FM, Attwell D. A role for pericytes in coronary no-reflow. Nat Rev Cardiol 2014; 11(7):427–432. DOI: 10.1038/nrcardio.2014.58

[2] Pries AR, Badimon L, Bugiardini R, Camici PG, Dorobantu M, Duncker DJ, et al. Coronary vascular regulation, remodelling, and collateralization: mechanisms and clinical implications on behalf of the working group on coronary pathophysiology and microcirculation. Eur Heart J 2015; 36(45):3134–3146. DOI: 10.1093/eurheartj/ehv100

[3] Deussen A, Ohanyan V, Jannasch A, Yin L, Chilian W. Mechanisms of metabolic coronary flow regulation. J Mol Cell Cardiol 2012; 52(4):794–801. DOI: 10.1016/j.yjmcc.2011.10.001

[4] Crea F, Camici PG, Bairey Merz CN. Coronary microvascular dysfunction: an update. Eur Heart J 2014; 35(17):1101–1111.DOI: 10.1093/eurheartj/eht513

[5] van den Akker J, Schoorl MJ, Bakker EN, Vanbavel E. Small artery remodeling: current concepts and questions. J Vasc Res 2010; 47(3):183–202. DOI: 10.1159/000255962

[6] Korthuis RJ. Exercise Hyperemia and Regulation of Tissue Oxygenation During Muscular Activity. Skeletal Muscle Circulation. San Rafael (CA): Morgan and Claypool Life Sciences, 2011.

[7] Kolka CM, Richey JM, Castro AV, Broussard JL, Ionut V, Bergman RN. Lipid-induced insulin resistance does not impair insulin access to skeletal muscle. Am J Physiol Endocrinol Metab 2015; 308(11):E1001–E1009.

[8] Richey JM, Ader M, Moore D, Bergman RN. Angiotensin II induces insulin resistance independent of changes in interstitial insulin. Am J Physiol 1999; 277(5 Pt 1):E920–E926.

[9] Karaca U, Schram MT, Houben AJ, Muris DM, Stehouwer CD. Microvascular dysfunction as a link between obesity, insulin resistance and hypertension. Diabetes Res Clin Pract 2014; 103(3):382–387.

[10] Heinonen I, Saltin B, Kemppainen J, Sipila HT, Oikonen V, Nuutila P, et al. Skeletal muscle blood flow and oxygen uptake at rest and during exercise in humans: a pet study with nitric oxide and cyclooxygenase inhibition. Am J Physiol Heart Circ Physiol 2011; 300(4):H1510–H1517.

[11] Sjoberg KA, Holst JJ, Rattigan S, Richter EA, Kiens B. GLP-1 increases microvascular recruitment but not glucose uptake in human and rat skeletal muscle. Am J Physiol Endocrinol Metab 2014; 306(4):E355–E362.

[12] Aronis KN, Chamberland JP, Mantzoros CS. GLP-1 promotes angiogenesis in human endothelial cells in a dose-dependent manner, through the Akt, Src and PKC pathways. Metabolism 2013; 62(9):1279–1286.

[13] Kolka CM, Rattigan S, Richards S, Clark MG. Metabolic and vascular actions of endothelin-1 are inhibited by insulin-mediated vasodilation in perfused rat hindlimb muscle. Br J Pharmacol 2005; 145(7):992–1000.

[14] Bussey CT, Kolka CM, Rattigan S, Richards SM. Adiponectin opposes endothelin-1-mediated vasoconstriction in the perfused rat hindlimb. Am J Physiol Heart Circ Physiol 2011; 301(1):H79–H86.

[15] Serne EH, Ijzerman RG, Gans RO, Nijveldt R, de Vries G, Evertz R, et al. Direct evidence for insulin-induced capillary recruitment in skin of healthy subjects during physiological hyperinsulinemia. Diabetes 2002; 51(5):1515–1522.

[16] Vincent MA, Clerk LH, Lindner JR, Klibanov AL, Clark MG, Rattigan S, et al. Microvascular recruitment is an early insulin effect that regulates skeletal muscle glucose uptake in vivo. Diabetes 2004; 53(6):1418–1423.

[17] Becker BF, Chappell D, Bruegger D, Annecke T, Jacob M. Therapeutic strategies targeting the endothelial glycocalyx: acute deficits, but great potential. Cardiovasc Res 2010; 87:300–310.

[18] Chen JX, et al. Isoprostanes as physiological mediators of transition to newborn life: novel mechanisms regulating patency of the term and preterm ductus arteriosus. Pediatr Res 2012; 72(2):122–128.

[19] Schwepcke A, et al. Microcirculatory mechanisms in postnatal hypotension affecting premature infants. Pediat Res 2013; 74(2):186–190.

[20] Kent AL, Wright IM, Abdel-Latif ME. Mortality and adverse neurologic outcomes are greater in preterm male infants. Pediatrics 2012; 129(1):124–131.

[21] Dyson RM, et al. A role for H2S in the microcirculation of newborns: the major metabolite of H2S (thiosulphate) is increased in preterm infants. PLoS One 2014; 9(8):e105085.

[22] Stark MJ, et al. The influence of sex and antenatal betamethasone exposure on vasoconstrictors and the preterm microvasculature. J Matern Fetal Neonatal Med 2011; 24(10):1215–1220.

[23] Dyson RM, et al. Interactions of the gasotransmitters contribute to microvascular tone (dys)regulation in the preterm neonate. PLoS One 2015; 10(3): e0121621.

[24] Knecht KR, et al. Time-dependent action of carbon monoxide on the newborn cerebrovascular circulation. Am J Physiol Heart Circ Physiol 2010; 299:H70–H75.

[25] Zinkevich NS, Wittenburg AL, Gutterman DD. Abstract 15764: role of cyclooxygenase in flow-induced dilation of human coronary arterioles depends upon age. Circulation 2010; 122(Suppl 21):A15764.

[26] Tacconelli S, Patrignani P. Inside epoxyeicosatrienoic acids and cardiovascular disease. Front Pharmacol 2014; 10(5):239.

[27] Droge W. Free radicals in the physiological control of cell function. Physiol Rev 2002; 82:47–95.

[28] Boegehold MA, Drenjancevic I, Lombard JH. Salt, angiotensin II, superoxide, and endothelial function. Compr Physiol 2015; 6(1):215–254.

[29] Williams B, Baker AQ, Gallacher B, Lodwick D. Angiotensin II increases vascular permeability factor gene expression by human vascular smooth muscle cells. Hypertension 1995; 25(5):913–917.

[30] Riedel B, Schier R. Endothelial dysfunction in the perioperative setting. Semin Cardiothorac Vasc Anesth 2010; 14:41–43.

[31] Schier R, El-Zein R, Cortes A, et al. Endothelial progenitor cell mobilization by preoperative exercise: a bone marrow response associated with postoperative outcome. Br J Anaesthesia 2014; 113:652–660

[32] Grueter BE, Schulz UG. Age-related cerebral white matter disease (leukoaraiosis): a review. Postgrad Med J 2012; 1036:79–87. DOI: 10.1136/postgradmedj-2011-130307.

[33] Zupan M, Šabović M, Zaletel M, et al. The presence of cerebral and/or systemic endothelial dysfunction in patients with leukoaraiosis – a case control pilot study. BMC Neurol 2015; 15:158. DOI: 10.1186/s12883-015-0416-z.

[34] Birns J, Jarosz J, Markus HS, et al. Cerebrovascular reactivity and dynamic autoregulation in ischaemic subcortical white matter disease. J Neurol Neurosurg Psychiat 2009: 80:1093–1098.

[35] Malan L, Hamer, M, Frasure-Smith N, et al. COHORT PROFILE: Sympathetic activity and Ambulatory Blood Pressure in Africans (SABPA) Prospective Cohort Study. Int J Epidemiol 2015;44:1814–1822. DOI:10.1093/ije/dyu199.

[36] Malan L, Hamer M, von Känel R, et al. Chronic depression symptoms and salivary NOx associated with retinal vascular dysregulation: the SABPA study. Nitric Oxide. DOI: 1016/j.niox.2016.02.008.

[37] Hellhammer DH, Wüst S, Kudielka BM. Salivary cortisol as a marker in stress research. Psychoneuroendocrinology 2009;34:163–171.

[38] Cavka A, Cosic A, Jukic I, Jelakovic B, Lombard JH, Phillips SA, Seric V, Mihaljevic I, Drenjancevic I. The role of cyclo-oxygenase-1 in high-salt diet-induced microvascular dysfunction in humans. J Physiol 2015; 593(24):5313–5324.

[39] Lal C, Leahy MJ. An Updated Review of Methods and Advancements in Microvascular Blood Flow Imaging 2016 Microcirculation. Apr 20. DOI: 10.1111/micc.12284. [Epub ahead of print].

[40] Claudon M, Dietrich CF, Choi BI, Cosgrove DO, Kudo M, Nolsoe CP, et al. Guidelines and good clinical practice recommendations for Contrast Enhanced Ultrasound (CEUS) in the liver – update 2012. Ultrasound Med Biol 2013;34(1):11–29. DOI: 10.1016/j.ultrasmedbio.2012.09.002.

[41] Heine GH, Gerhart MK, Ulrich C, Kaler H, Girndt M. Renal Doppler resistance indices are associated with systemic atherosclerosis in kidney transplant recipients. Kidney Intl 2005; 68(2):878–885. DOI: 10.1111/j.1523-1755.2005.00470.x.

[42] Kupeli A, Kul S, Eyuboglu I, Oguz S, Mungan S. Role of 3D power Doppler ultrasound in the further characterization of suspicious breast masses. Eur J Radiol 2016; 0(1):1–6. DOI: 10.1016/j.ejrad.2015.10.019.

[43] Lassau N, Paturel-Asselin C, Guinebretiere JM, Leclere J, Koscielny S, Roche A, et al. New hemodynamic approach to angiogenesis: color and pulsed Doppler ultrasonography. Invest Radiol 1999;34(3):194–198. DOI: 10.1097/00004424-199903000-00007.

[44] Schmidt WA. Technology insight: the role of color and power Doppler ultrasonography in rheumatology. Nat Clin Pract Rheum 2007;3(1):35–42. DOI: 10.1038/ncprheum0377.

[45] Noditi G, Todea C. Laser Doppler imaging – as a non-invasive method for assessing regional microcirculation when using plastic materials for guided healing. Mater Plast 2013; 1(50):40–43.

[46] Miron MI, Dodenciu D, Calniceanu M, Lungeanu D, Filip LM, Balabuc CA, Todea C. Evaluation of the effect of ambient light on laser Doppler flowmetry recordings in anterior teeth. Arch Balkan Medical Union 2009; 44(4):265–270.

[47] Todea C, Canjau S, Dodenciu D, Miron MI, Tudor A, Bălăbuc C. Laser Doppler flowmetry evaluation of gingival recovery response after laser treatment. Head and Neck Optical Diagnostics, Proc. SPIE 8805 2013; 880508: DOI: 10.1117/12.2034038.

[48] Tocci G, Paneni F, Palano F, Sciarretta S, Ferrucci A, Kurtz T, et al. Angiotensin-converting enzyme inhibitors, angiotensin II receptor blockers and diabetes: a meta-analysis of placebo-controlled clinical trials. Am J Hypertens 2011; 24(5): 582–590.

[49] Blondin DP, Labbe SM, Phoenix S, Guerin B, Turcotte EE, Richard D, et al. Contributions of white and brown adipose tissues and skeletal muscles to acute cold-induced metabolic responses in healthy men. J Physiol 2015; 593(3):701–714.

[50] Calabro RS, Gervasi G, Baglieri A, et al. Is high oral dose L-arginine intake effective in leukoaraiosis? Preliminary data, study protocol and expert's opinion. Curr Aging Sci 2013; 6(2):170–177.

[51] Luppi P, Powers RW, Verma V, Edmunds L, Plymire D, Hubel CA. Maternal circulating CD34+VEGFR-2+ and CD133+VEGFR-2+ progenitor cells increase during normal pregnancy but are reduced in women with preeclampsia. Reproduct Sci 2010; 17(7): 643–652.

[52] Rehman J, Li J, Parvathaneni L, et al. Exercise acutely increases circulating endothelial progenitor cells and monocyte-/macrophage-derived angiogenic cells. J Am Coll Cardiol 2004; 43:2314–2318.

[53] Ott I, Keller U, Knoedler M, Gotze KS, Doss K, Fischer P, et al. Endothelial-like cells expanded from CD34+ blood cells improve left ventricular function after experimental myocardial infarction. FASEB J 2005; 19(8):992–994.

[54] Alessio AM, Beltrame MP, Nascimento MC, Vicente CP, de Godoy JA, Silva JC, et al. Circulating progenitor and mature endothelial cells in deep vein thrombosis. Intl J Med Sci 2013; 10(12):1746–1754.

[55] Ikutomi M, Sahara M, Nakajima T, Minami Y, Morita T, Hirata Y, et al. Diverse contribution of bone marrow-derived late-outgrowth endothelial progenitor cells to vascular repair under pulmonary arterial hypertension and arterial neointimal formation. J Mol Cell Cardiol 2015; 86:121–135.

[56] Lara-Hernandez R, Lozano-Vilardell P, Blanes P, Torreguitart-Mirada N, Galmes A, Besalduch J. Safety and efficacy of therapeutic angiogenesis as a novel treatment in patients with critical limb ischemia. Ann Vascular Surg 2010; 24(2):287–294.

[57] Gutierrez-Grobe Y, Gavilanes-Espinar JG, Masso-Rojas FA, Sanchez-Valle V, Paez-Arenas A, Ponciano-Rodriguez G, et al. Metabolic syndrome and nonalcoholic fatty liver disease. The role of endothelial progenitor cells. Ann Hepatol 2013; 12(6):908–914.

Chapter 2

The Morphology, Physiology and Pathophysiology of Coronary Microcirculation

Diogo André Fonseca, Pedro Engrácia Antunes and
Maria Dulce Cotrim

Additional information is available at the end of the chapter

http://dx.doi.org/10.5772/64537

Abstract

The heart is one of the most demanding organs of the human body. The high nutrient and oxygen demands need to be met through an adequate vascularization of the myocardium. In fact, the myocardium vascular supply is achieved through an extensive vascular network that includes larger arteries, also known as coronary arteries, smaller arteries (arterioles) and capillaries. This set of arterioles and capillaries is known as microcirculation. Coronary artery disease is usually associated with larger epicardial coronary arteries. However, several studies have shown an important role of coronary microvascular dysfunction. This review aimed to explore the (a) morphology, with particular interest on the anatomical and histological aspects; (b) physiology, providing an insight on the several endothelium-dependent and endothelium-independent regulatory mechanisms; and (c) pathophysiology of the cardiac microcirculation, with a special focus on the changes in the regulatory mechanisms, on the atherogenesis and on the correlation to the systemic cardiovascular disease.

Keywords: coronary microcirculation, coronary microvascular morphology, coronary microvascular physiology, microcirculation regulatory mechanisms, coronary microvascular dysfunction, coronary microvascular pathology

1. Introduction

The heart is one of the most demanding organs of the human body as it presents high demands for nutrients and oxygen. These demands are physiologically met through an extensive and unique vascular network, which is usually known as *coronary circulation*. The coronary circulation includes larger arteries, also known as coronary arteries, smaller vessels (with a diameter below 100 μm), such as arterioles, capillaries and venules, that together form the coronary microcirculation and larger epicardial veins [1].

Historically, the large epicardial arteries were considered the coronary circulation. Nowadays, the scientific reports suggest the coronary circulation is characterized by an extreme complexity in terms of morphology but also physiology. Moreover, the theory that the coronary circulation involves the larger epicardial arteries is no longer acceptable given the extensive vascular network present in the myocardium.

Coronary artery disease (CAD) is usually associated with larger epicardial coronary arteries. However, previous studies have shown an important link between microcirculatory dysfunction and cardiovascular disease. In fact, pathological changes in smaller vessels have been detected prior to clinical manifestations of cardiovascular disease [1]. Moreover, microcirculatory dysfunction may even be a risk indicator for metabolic syndrome and associated cardiovascular disease [1, 2].

This review aimed to explore the (a) morphology, with particular interest on the anatomical and histological aspects; (b) physiology, providing an insight on the several endothelium-dependent and endothelium-independent regulatory mechanisms; and (c) pathophysiology of the cardiac microcirculation, with a special focus on the changes in the regulatory mechanisms, on the atherogenesis and on the correlation to the systemic cardiovascular disease.

2. Morphology and basic function

Based on the morphology and function, the coronary circulation involves several types of vessels as follows (from the larger arteries to the largest veins): epicardial arteries or coronary arteries, small arteries or intramural arteries, arterioles, capillaries, venules and epicardial veins. These vessels may be grouped according to their size into (a) *coronary macrocirculation*, referring to vessels with diameter higher than 100 μm (which includes the coronary arteries, the intramural arteries and the epicardial veins) and (b) *coronary microcirculation*, for vessels with a diameter lower than 100 μm, where the arterioles, capillaries and venules may be included.

2.1. Arterioles

The *arterioles* are smaller arteries that originate from the intramural arteries and run parallel to the myocardial fibres [3–5]. These vessels are characterized by a marked decrease in blood pressure, contributing to the blood flow resistance, along their length and by an increasing responsiveness to metabolites, for example hydrogen peroxide, adenosine, among others [3, 4, 6]. Therefore, arterioles represent the main metabolic regulation component of the myocardial blood flow and aim at controlling the blood flow to the capillary network [3, 4, 7].

The anatomy of these vessels varies along their length: the proximal and middle portions tend to present similar characteristics to the larger arteries, although with a thick tunica media [several layers of vascular smooth muscle cells (VSMCs)], while the distal portions, also termed terminal or precapillary arterioles, may present a thinner tunica media (one to two layers of VSMCs) or not even present any VSMC layer, which is replaced by small unique cells that will be explored in the following subsection, the *pericytes* (**Figure 1**) [8]. Moreover, the internal elastic membrane, in the tunica intima, may not be present [6]. The tunica adventitia is usually thinner in these vessels [6].

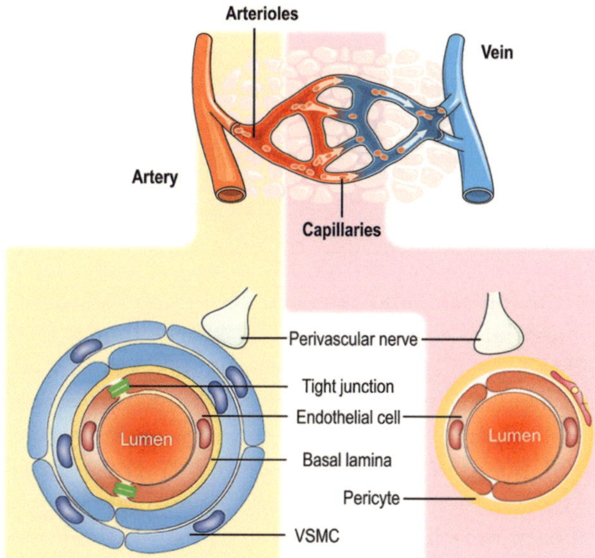

Figure 1. Vascular network and capillary neurovascular unit. As presented in the figure, the larger arteries (with a well-defined smooth muscle layer that may vary in size) present morphological differences to the capillaries, which do not present smooth muscle layer, being substituted by pericytes. The capillary neurovascular unit then includes the endothelium, basal lamina and pericytes, which are surrounded by neuron terminals. Moreover, the vascular network also includes other cell types, such as fibroblasts, collateral blood vessels, among others. Adapted from Zhang et al. [9] and prepared using Servier Medical Art (http://www.servier.com/).

2.2. Capillaries

The connection between the arterial and the venous systems is fundamentally achieved by a capillary network placed amid the arterioles and the venules (**Figure 1**).

The *capillaries*, with a diameter lower than 10 μm (average of 5.7 μm), are microscopic vessels that present numerous anastomotic loops (connections between the arterial and the venous systems), playing a crucial role in the exchange of nutrients and oxygen between the blood and the myocardium [5]. The capillary density may average up to 3500/mm^2 in the healthy myocardium and seems to vary from the subendocardium, which presents a higher oxygen-transport, to the subepicardium [5, 10, 11].

These vessels present structural differences to other vessels as the wall is essentially composed of two layers: an inner layer, the *endothelium*, and its *basal lamina* (**Figure 1**) [6]. In the inner layer, the endothelial cell junctions may be smaller, forming intercellular clefts, or larger, creating intercellular gaps.

According to their morphology, capillaries may be classified into three main categories: (a) continuous capillaries, (b) fenestrated capillaries and (c) discontinuous capillaries [6]. In the coronary microcirculation, the *continuous capillaries* are the most prevalent type. These vessels are commonly found in muscle, lung and central nervous system and are characterized by the presence of numerous pinocytotic vesicles and the absence of fenestrations [6]. These fenestrations, present in the *fenestrated capillaries*, are microscopic pores (80–100 nm in diameter) that allow the rapid diffusion of smaller molecules or proteins, which is particularly important in some tissues, such as the intestine and endocrine glands [6]. The *discontinuous capillaries*, also known as *sinusoidal capillaries or sinusoids*, present a higher diameter than other capillaries as well as an irregular shape and may be found in the liver, among other tissues [6].

Embedded in the basal membrane of capillaries, between the endothelium and the parenchyma, small contractile cells called *pericytes* may be found (**Figure 1**) [12, 13].

Pericytes may vary morphologically and physiologically depending on the vascular bed and on the position in the vascular bed itself [13]. Nevertheless, they generally extend processes along and around capillaries [12, 13]. In the central nervous system and kidneys, pericytes play an important role in angiogenesis, regulation of the endothelium, among other functions [12, 13]. These cells seem to be particularly relevant in the central nervous system where the regional blood flow regulation is of crucial importance [13]. These pericytes may also present contractile properties [12, 13]. Several proteins have been suggested to confer contractility to pericytes, such as α-smooth muscle actin and tropomyosin [13]. However, previous studies suggest that the contractile mechanisms differ from the VSMCs [13].

Although the role of pericytes in coronary physiology is not yet fully understood, the high number of these cells in cardiac capillaries and the similar characteristics to the central nervous system pericytes indicates these cells may play an important role in the regulation of the vessel diameter as well as permeability [12].

In the capillary network, other structures may be found such as *capillary sinuses*, which consist of reservoir-like spaces that could behave as micropumps [8].

2.3. Venules

After the exchange of nutrients and oxygen at the capillary level, the deoxygenated blood, containing metabolic products, proceeds to the *venules*, which present numerous intercommunications, through confluence of capillaries and postcapillary vessels [5]. Although the coronary circulation has been extensively studied over the years, little is known about the intramural venous system. Nevertheless, previous studies have suggested a larger venous network comparatively to the arterial network in the myocardium [5]. In fact, the existence of two veins per artery has been suggested [5].

The venules usually present a diameter ranging from 10 to 50 μm and similar anatomical characteristics to the arterioles [8]. The proximal venules, that is postcapillary venules, usually

http://dx.doi.org/10.5772/64537

exhibit only two layers: an inner layer, the *endothelium* and an outer layer, the *basal membrane* [6, 8]. The endothelium of the venules seems to be highly responsive to vasoactive agents, namely histamine and 5-hydroxytryptamine, commonly known as serotonin [6]. As well as in terminal arterioles and capillaries, *pericytes* may also be found in the venular wall in a particularly higher extent than in arterioles or capillaries [6, 8].

The distal venules are morphologically different relatively to the postcapillary venules, as they may present a thin tunica media (one to two layers of VSMCs) and a thin tunica adventitia on the outer side of the vessel [6]. The absence of pericytes is a key characteristic of these distal venules [6]. These venules initially course parallel to the muscle fibres, accompanying the arterioles and capillaries, then changing their position and configuration to meet the larger coronary veins [5].

2.4. Special circulatory considerations

2.4.1. Arteriovenous shunts

In healthy conditions, the myocardial blood supply is fundamentally provided through the normal coronary circulation. However, in the presence of cardiac disease, such as chronic cardiac disease or regional ischemic injuries, the myocardial perfusion may be compromised [4, 5]. Compensatory circulatory communications named *arteriovenous anastomoses or shunts* seem to play a key role in the preservation of the myocardial perfusion in these situations [4, 5, 14]. This collateral circulation links directly the arteries or arterioles to the veins or venules, bypassing the capillary bed [14]. The arteriole of these shunts frequently presents morphological particularities: a *thicker tunica media* with a higher content in VSMCs, a more *developed tunica adventitia,* forming a capsule of connective tissue, *abundant innervation* and are frequently *coiled* [6].

2.4.2. Heart chamber-coronary circulation direct communication

The direct communication between the heart chamber and the coronary circulation is generally referred to *Thebesian vessels* [5]. These vessels were first described by Thebesius in 1708 [15] and involve the communication between the heart chamber and the capillaries and venules, referring to a venular connection [5, 16, 17]. These veins usually present a diameter of 200–400 μm and are more frequent in the right ventricle [5]. This type of chamber-vessel communication was later studied by Wearn et al. [18] who further described and defined this and other types of vessels, namely the arteriosinusoidal vessels and the arterioluminal vessels [5, 16, 18]. The *arteriosinusoidal vessels* provide a communication between a heart chamber and a myocardial sinusoid and are irregularly shaped short branches (diameter from 50 to 350 μm) composed of just an endothelial layer [5, 18]. The *arterioluminal vessels* are smaller vessels (diameter from 40 to 200 μm) that provide a direct communication to a heart chamber (more frequently the left ventricle), presenting a morphology similar to arterioles [5, 18]. Although previous studies have demonstrated the presence of these special vessels, their clinical significance is still debatable [5].

3. Microcirculatory physiology

3.1. General considerations

The physiologic behaviour of the coronary circulation is inherently linked to a balance between the blood supply and the metabolic demand of the heart [19]. Furthermore, the physiological responses in the microcirculation seem to depend on the vessel size and type and appear to vary within the microcirculation itself and from those in the macrocirculation [19–21]. Physiologically, the coronary microcirculation is able to respond to a wide range of stimuli, such as growth and physical exercise, through adaptive processes, essential to the maintenance of its physiology [19]. In fact, vessels present a high adaptation ability and may undergo both acute and chronic adjustments. The acute adjustments involve changes in the vascular smooth muscle tone, while the chronic adjustments involve wall structure changes [19].

The *vascular tone* is defined as the ratio between baseline and maximal vessel diameter and is determined by the vascular smooth muscle function [19]. In turn, this is regulated by several mechanisms, such as (a) the myogenic tone, which is an intrinsic property of the VSMC, (b) the metabolic control exerted by adjacent cells, (c) the endothelial function responding to changes in the shear stress and (d) autonomic innervation and circulating factors, such as hormones [19].

3.2. Myogenic tone

The *myogenic tone* is produced by the response of the VSMCs to changes in transmural pressure that leads to stretching of the vessel wall [19, 22, 23]. This relation seems to be linear, that is increasing transmural pressure leads to higher vasoconstriction (reduction in the lumen diameter) [19]. The mechanism underlying this response appears to involve the opening of ion channels, namely nonspecific cation channels, with an increase in intracellular sodium and calcium and consequently the depolarization of the VSMCs [19]. Several receptors have been implicated in the myogenic response, such as (a) integrins [24], (b) transient-receptor potential channels (TRPs) [25, 26] and (c) G protein-coupled receptors [27].

3.3. Metabolic regulation

The coronary blood flow is intrinsically linked with metabolic demands of the myocardium, namely of oxygen. At rest, the myocardial oxygen extraction averages 60–70%, which leads to the coronary venous pO_2 of about 20 mmHg [28]. During physical exercise, several mechanisms of adaptation are triggered in the myocardium, pO_2 seems to be kept constant, which highlights the role of several pathways, namely the myocardial aerobic metabolism [28]. This energy production is generally dependent on mitochondrial oxidative phosphorylation pathways [19]. Among several metabolites produced in these intracellular pathways, carbon dioxide (CO_2) and reactive oxygen species (ROS) seem to play an important role in physiological conditions [19, 28].

As previously mentioned, *CO_2* production is linked to metabolic demands and therefore dependent on the myocardium oxygen consumption [19, 28]. This metabolite results from two main metabolic pathways: (a) the pyruvate dehydrogenase reaction and (b) the citric acid cycle [28]. The pyruvate dehydrogenase reaction converts pyruvate into acetyl-CoA, which is a substrate for the production of citrate, according to the following reaction:

$$\text{Pyruvate} + \text{CoA} + \text{NAD}^+ \xrightarrow{\text{Pyruvate dehydrogenase}} \text{Acetyl} - \text{CoA} + \text{CO}_2 + \text{NADH} + \text{H}^+ \quad (1)$$

After the conversion of oxaloacetate into citrate, the citric acid cycle involves several reactions in chain. Some of them also involve the production of CO_2, such as the production of α-ketoglutarate (reaction 2) and succinyl-CoA (reaction 3).

$$\text{D - Isocotrate} + \text{NAD}^+ \xrightarrow{\text{Isocitrate dehydrogenase}} \alpha - \text{Ketoglutarate+CO}_2 + \text{NADH+H}^+ \quad (2)$$

$$\alpha - \text{Ketoglutarate} + \text{CoA} + \text{NAD}^+ \xrightarrow{\alpha-\text{Ketoglutarate dehydrogenase}} \text{Succinyl} - \text{CoA} + \text{CO}_2 + \text{NADH} + \text{H}^+ \quad (3)$$

The increased production of CO_2 may also induce a decrease in pH due to the increase in proton concentration, as presented in the following reaction:

$$\text{CO}_2 + \text{H}_2\text{O} \leftrightarrow \text{H}^+ + \text{HCO}_3^- \quad (4)$$

This change in pH seems to promote the coronary vasodilation [28–30].

As can be seen in **Figure 2**, the metabolic production of *ROS* also plays an important role in the metabolic regulation of the coronary blood flow involving a feedforward mechanism [19, 28]. Among the several ROS, hydrogen peroxide (H_2O_2) seems to be one of the most important metabolites being considered a feedforward vasodilator [31]. H_2O_2 results from the conversion of superoxide anions ($O_2^{\cdot -}$) by the superoxide dismutase (SOD) [28]. In turn, the superoxide anions result from the reduction in O_2 by electrons released from mitochondrial complexes (I and III) [28]. This pathway may be stimulated by shear stress in human coronary resistance arteries [32].

The vasodilator properties of H_2O_2 have long been studied, but the precise underlying mechanisms are not yet fully established [28]. Previous studies suggested H_2O_2 behaves as an endothelium-derived hyperpolarizing factor (EDHF) [34, 35], as described in the following subsection. However, other previous studies suggested the mechanism may involve the stimulation of the nitric oxide (NO) production or be mediated by the guanylyl cyclase in human coronary arterioles [36]. These pathways will be further discussed in the following subsections.

Other studies have suggested additional mechanisms involved in the metabolic regulation exerted by H_2O_2 on the coronary blood flow. The involvement of oxidation of thiol groups as a pathway of coronary metabolic dilation in isolated coronary arterioles has been previously proposed [37]. The thiol groups are involved in many pathophysiological mechanisms and play a key role in the biological protection against oxidative injuries [38, 39]. This oxidation process promotes modifications in the protein conformation and includes the conversion of protein-bound thiols (-SH) into sulfenic (SO^-, reaction 5), sulphinic (SOO^-) and sulphonic ($SOOO^-$) acids as well as disulphide bridges (S-S, reaction 6) [37, 39].

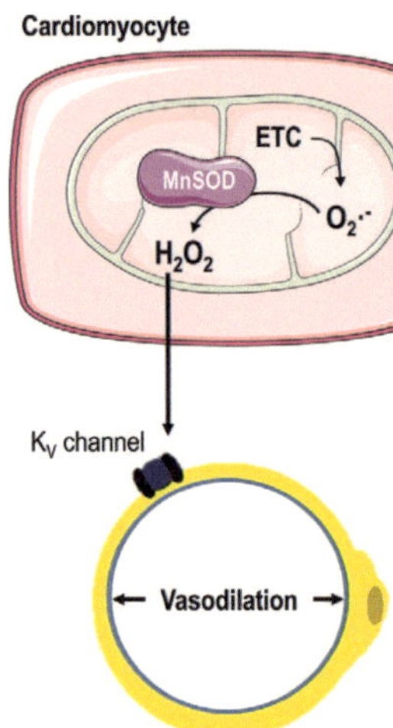

Figure 2. Feedforward reactive oxygen species-dependent metabolic regulation of coronary blood flow. The increased metabolic demands of the myocardium trigger an increase in mitochondrial metabolism and flux, through the electron transport chain (ETC), increasing the production of $O_2 \cdot -$ and subsequently of H_2O_2 by manganese SOD (MnSOD). H_2O_2 then diffuses to the VSMC and activates voltage-dependent K^+ (K_V) channels promoting the hyperpolarization of the VSMCs and thus the vasodilation in the coronary microcirculation. Adapted from Muller-Delp [33] and prepared using Servier Medical Art (http://www.servier.com/).

$$R - SH + H_2O_2 \rightarrow R - SOH + H_2O \tag{5}$$

$$R - SOH + RSH \rightarrow R - SS - R + H_2O \tag{6}$$

Furthermore, these modifications in the redox state of the cell may also affect the hyperpolarization mediated by thiol-dependent voltage-dependent K^+ (K_V) channels, which will be further explored in the following subsection [40].

Other metabolic vasodilators may also be involved, such as adenosine (which concentration is dependent on the metabolism) and potassium ions, which will be explored further below.

3.4. Endothelial function

The *endothelial function* plays a crucial role in the vascular physiology, especially in the regulation of the vascular tone. The endothelium is responsible for the production of a number of different vasoactive substances, such as: (a) *endothelium-derived contracting factors* (EDCFs), such as endothelin, prostanoids and 20-hydroxyeicosatetraenoic acid (20-HETE) and (b) *endothelium-derived relaxing factors* (EDRFs), such as NO, prostaglandins (e.g. prostacyclin) and EDHFs, for example H_2O_2 and epoxyeicosatrienoic acids (EETs) [35, 41–47].

Vasoconstrictors. The stimulation of receptors in the endothelial cell membrane may trigger the production of several EDCFs, namely prostanoids and endothelin, particularly endothelin-1, among others (**Figure 3**) [35, 41]. The *prostanoids* are vasoactive substances that result from the arachidonic acid pathway. Following the stimulation of specific membrane receptors, such as muscarinic receptors for acetylcholine and purinergic (P_2Y) receptors for adenosine triphosphate (ATP), the increase in intracellular Ca^{2+} promotes the production of arachidonic acid from membrane phospholipids by phospholipase A_2 [41]. The arachidonic acid is then converted by the endothelial cyclooxygenase-1 (COX-1) to endoperoxides and ultimately to prostanoids, namely thromboxane A_2 (TXA_2) and prostaglandins, such as prostacyclin (PGI_2) [41]. Additionally, the COX-1 activity might also promote the production of ROS [41]. Those vasoactive substances (i.e. TXA_2 and prostaglandins) may then diffuse to the smooth muscle layer where they activate thromboxane-prostanoid (TP) receptors, promoting the contraction of the VSMCs [41].

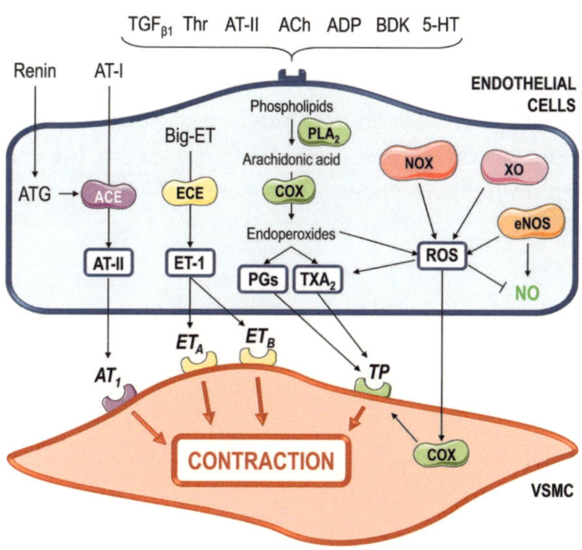

Figure 3. Multitude of pathways involved in the endothelium-dependent contraction. Abbreviations: 5-HT, 5-hydrotryptamine; ACE, angiotensin-converting enzyme; ACh, acetylcholine; ADP, adenosine diphosphate; AT-I, angiotensin-I; AT_1, angiotensin receptor; AT-II, angiotensin-II; ATG, angiotensinogen; BDK, bradykinin; COX, cyclooxygenases; ECE, endothelin-converting enzyme; ET-1, endothelin-1; ET_A, endothelin receptor A; ET_B, endothelin receptor B; NO, nitric oxide; eNOS, endothelial nitric oxide synthase; NOX, NADPH oxidase; PGs, prostaglandins; PLA_2, phospholipase A_2; ROS, reactive oxygen species; $TGF_{\beta1}$, transforming growth factor; Thr, thrombin; TP, thromboxane-prostanoid receptor; TXA_2, thromboxane A_2; VSMC, vascular smooth muscle cell; XO, xanthine oxidase. Adapted from Virdis et al. [49] and prepared using Servier Medical Art (http://www.servier.com/).

Endothelin (ET) is considered a major vasoactive substance in the EDCF family and a major vascular function regulator. In fact, this term refers to a group of peptides synthesized by the endothelin-converting enzyme (ECE) that may mediate vasoconstriction through the stimulation of receptors, namely ET_A and ET_B receptors, in the VSMC membrane [48, 49]. Among the several peptides, ET-1 is the most known, and its vasoactive properties have been extensively researched. This peptide promotes a long-lasting vasoconstriction essential to the vessel tone control in coronary arterioles, as reduction ET-1 induces an elevation of coronary blood flow in increased demand situations, that is increased metabolism [50, 51].

20-HETE is a metabolite that results from the conversion of arachidonic acid by the 4A and 4F families of cytochrome P450 mono-oxygenases (CYP), particularly in the VSMCs but also in the endothelial cells [35]. This metabolite seems to play an important role in the regulation of the vascular tone, behaving as a potent endogenous vasoconstrictor in several vascular tissues, namely in the brain and in the heart [35, 52].

Vasodilators. NO is the most researched EDRF worldwide and is produced in the endothelial cells by the endothelial nitric oxide synthase (eNOS). This constitutive enzyme converts L-arginine to L-citrulline and requires several cofactors, such as calcium, calmodulin, 3,4-tetrahydrobiopterin (BH_4) and nicotinamide adenine dinucleotide phosphate (NADPH) [53]. The NO-mediated vasodilation primarily involves the conversion of guanosine triphosphate (GTP) to cGMP by soluble guanylyl cyclase (solGC) [34]. However, other mechanisms may also be involved in the NO-mediated vasodilation, namely the hyperpolarization of the VSMCs [34, 54], which will be further explored below. The production of NO may be regulated by several mechanisms, which have been previously explored and published [55]. In addition to the stimulation of receptors on the endothelial cell membrane, the eNOS-mediated production of NO may also be stimulated by shear forces exerted by the blood flow on the vessel wall, as explored further below.

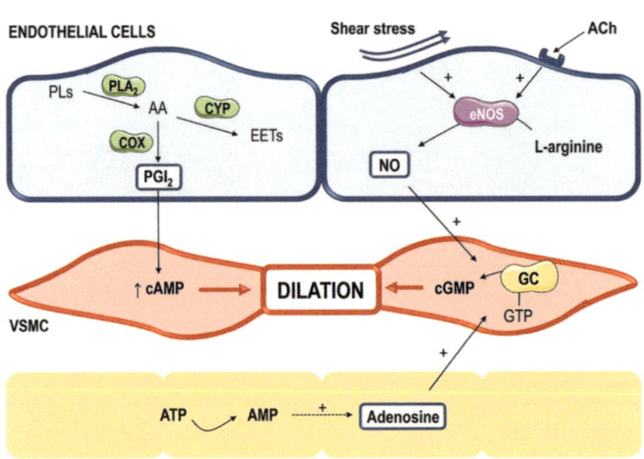

Figure 4. Pathways involved in the endothelium-dependent and endothelium-independent relaxation of the VSMC. Stimulation of the endothelial cells by acetylcholine (ACh) or other agents (e.g. bradykinin and shear stress) results in the formation and release of an EDRF identified as nitric oxide (NO). Substances such as adenosine, nitroprusside (NP), H^+, CO_2 and K^+ can be produced in the parenchymal tissue and elicit vasodilation by direct action on vascular smooth muscle. Adapted from Koeppen et al. [58] and prepared using Servier Medical Art (http://www.servier.com/).

http://dx.doi.org/10.5772/64537

Although NO is considered the major pathway of endothelium-mediated vasodilation in the systemic circulation, multiple pathways may be involved in this physiological response, such as the prostaglandins-induced vasodilation (**Figure 4**). The *prostaglandins* are constitutively produced by cyclooxygenases (COX) [34]. The main substrate of these enzymes is arachidonic acid, which is converted from diacylglycerol or phospholipids, respectively, by phospholipase A_2 and phospholipase C [34]. Several prostaglandins are produced by COX, although the main vasoactive prostaglandin produced in the endothelium is PGI_2 [35, 56, 57]. Similarly to NO, PGI_2 may diffuse from the endothelial cells to the VSMCs where they activate their (IP) receptors and trigger the conversion of ATP into cyclic adenosine monophosphate (cAMP) by adenylyl cyclase (AC) [34, 57]. This activation promotes the hyperpolarization of the VSMCs and hence the vasodilation [34, 57]. However, these prostaglandins, namely PGI_2, may also elicit vasoconstriction in disease, as previously discussed [35, 41].

Several vasoactive substances have been included in the *EDHFs* family, such as H_2O_2, carbon dioxide (CO_2), hydrogen sulphide (H_2S), C-natriuretic peptide (CNP), EETs, potassium ion (K^+), among others [34, 35, 54, 59]. Previous studies suggested these factors play a key role in the VSMC hyperpolarization in smaller vessels rather than in larger ones [19, 34].

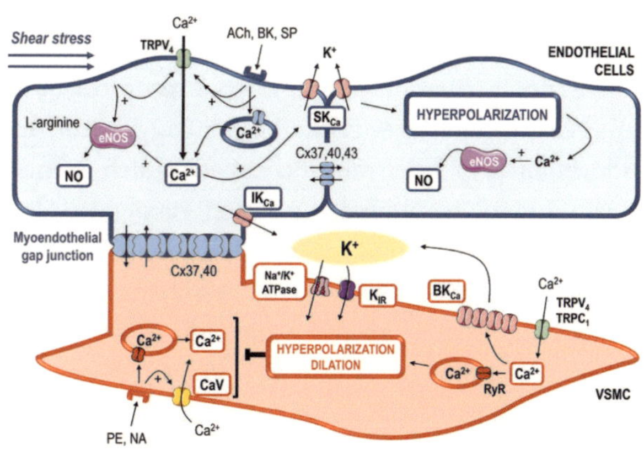

Figure 5. Hyperpolarization of the VSMC. Abbreviations: ACh, acetylcholine; BK, bradykinin; BK_{Ca}, large conductance Ca^{2+}-activated K^+ channels; Ca_V, voltage-activated Ca^{2+} channels; Cx, connexin; EC, endothelial cell; eNOS, endothelial nitric oxide synthase; IK_{Ca}, intermediate conductance Ca^{2+}-activated K^+ channels; K_{IR}, inwardly rectifying K^+ channels; NO, nitric oxide; PE, phenylephrine; RyR, ryanodine receptor; SK_{Ca}, small conductance Ca^{2+}-activated K^+ channels; SP, substance P, TRPC1, transient receptor potential canonical channel 1; TRPV4, transient receptor potential vanilloid channel 4; VSMC, vascular smooth muscle cell. Adapted from Félétou et al. [35] and prepared using Servier Medical Art (http://www.servier.com/).

The hyperpolarization of the VSMC may involve several ionic channels, such as the voltage-activated Ca^{2+} (Ca_V) channels, which regulate the intracellular Ca^{2+} concentration, the K_V channels and the Ca^{2+}-activated K^+ (K_{Ca}) channels [35, 40]. The K_{Ca} channels may be subdivided into small (SK_{Ca} or K_{Ca} 2.3 isoform), intermediate (IK_{Ca} or K_{Ca} 3.1 isoform) and large (BK_{Ca}) conductance Ca^{2+}-activated K^+ channels, which are located in specific cellular and subcellular sites [35]. The hyperpolarization of the VSMCs may be triggered directly, through receptors on the VSMC membrane, or indirectly, through the hyperpolarization of the endothelial cells [35].

As can be seen in **Figure 5**, the *direct hyperpolarization* may be promoted through the stimulation of BK_{Ca} channels on discrete locations of the VSMC layer, that is smooth muscle plasmerosome, associated with the TRP canonical channel 1 (TRPC1) and the TRP vanilloid channel 4 (TRPV4). These signal complexes promote (a) the influx of Ca^{2+}, which is then stored through ryanodine receptor (RyR) on the endoplasmic reticulum and (b) the efflux of K^+, contributing to the formation of a potassium cloud in the intercellular space, which functions as a negative-feedback mechanism. This ionic cloud may activate inwardly rectifying K^+ (K_{IR}) channels and Na^+/K^+-ATPase promoting the influx of K^+ to the VSMC, thus leading to the hyperpolarization and vasodilation. This hyperpolarization also inhibits the Ca^{2+} influx through Ca_V channels that may be stimulated by the binding of noradrenaline or phenylephrine to the adrenergic receptors on the membrane of VSMCs. The stimulation of these receptors leads to the increase in the intracellular Ca^{2+} concentration triggering the depolarization of the VSMC. Furthermore, this increase in intracellular Ca^{2+} may subsequently activate K_V and BK_{Ca} channels, which then promote the efflux of K^+ ions to the intercellular space, thus controlling the ionic balance and contributing to the formation of the potassium cloud [35, 57].

Moreover, the VSMCs may be *indirectly hyperpolarized* through the hyperpolarization of the endothelial cells [35]. Following activation of endothelial receptors and action of shear stress, the increased intracellular calcium in the endothelial cell triggers the opening of SK_{Ca} (located at the homocellular endothelial gap junctions and caveolin-rich domains) and IK_{Ca} channels (preferentially located at the myoendothelial gap junctions or MEJ) leading to K^+ efflux and consequently to the hyperpolarization of the endothelial cell [35]. In turn, this may ultimately lead to the hyperpolarization of the VSMCs by direct electric coupling through MEJs, which consist of a cell-cell contact resulting from the projection of an endothelial cell or a VSMC through the internal elastic membrane (**Figure 5**) [35, 60]. These contacts are essentially established through connexins (Cx), namely Cx40 and Cx37 [35, 61]. Particularly, at the level of the MEJs, the IK_{Ca} channels may be activated directly or through the generation of Ca^{2+} pulsars, contributing further to the potassium cloud in the intercellular space, eventually promoting the activation of K_{IR} channels and Na^+/K^+-ATPase involved in the hyperpolarization of the VSMCs. The influx of Ca^{2+} from the intercellular space to the VSMC, through Ca_V channels may be detected by Ca^{2+}-sensing receptors (CaSR), which may activate IK1 gene, involved in the hyperpolarization of the VSMC [35, 57].

Besides the hyperpolarization of the VSMCs, the EDHFs, particularly H_2O_2, may also promote vasodilation through other mechanisms, namely by stimulating the production of prostaglandin E_2 in the endothelial cell, thus promoting the endothelium-dependent vasodilation [62].

The relative importance of each pathway is still unestablished, but it has been proposed to depend for example on the activation state of the VSMCs, the density of MEJs and the expression of K_{IR} and Na^+/K^+-ATPase [57].

http://dx.doi.org/10.5772/64537

3.4.1. Shear stress

As previously mentioned, in addition to the stimulation of receptors on the endothelial cell membrane, other factors may modulate the endothelial function, namely the forces exerted by the blood flow on the vessel wall. There are two major forces: (a) one perpendicular to the wall and (b) another parallel to the wall, known as *wall shear stress* that results from the friction of blood flow on the endothelial cells [63]. These shear forces trigger several pathways, such as (a) production, release and binding of bradykinin to endothelial cell membrane receptors and (b) bradykinin-independent pathways, namely the activation of the Akt phosphorylation pathway and the ROS-mediated hyperpolarization of the VSMC. The production and release of *bradykinin*, which may bind to its G_q-coupled endothelial receptors, increases the activity of eNOS thus promoting the synthesis of NO [64]. The activation of the *Akt phosphorylation* pathway also promotes the production of NO by eNOS [64, 65]. In human coronary arterioles, the shear forces exerted on the vessel wall may also promote the *ROS-mediated hyperpolarization of the VSMC* through two main mechanisms: one involving the EETs and other involving the direct stimulation of ROS production (**Figure 6**). First, the shear stress may induce the production of EETs by triggering the cleavage of arachidonic acid from the cellular membrane by phospholipases. The arachidonic acid then works as a substrate to CYP for the production of EETs, which may activate the $TRPV_4$ channels promoting an increase in intracellular Ca^{2+}, thus stimulating the mitochondrial production of $O_2{\cdot}^-$. The production of ROS may also result

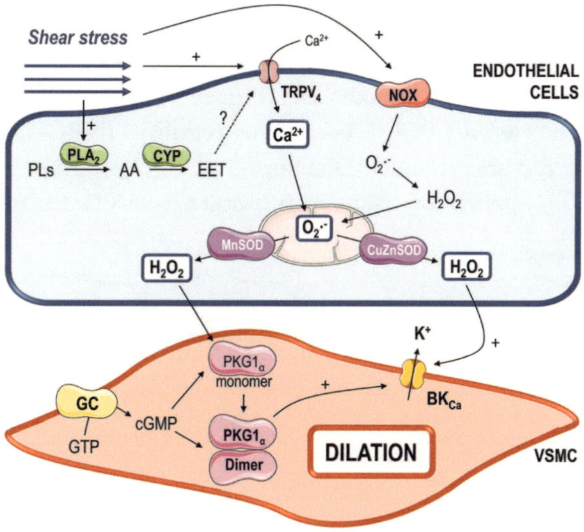

Figure 6. Flow-mediated dilation in the human coronary arterioles. Abbreviations: AA, arachidonic acid; BK_{Ca}, large conductance Ca^{2+}-activated K^+ channels; cGMP, cyclic guanosine monophosphate; CuZnSOD, copper-zinc superoxide dismutase; CYP, cytochrome P450; CYS 42, cysteine residue; EETs, epoxyeicosatrienoic acids; GC, guanylyl cyclase; GTP; guanosine triphosphate; H_2O_2, hydrogen peroxide; K_{Ca}, Ca^{2+}-activated K^+ channels; MnSOD, manganese superoxide dismutase; NADPH, nicotinamide adenine dinucleotide phosphate; NOX, NADPH oxidase; $O_2{\cdot}-$, superoxide anion; $PKG1_\alpha$, protein kinase G 1_α; PLA_2, phospholipase A_2; PLs, phospholipids; $TRPV_4$, transient receptor potential vanilloid channel 4. Adapted from Durand et al. [34] and prepared using Servier Medical Art (http://www.servier.com/).

from the direct stimulation of $TRPV_4$ channels and NADPH oxidases. The $O_2\cdot^-$ produced through both these mechanisms is then dismutated to H_2O_2, which diffuses to the VSMCs to oxidize cysteine residues of protein kinase G 1_α ($PKG1_\alpha$), activating this enzyme. The activation of this enzyme promotes the opening of BK_{Ca} channels and the hyperpolarization of the VSMCs resulting in vasodilation of coronary arterioles [32, 34, 66, 67].

Previous studies showed the sensitivity to these pathways of vasodilation increases with decreasing vessel diameter thus assuming a particularly important role in the coronary microcirculation [19]. Previous studies have also suggested the relative weight of these pathways changes from childhood to adulthood and between healthy and pathological conditions. In a preliminary study with human-isolated arterioles, Zinkevich et al. [68] proposed the flow-mediated dilation (FMD) in infants was exclusively COX-dependent, that is mediated by prostaglandins, while in adulthood the main pathway involved the NO. However, in the presence of coronary artery disease (CAD), both these mechanisms seem to remain as secondary pathways as the EDHF-mediated vasodilation (especially by H_2O_2) gains importance, serving as backup mechanisms in disease [66]. In fact, low response to shear forces and high mechanical stress seem to predispose to vascular dysfunction and disease [63].

3.4.2. *Endothelium-cardiomyocyte interaction*

The heart is a highly organized organ where several cells may be found, namely endothelial cells and cardiomyocytes. Therefore, the physiological mechanisms depend on the communication between the several types of cells. Until today, many endothelial-derived cardio-active factors have been identified and characterized (**Figure 7**). The cardiac modulator effects of some of these factors, such as NO, PGI_2, ET-1 and neuregulin-1 (NRG-1), have been previously acknowledged. Other factors, namely Dickkopf-3 (DKK3), periostin, thrombospondin-1 (TSP-1), follistatin (FST), apelin and connective tissue growth factor (CTGF), also appear to

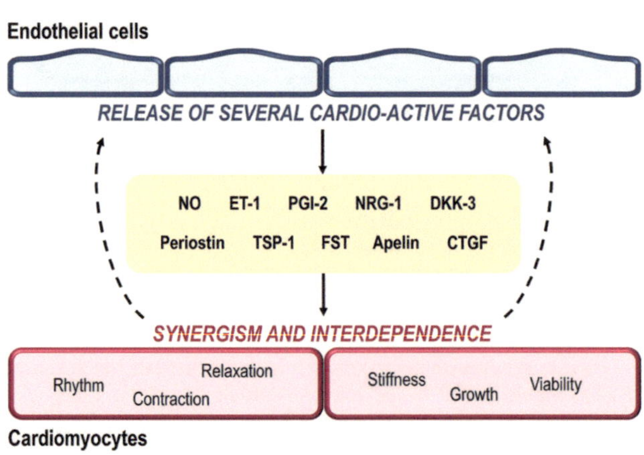

Figure 7. Communication between endothelial cells and cardiomyocytes. Abbreviations: CTGF, connective tissue growth factor; DKK3, Dickkopf-3; ET-1, endothelin; FST, follistatin; NO, nitric oxide; NRG-1, neuregulin-1; PGI-2, prostacyclin; TSP-1, thrombospondin. Adapted from Lim et al. [69].

modulate the cardiomyocyte function, though with little evidence so far. These cardio-active factors seem to be interdependent (additive, synergistic or inhibitory) as their modulator effects may be exerted on the same target cell [69].

3.5. Autonomic innervation and circulating factors

The previously explored pathways are nowadays considered the major pathways of regulation of the vessel tone. However, other mechanisms may also come into play, such as the autonomic nervous system and circulating factors.

The innervation of the coronary circulation by the sympathetic and the parasympathetic divisions of the *autonomic nervous system* have been previously shown [70]. The endothelial production of vasoactive substances, namely NO, may be influenced by the stimulation of specific receptors in the endothelial cell membrane, such as muscarinic receptors for acetylcholine [41, 70]. Furthermore, the coronary circulation may also be regulated through adrenergic receptors (i.e. α- and β-adrenergic receptors) in both the endothelial cell and the VSMC membranes [70]. In general, the stimulation of the α-adrenergic stimulation seems to induce vasoconstriction, with the exception for the α_2 receptors which seem to elicit vasodilation. Moreover, the stimulation of β-adrenergic receptors generally induces vasodilation with β_2 receptors being the main population in the coronary microcirculation [19, 70, 71]. This autonomic innervation provides a mechanism for vessel tone regulation, particularly important during exercise. However, the role of the parasympathetic innervation remains debatable in the human coronary microcirculation [70].

Moreover, several *circulating factors* may also modulate the coronary blood flow through the regulation of the vessel tone, such as angiotensin II and other hormones (e.g. cortisol and tiroxine, among others), adipokines (particularly adiponectin) and growth factors among many others [19, 72].

4. Microcirculation pathophysiology

As previously discussed, the coronary microcirculation plays a key role in the myocardial perfusion. Therefore, the presence of functional and/or structural abnormalities of this circulatory pathway may impair the myocardial perfusion and be involved alone as the main mechanism of myocardial ischaemia. These abnormalities are normally designated as *coronary microvascular dysfunction* (CMD) [3]. The CMD may be assessed by several methods, though one of the most used methods is through the determination of the coronary flow reserve (CFR), which represents an integrated measure of coronary blood flow in both the macro- and microcirculation. The CFR involves the maximal vasodilation of a vessel in response to an endothelium-independent vasodilator, such as adenosine, thus reflecting the ratio of hyperaemic to baseline blood flow. This ratio may be measured through several methods, namely echocardiography and positron emission tomography (PET) [3].

CMD type	Clinical setting	Pathogenic mechanisms
In the absence of myocardial disease or obstructive CAD	Cardiovascular risk factors (e.g. ageing, arterial hypertension, smoking, diabetes) Microvascular angina	Endothelial dysfunction VSMC dysfunction Vascular wall remodeling
In the presence of myocardial disease	Cardiomyopathies (e.g. HCM, DCM) Aortic stenosis	Vascular wall remodeling VSMC dysfunction Extramural compression Luminal obstruction
In the presence of obstructive CAD	Acute coronary syndrome AMI	Endothelial dysfunction VSMC dysfunction Luminal obstruction
Iatrogenic microembolization	Coronary reperfusion procedures (e.g. PCI) Revascularization (i.e. CABG)	Luminal obstruction Autonomic dysfunction

Abbreviations: AMI, acute myocardial infarction; CABG, coronary artery bypass grafting; DCM, dilated cardiomyopathy; HCM, hypertrophic cardiomyopathy; PCI, percutaneous coronary intervention; VSMC, vascular smooth muscle cell. Adapted from Crea et al. [20].

Table 1. Classification of CMD according to the involvement of pathogenic mechanisms and the clinical setting.

CMD may present several pathogenic underlying mechanisms, depending on the source of the abnormality, namely structural and functional (**Table 1**), which will be discussed in this section. According to the underlying clinical setting, the CMD may also be classified into four types: type 1, in the absence of cardiomyopathies or obstructive CAD; type 2, in the presence of cardiomyopathies; type 3, in the presence of CAD; and type 4, iatrogenic [3, 20, 73, 74].

4.1. Functional abnormalities

The most common functional abnormalities are the *dysfunction of the endothelial cells and/or the VSMCs*, involving cardiovascular risk factors or cardiomyopathies, and the *autonomic nervous system dysfunction*, secondary to coronary reperfusion procedures.

4.1.1. Endothelial and/or VSMC dysfunction

As presented in **Table 1**, the traditional cardiovascular risk factors (i.e. ageing, gender, obesity, smoking, hypertension, dyslipidaemia and diabetes) may impair the endothelial function by several mechanisms, namely increased production of EDCFs and/or decreased production of EDRFs [3, 73]. Furthermore, this impairment may also contribute to the dysfunction of the VSMCs, which may also result from structural changes, derived from cardiomyopathies or arterial hypertension, described further below.

Ageing is considered as one of the major cardiovascular risk factors that may influence the endothelial function. This influence seems to primarily involve both functional and structural changes, which will be discussed further below [42, 75]. Several mechanisms have been identified to mediate these changes and have been previously reviewed [55, 64, 76, 77]. In fact, the imbalance between vasoconstriction and vasodilation seems to be a key mechanism underlying ageing-induced vascular dysfunction.

Gender-associated differences related to hormones (i.e. oestrogens) have been previously described for the vascular reactivity in several vascular beds [42, 65]. The stimulation of G protein-coupled receptors by these hormones seems to promote an increased production of EDRFs, especially NO, which could elucidate the lower incidence of coronary disease and atherosclerosis in premenopausal women compared to men of the same age and postmenopausal women. In fact, impaired expression of eNOS was previously reported in postmenopausal women and suggested as a gender-specific risk factor in coronary surgery [78]. Moreover, Muir et al. [79] also showed differences in the endothelium-dependent vasodilation between males and females. In the coronary circulation, oestrogens seem to promote a decreased vascular tone, which promotes a reduced blood flow resistance and thus a higher coronary blood flow [80].

Obesity has also been considered an important cardiovascular risk factor; thus, a healthy diet and the regular practice of exercise have been proposed as important preventive measures. The influence of obesity in the vasoreactivity involves several mechanisms, namely an impaired regulation of vascular tone, a systemic chronic inflammation, induced by adipokines, which are involved in CMD, an altered lipidic profile (i.e. dyslipidaemia) and increased incidence of atherosclerosis and vascular oxidative stress [55, 80–82].

Cigarette smoking has been widely recognized as a major cardiovascular risk factor that induces endothelial dysfunction. In the peripheral circulation, this effect primarily involves the decreased production of EDRFs, namely NO, mainly through the impairment of eNOS activity [79, 83]. Interestingly, this downregulation of NO-mediated vasodilation seems to be exposure-dependent [84]. The ability to induce endothelial dysfunction may also manifest in the coronary circulation, particularly in long-term smokers, independently of the presence of atherosclerotic plaques [85]. Moreover, Kaufmann et al. [86] found CMD in asymptomatic smokers in the absence of CAD. These patients presented a reduction in 21% of the CFR, which could be restored with the short-term administration of vitamin C. These findings suggested that the smoking-associated CMD may involve an increase in oxidative stress in the coronary microcirculation [86].

Similarly to smoking, *arterial hypertension* is also considered a major cardiovascular risk factor. Previous studies suggested the increased production of EDCFs as the main mechanism underlying the hypertension-induced endothelial dysfunction [41]. This effect is primarily triggered by an increase in intracellular Ca^{2+}, stimulating a higher production of COX-derived prostanoids (e.g. TXA_2 and PGI_2) and ROS, namely $O_2 \cdot^-$ [41]. The prostanoids may then diffuse to the VSMCs activating TP receptors, with subsequent influx of Ca^{2+}, creating the conditions to a predominant vasoconstriction [41]. The ROS may also influence the vascular function since they may react with NO, reducing its availability, or even stimulate the influx of Ca^{2+} [41].

The vascular effects of *dyslipidaemia,* namely hypercholesterolaemia, are dependent on the degree of atherogenesis. In fact, the accumulation and oxidation of low-density lipoproteins

(LDLs) are considered major steps in the development of the chronic inflammatory process that is atherosclerosis [87]. The accumulation of LDL in the subendothelial matrix depends on the circulating LDL levels as the LDLs diffuse from the lumen to the vessel wall through endothelial cell junctions [87]. Once in the subendothelial matrix, the LDLs may undergo oxidation by reacting with endothelium-derived ROS, producing oxidized LDLs [87]. These proinflammatory factors may mediate several effects on the vessel wall, mainly the impairment of NO-mediated vasodilation and the atherogenesis [64]. In fact, oxidized LDLs may (a) trigger the influx of asymmetric dimethyl-L-arginine (ADMA), which is a competitor substrate for eNOS, (b) downregulate the NO production through the Rho kinase and protein kinase C pathways and (c) promote the uncoupling of eNOS by upregulating the NADPH oxidase production of ROS [64]. Previous studies in the human coronary circulation have revealed a reduced CFR in asymptomatic patients with hypercholesterolaemia, which seems to be reversible with a cholesterol-lowering therapy [88–91].

Diabetes is a known cardiovascular risk factor responsible for several effects on the cardiac and peripheral vascular systems, which intermediate an increased morbidity and mortality [92]. In spite of the array of mechanisms involved, the relation between diabetes and CMD is not yet fully understood [93]. Previous studies suggested several mechanisms involved in the diabetes-induced vascular dysfunction, namely (a) impaired production of NO, due to BH_4 deficiency, increased arginase activity, increased ADMA influx or downregulation of the Akt phosphorylation pathway; (b) increased production of EDCFs, namely endothelin; and (c) other NO-independent mechanisms, such as hyperglycaemia [55]. Chronic hyperglycaemia has been previously suggested to play a key role in the diabetes-related CMD, as several mechanisms may be involved [55], namely the endothelial-protein glycation through the formation of advanced glycation end-products (AGEs) and subsequent stimulation of the respective receptors (RAGE). In fact, previous studies suggested that diabetic patients (both type 1 and type 2) present a marked reduction in the endothelium-dependent and endothelium-independent coronary vasodilation [94].

The impairment of the vasodilator response of the coronary microcirculation may also be present in patients with angina-like chest pain but without evidence of obstructive CAD or myocardial disease. This situation is usually known as *microvascular angina* or *coronary syndrome X*. The literature seems to be contradictory as some studies suggest no changes in the coronary blood flow and in the CFR [73], while others showed the presence of CMD through impairment of the endothelium-dependent and endothelium-independent vasodilation [95], reduction in the coronary blood flow and CFR [96] and evidence of myocardial ischaemia [97, 98]. However, the precise pathogenic mechanisms involved in these changes are not yet completely understood as this situation seems to be multifactorial [99].

4.1.2. Autonomic nervous system dysfunction

The autonomic nervous system dysfunction, following acute myocardial infarction (AMI) and/or coronary reperfusion procedures, may also contribute to the CMD. In fact, increased coronary vasoconstriction has been previously shown, after AMI and successful percutaneous coronary angioplasty, both at the site of stenosis and distal to it, suggesting abnormal coronary vasodilator response [73, 100].

After AMI, the CMD may result from autonomic dysfunction and luminal obstruction, discussed further below. The autonomic dysfunction in the AMI-associated CMD involves increased sympathetic activation with increased vasoconstriction. These findings were confirmed by Gregorini et al. [101], who showed this impaired autonomic function might be reverted with α-blockers, such as phentolamine (nonselective α-blocker) and urapidil (α_1-selective blocker), which may improve the recovery of myocardial perfusion after coronary stenting in patients with AMI [101–103]. Autonomic dysfunction secondary to percutaneous coronary angioplasty was also showed by Gregorini et al. [104] who linked the left ventricular macro- and microcirculatory dysfunction in patients with transient ischaemia. In this study, phentolamine and urapidil were similarly used to block the α-adrenergic neurotransmission and propranolol (nonselective β-blocker) and the β-adrenergic neurotransmission, and the results showed that the increased coronary vasoconstriction, secondary to percutaneous coronary angioplasty, may be prevented with α-adrenergic receptor antagonists as no effect was demonstrated for the β-adrenergic blockade. Moreover, this study suggested that CFR may still be decreased for 7 days to 3 months after the procedure [104]. In a similar study, Kozàkovà et al. [105] confirmed the potential usefulness of urapidil to improve the left ventricular function in the angioplasty follow-up. Moreover, persistent yet reversible CMD after coronary revascularization was also previously showed [106].

4.2. Structural abnormalities

In addition to functional abnormalities, structural abnormalities, namely vascular remodelling, vascular rarefaction, perivascular fibrosis, luminal obstruction and infiltration of the myocardium and vascular wall, may also contribute to CMD [3, 73].

4.2.1. Vascular wall remodelling

The remodelling of the vessel wall involves persistent modifications which may result from several *remodelling signals*, such as (a) the wall shear stress (which mechanisms have been previously discussed), (b) the circumferential wall stress (resulting from the stretch of the smooth muscle layer) and (c) specific metabolic signals [19, 107]. As mentioned above, the physiologic metabolic control of coronary blood flow mainly involves CO_2 and ROS. In a pathological setting (i.e. myocardial ischaemia) however, the metabolic control may involve several mediators, such as oxygen, adenosine, prostaglandins, nitric oxide and protons [28]. In the presence of myocardial ischaemia, the decreased pO_2 is detected by (a) the cardiomyocytes triggering the production of adenosine (which promotes the VSMC hyperpolarization through its receptors A_{2A} and A_{2B}) and NO, by (b) the endothelium, inducing the production of prostaglandins and by (c) the VSMCs, where K_{ATP} and Ca_V channels are activated leading to the hyperpolarization of these cells and to the vasodilation [28]. These remodelling signals promote, on one hand, the increase in the *luminal diameter* and, on the other hand, the *VSMC plasticity* and *matrix remodelling*, inducing the wall thickening [19, 108]. However, in the presence of certain factors, such as ageing, arterial hypertension and cardiomyopathies, these mechanisms of adaptation may be impaired leading to pathogenic changes.

In addition to the functional changes, *ageing* may induce these structural modifications, namely the proliferation of VSMCs and increase the inflammation status in the vascular wall, which is linked to atherogenesis, leading to the remodelling of the vessel wall and to the decrease in the luminal diameter [75].

Other situations may also contribute to the vascular remodelling, especially arterial hypertension and cardiomyopathies. Previous studies have suggested that *arterial hypertension* may promote the thickening of the smooth muscle layer, by stimulating the proliferation of VSMCs and collagen fibres [3, 73].

Furthermore, *cardiomyopathies* (especially hypertrophic cardiomyopathy) may also contribute to the vascular remodelling. According to Maron et al. [109], "cardiomyopathies are a heterogeneous group of diseases of the myocardium associated with mechanical and/or electrical dysfunction that usually (but not invariably) exhibit inappropriate ventricular hypertrophy or dilatation and are due to a variety of causes that frequently are genetic. Cardiomyopathies either are confined to the heart or are part of generalized systemic disorders, often leading to cardiovascular death or progressive heart failure-related disability". The cardiomyopathies are usually classified into primary and secondary, based on the American Heart Association classification [109]. On the basis of the management of cardiomyopathy with a morphofunctional phenotype, the European Society of Cardiology proposed in 2008 the classification of cardiomyopathies into the hypertrophic (HCM), dilated (DCM), restrictive (RCM), arrhytmogenic right ventricular (ARVC) and unclassified varieties [110]. Each of these groups was subdivided into familial or genetic and nonfamilial or nongenetic forms [110]. In 2014, another classification was proposed by the World Heart Federation, involving a descriptive genotype-phenotype nosology system, the MOGE(S) classification [111]. Vascular remodelling in coronary arterioles has been previously associated with both HCM and DCM [73]. Similarly to arterial hypertension, the remodelling of these vessels also involves the thickening of both the smooth muscle layer and the intimal layer. These morphological changes may contribute to the CMD associated with HCM, as patients with this cardiomyopathy showed a marked decrease in vasodilator response in the endocardium, proportional to the degree of hypertrophy [3, 73]. Relatively to DCM, the degree of CMD may be considered an independent prognostic factor for cardiac events [73, 112, 113].

4.2.2. *Vascular rarefaction and perivascular fibrosis*

The coronary microvascular function may also be influenced by modifications in the vascular density, particularly by vascular rarefaction, that is the reduction in the number of microcirculatory vessels, which may also be recognized as hypotrophic remodelling [19]. The presence of arterial hypertension and the extravascular compression, observed in aortic stenosis and cardiomyopathies, induces vascular rarefaction leading to the reduction in the CFR. In addition to the vascular rarefaction, both situations may also induce perivascular fibrosis promoting structural modifications of the vessel wall [73, 114].

4.2.3. *Luminal obstruction*

CMD may also be characterized by luminal obstruction originated from (a) obstructive CAD or (b) iatrogenic microembolization [73].

According to the mechanisms underlying the associated CMD as well as the clinical findings, the *obstructive CAD* may be divided into stable CAD, unstable CAD and AMI [73]. Changes in the CFR were previously showed in patients with both stable CAD and acute coronary syndromes.

In patients with *stable CAD*, the CMD distal to a coronary stenosis seems to be triggered through two main pathways: (a) increased prearteriolar and arteriolar constriction, increasing the blood flow resistance and decreasing the myocardial perfusion and (b) impaired prearteriolar dilation in the presence of increased myocardial oxygen demands [73]. Although in the presence of coronary stenosis (for example during exercise), the transmural myocardial perfusion tends to be redistributed, with an increase in the subendocardial perfusion. The impairment of this mechanism in patients with stable CAD may lead to increased microvascular vasoconstriction, which might promote a critical stenosis and thus capillary derecruitment distal to the stenosis, ultimately contributing to CMD [73].

Similarly to stable CAD, *unstable CAD* (i.e. acute coronary syndromes without ST-segment elevation) may also involve a CMD distal to a critical stenosis which might play a role in the severity of the myocardial ischaemia. In addition to the mechanisms described for stable CAD, this type of acute coronary syndromes also involves other mechanisms, such as thrombogenesis [73]. In fact, Marzilli et al. [115] suggested that the blockade of the platelet glycoprotein IIb/IIIa receptor with abciximab might improve the microvascular function in patients with unstable CAD. Moreover, the inflammation status may also come into play as suggested by previous studies that showed a direct relation between CMD and the systemic levels of C-reactive protein, a marker of inflammation independent of the cardiovascular risk factors [116, 117]. Both of these factors may contribute to the luminal obstruction observed in patients with unstable CAD.

Luminal obstruction is a key characteristic of the *AMI*. Early after a myocardial infarction, patients may present a marked reduction in the CFR that could significantly impair the contractility of the myocardium in the infarction region [73]. In addition to the autonomic dysfunction (previously explored), this impaired myocardial contractility might also be reverted with α-blockers [73, 101]. Even after reperfusion procedures, the CMD involving luminal obstruction in the stenotic and poststenotic areas may be responsible for the failure of the reperfusion, situation usually known as *"no-reflow" phenomenon*. This phenomenon is characterized by the lack of morphological and functional integrity in the microcirculation, in spite of successful reperfusion procedures [12, 73, 118, 119] and is associated with clinically significant decreased prognosis. The pathogenesis of the "no-reflow" phenomenon seems to be multifactorial; thus, a classification has been previously proposed which divides this phenomenon into (a) structural and (b) functional types. The structural type involves irreversible changes in the wall of the microvessels, while the functional type includes morphologically intact yet functionally compromised microvessels. The functional changes include impairment of the endothelium-dependent vasodilation, autonomic nervous system dysfunction and extravascular compression due to interstitial oedema, among others [73, 120, 121]. Recently, O'Farrell et al. [12] proposed a key role of pericytes in the pathogenesis of this phenomenon (**Figure 8**), suggesting that these cells irreversibly constrict the coronary microcirculation impeding the adequate reperfusion after AMI.

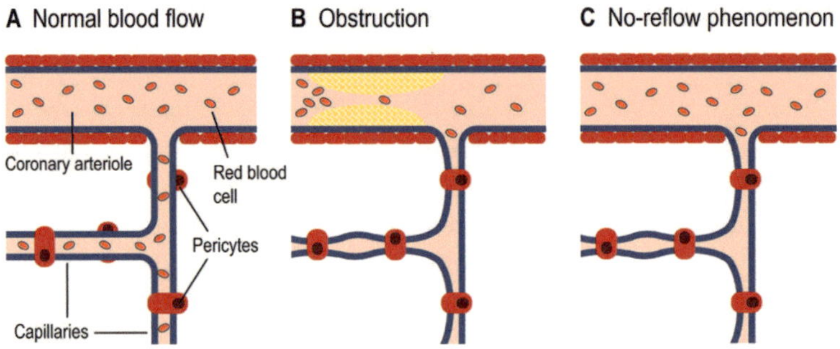

Figure 8. Role of pericytes in healthy and ischaemic microvessels: (a) normal blood flow in coronary arterioles and capillaries covered with pericytes; (b) in ischaemia, the pericytes may constrict the coronary microcirculation compromising the coronary blood flow and leading to coronary microvascular dysfunction; (c) after reperfusion procedures, the coronary microvascular dysfunction may block the re-establishment of the normal blood flow, situation usually known as no-reflow phenomenon.

As previously mentioned, CMD may also be originated from *iatrogenic microembolization* after coronary reperfusion procedures or coronary artery bypass grafting. During or after these procedures, plaque rupture may occur thus releasing plaque content into the blood which in turn might lead to luminal obstruction in the microcirculation [73].

4.2.4. Vascular wall infiltration

In addition to the previous explored structural changes, the infiltration of the vessel wall with metabolic deposits may also be found. This infiltration is commonly found in infiltrative diseases, such as Anderson-Fabry disease and other metabolic disorders. The Anderson-Fabry disease involves a genetically linked (X chromosome) deficiency of lysosomal α-galactosidase A, which leads to damages in several organs, namely the heart, through the deposition of glycosphingolipid in cardiomyocytes and in the vascular wall [73]. In turn, this infiltration promotes the hypertrophy and fibrosis of cardiomyocytes as well as CMD and perivascular fibrosis [73]. In fact, Elliott et al. [122] demonstrated these patients present a marked decrease in CFR, confirming the presence of CMD in the pathogenesis of the cardiomyopathy induced by this disease.

5. Conclusions

This review provides an insight on the morphology, physiology and pathophysiology of the cardiac microcirculation. As discussed, the heart is one of the most nutrient and oxygen

http://dx.doi.org/10.5772/64537

demanding organs as this demand needs to be satisfied with an adequate vascularization of the myocardium through an extensive macro- and microvascular network. Although most of the cardiac diseases, such as the acute coronary syndrome, are commonly associated with the coronary macrocirculation (i.e. epicardial coronary arteries), the coronary microcirculation also seems to play a key role in the coronary pathophysiology. This role involves both molecular and clinical aspects that should not be overlooked and that constitute potential diagnostic and therapeutic targets, particularly important in the early pathogenesis of these diseases.

Author details

Diogo André Fonseca[1,2,3*], Pedro Engrácia Antunes[4] and Maria Dulce Cotrim[1,2,3]

*Address all correspondence to: diogo.andre.fonseca@gmail.com

1 Pharmacology and Pharmaceutical Care Group, Faculty of Pharmacy, University of Coimbra, Coimbra, Portugal

2 Institute for Biomedical Imaging and Life Sciences (IBILI), Faculty of Medicine, University of Coimbra, Coimbra, Portugal

3 CNC.IBILI, University of Coimbra, Coimbra, Portugal

4 Centre of Cardiothoracic Surgery, Coimbra University Hospitals, Coimbra, Portugal

References

[1] Clough, G. and Cracowski, J.-L. Spotlight issue: microcirculation-from a clinical perspective. Microcirculation, 2012; 19(1): p. 1–4. doi:10.1111/j.1549-8719.2011.00142.x

[2] De Boer, M.P., Meijer, R.I., Wijnstok, N.J., Jonk, A.M., Houben, A.J., Stehouwer, C.D., et al. Microvascular dysfunction: a potential mechanism in the pathogenesis of obesity-associated insulin resistance and hypertension. Microcirculation, 2012; 19(1): p. 5–18. doi:10.1111/j.1549-8719.2011.00130.x

[3] Camici, P.G., d'Amati, G. and Rimoldi, O. Coronary microvascular dysfunction: mechanisms and functional assessment. Nature Reviews. Cardiology., 2015; 12(1): p. 48–62. doi:10.1038/nrcardio.2014.160

[4] Duncker, D.J. and Bache, R.J. Regulation of coronary vasomotor tone under normal conditions and during acute myocardial hypoperfusion. Pharmacology & Therapeutics, 2000; 86(1): p. 87–110

[5] Meerbaum, S. Myocardial perfusion. In *Myocardial Perfusion, Reperfusion, Coronary Venous Retroperfusion*, S. Meerbaum, Editor. 1990, Berlin, Heidelberg: Springer-Verlag. p. 1–17.

[6] Ross, M.H. and Pawlina, W. *Histology – A Text and Atlas: With Correlated Cell and Molecular Biology*. 6th edn. 2011, Philadelphia, PA: Lippincott Williams & Wilkins. p. 974.

[7] Camici, P.G., Olivotto, I. and Rimoldi, O.E. The coronary circulation and blood flow in left ventricular hypertrophy. Journal of Molecular and Cellular Cardiology, 2012; 52(4): p. 857–864. doi: doi:10.1016/j.yjmcc.2011.08.028

[8] Lee, J. and Smith, N.P. The multi-scale modelling of coronary blood flow. Annals of Biomedical Engineering, 2012; 40(11): p. 2399–2413. doi:10.1007/s10439-012-0583-7

[9] Zhang, J.H., Badaut, J., Tang, J., Obenaus, A., Hartman, R. and Pearce, W.J. The vascular neural network – a new paradigm in stroke pathophysiology. Nature Reviews. Neurology, 2012; 8(12): p. 711–716.

[10] Duncker, D.J., Koller, A., Merkus, D. and Canty, J.M., Jr. Regulation of coronary blood flow in health and ischemic heart disease. Progress in Cardiovascular Diseases, 2015; 57(5): p. 409–422. doi:10.1016/j.pcad.2014.12.002

[11] Weiss, H.R. and Sinha, A.K. Regional oxygen saturation of small arteries and veins in the canine myocardium. Circulation Research, 1978; 42(1): p. 119–126. doi: 10.1161/01.res.42.1.119

[12] O'Farrell, F.M. and Attwell, D. A role for pericytes in coronary no-reflow. Nature Reviews. Cardiology, 2014; 11(7): p. 427–432. doi:10.1038/nrcardio.2014.58

[13] Hamilton, N.B., Attwell, D. and Hall, C.N. Pericyte-mediated regulation of capillary diameter: a component of neurovascular coupling in health and disease. Frontiers in Neuroenergetics, 2010; 2: 5. doi:10.3389/fnene.2010.00005

[14] Berry, C., Balachandran, K.P., L'Allier, P.L., Lespérance, J., Bonan, R. and Oldroyd, K.G. Importance of collateral circulation in coronary heart disease. European Heart Journal, 2007; 28(3): p. 278–291. doi:10.1093/eurheartj/ehl446

[15] Thebessius, A. *Dissertatio Medica de Circulo Sanguinis in Corde*. 1708, Lagdumi Batavorium, Amsterdam: Elsevier.

[16] Snodgrass, B.T. Vessels described by Thebesius and Pratt are distinct from those described by Vieussens and Wearn. American Journal of Cardiology, 2012; 110(1): p. 160. doi:10.1016/j.amjcard.2012.04.005

[17] Wearn, J. The role of the Thebessian vessels in the circulation of the heart. Journal of Experimental Medicine, 1928; 47: p. 293–304.

[18] Wearn, J.T., Mettier, S.R., Klumpp, T.G. and Zschiesche, L.J. The nature of the vascular communications between the coronary arteries and the chambers of the heart. American Heart Journal, 1933; 9(2): p. 143–146. doi:10.1016/S0002-8703(33)90711-5

[19] Pries, A.R., Badimon, L., Bugiardini, R., Camici, P.G., Dorobantu, M., Duncker, D.J., et al. Coronary vascular regulation, remodelling, and collateralization: mechanisms and clinical implications on behalf of the working group on coronary pathophysiology and microcirculation. European Heart Journal, 2015; 36(45): p. 3134–3146. doi:10.1093/eurheartj/ehv100

[20] Crea, F., Camici, P.G. and Bairey Merz, C.N. Coronary microvascular dysfunction: an update. European Heart Journal, 2014; 35(17): p. 1101–1111. doi:10.1093/eurheartj/eht513

[21] Levy, B.I., Ambrosio, G., Pries, A.R. and Struijker-Boudier, H.A. Microcirculation in hypertension: a new target for treatment? Circulation, 2001; 104(6): p. 735–740.

[22] Davis, M.J. and Hill, M.A. Signaling mechanisms underlying the vascular myogenic response. Physiological Reviews, 1999; 79(2): p. 387–423.

[23] Kuo, L., Davis, M.J. and Chilian, W.M. Myogenic activity in isolated subepicardial and subendocardial coronary arterioles. American Journal of Physiology, 1988; 255(6 Pt 2): p. H1558–H1562.

[24] Davis, M.J., Wu, X., Nurkiewicz, T.R., Kawasaki, J., Davis, G.E., Hill, M.A., et al. Integrins and mechanotransduction of the vascular myogenic response. American Journal of Physiology. Heart and Circulatory Physiology, 2001; 280(4): p. H1427–H1433.

[25] Baylie, R.L. and Brayden, J.E. TRPV channels and vascular function. Acta Physiol (Oxf), 2011; 203(1): p. 99–116. doi:10.1111/j.1748-1716.2010.02217.x

[26] Brayden, J.E., Earley, S., Nelson, M.T. and Reading, S. Transient receptor potential (TRP) channels, vascular tone and autoregulation of cerebral blood flow. Clinical and Experimental Pharmacology & Physiology, 2008; 35(9): p. 1116–1120. doi:10.1111/j.1440-1681.2007.04855.x

[27] Kauffenstein, G., Laher, I., Matrougui, K., Guerineau, N.C. and Henrion, D. Emerging role of G protein-coupled receptors in microvascular myogenic tone. Cardiovascualr Research, 2012; 95(2): p. 223–232. doi:10.1093/cvr/cvs152

[28] Deussen, A., Ohanyan, V., Jannasch, A., Yin, L. and Chilian, W. Mechanisms of metabolic coronary flow regulation. Journal of Molecular and Cellular Cardiology, 2012; 52(4): p. 794–801. doi:10.1016/j.yjmcc.2011.10.001

[29] Wexels, J.C., Myhre, E.S. and Mjos, O.D. Effects of carbon dioxide and pH on myocardial blood-flow and metabolism in the dog. Clinical Physiology, 1985; 5(6): p. 575–588.

[30] Feigl, E.O. Coronary physiology. Physiological Reviews, 1983; 63(1): p. 1–205.

[31] Saitoh, S., Zhang, C., Tune, J.D., Potter, B., Kiyooka, T., Rogers, P.A., et al. Hydrogen peroxide: a feed-forward dilator that couples myocardial metabolism to coronary blood

flow. Arteriosclerosis, Thrombosis, and Vascular Biology, 2006; 26(12): p. 2614–2621. doi:10.1161/01.ATV.0000249408.55796.da

[32] Liu, Y., Zhao, H., Li, H., Kalyanaraman, B., Nicolosi, A.C. and Gutterman, D.D. Mitochondrial sources of H_2O_2 generation play a key role in flow-mediated dilation in human coronary resistance arteries. Circulation Research, 2003; 93(6): p. 573–580. doi: 10.1161/01.res.0000091261.19387.ae

[33] Muller-Delp, J.M. The coronary microcirculation in health and disease. ISRN Physiology, 2013; 2013: p. 24. doi:10.1155/2013/238979

[34] Durand, M.J. and Gutterman, D.D. Diversity in mechanisms of endothelium-dependent vasodilation in health and disease. Microcirculation, 2013; 20(3): p. 239–247. doi: 10.1111/micc.12040

[35] Félétou, M. and Vanhoutte, P.M. EDHF: an update. Clinical Sciences (London), 2009; 117(4): p. 139–155. doi:10.1042/cs20090096

[36] Sato, A., Sakuma, I. and Gutterman, D.D. Mechanism of dilation to reactive oxygen species in human coronary arterioles. American Journal of Physiology. Heart and Circulatory Physiology, 2003; 285(6): p. H2345–H2354. doi:10.1152/ajpheart.00458.2003

[37] Saitoh, S., Kiyooka, T., Rocic, P., Rogers, P.A., Zhang, C., Swafford, A., et al. Redox-dependent coronary metabolic dilation. American Journal of Physiology. Heart and Circulatory Physiology, 2007; 293(6): p. H3720–H3725. doi:10.1152/ajpheart.00436.2007

[38] Shan, X.Q., Aw, T.Y. and Jones, D.P. Glutathione-dependent protection against oxidative injury. Pharmacology & Therapeutics, 1990; 47(1): p. 61–71.

[39] Winterbourn, C.C. and Metodiewa, D. Reactivity of biologically important thiol compounds with superoxide and hydrogen peroxide. Free Radical Biology & Medicine, 1999; 27(3–4): p. 322–328.

[40] Rogers, P.A., Chilian, W.M., Bratz, I.N., Bryan, R.M., Jr. and Dick, G.M. H_2O_2 activates redox- and 4-aminopyridine-sensitive Kv channels in coronary vascular smooth muscle. American Journal of Physiology. Heart and Circulatory Physiology, 2007; 292(3): p. H1404–H1411. doi:10.1152/ajpheart.00696.2006

[41] Vanhoutte, P.M. Endothelium-dependent contractions in hypertension: when prostacyclin becomes ugly. Hypertension, 2011; 57(3): p. 526–531. doi:10.1161/hypertensionaha.110.165100

[42] Virdis, A. and Taddei, S. Endothelial aging and gender. Maturitas, 2012; 71(4): p. 326–330. doi:10.1016/j.maturitas.2012.01.010

[43] Moncada, S., Palmer, R.M. and Higgs, E.A. The discovery of nitric oxide as the endogenous nitrovasodilator. Hypertension, 1988; 12(4): p. 365–372.

[44] Lüscher, T.F. The endothelium and cardiovascular disease—a complex relation. New England Journal of Medicine, 1994; 330(15): p. 1081–1083. doi:10.1056/nejm199404143301511

[45] Ruschitzka, F.T., Noll, G. and Lüscher, T.F. The endothelium in coronary artery disease. Cardiology, 1997; 88(Suppl. 3): p. 3–19.

[46] Flammer, A.J. and Lüscher, T.F. Human endothelial dysfunction: EDRFs. Pflugers Archiv, 2010; 459(6): p. 1005–1013. doi:10.1007/s00424-010-0822-4

[47] Félétou, M., Köhler, R. and Vanhoutte, P.M. Nitric oxide: orchestrator of endothelium-dependent responses. Annals of Medicine, 2012; 44(7): p. 694–716. doi:10.3109/07853890.2011.585658

[48] Mazzuca, M.Q. and Khalil, R.A. Vascular endothelin receptor type B: structure, function and dysregulation in vascular disease. Biochemistry and Pharmacology, 2012; 84(2): p. 147–162. doi:10.1016/j.bcp.2012.03.020

[49] Virdis, A., Ghiadoni, L. and Taddei, S. Human endothelial dysfunction: EDCFs. Pflugers Archiv, 2010; 459(6): p. 1015–1023. doi:10.1007/s00424-009-0783-7

[50] Leblanc, A.J., Chen, B., Dougherty, P.J., Reyes, R.A., Shipley, R.D., Korzick, D.H., et al. Divergent effects of aging and sex on vasoconstriction to endothelin in coronary arterioles. Microcirculation, 2013; 20(5): p. 365–376. doi:10.1111/micc.12028

[51] Merkus, D., Duncker, D.J. and Chilian, W.M. Metabolic regulation of coronary vascular tone: role of endothelin-1. American Journal of Physiology. Heart and Circulatory Physiology, 2002; 283(5): p. H1915–H1921. doi:10.1152/ajpheart.00223.2002

[52] Miyata, N. and Roman, R.J. Role of 20-hydroxyeicosatetraenoic acid (20-HETE) in vascular system. Journal of Smooth Muscle Research, 2005; 41(4): p. 175–193.

[53] Förstermann, U. and Sessa, W.C. Nitric oxide synthases: regulation and function. European Heart Journal, 2012; 33(7): p. 829–837, 837a–837d. doi:10.1093/eurheartj/ehr304

[54] Félétou, M. and Vanhoutte, P.M. *EDHF: the Complete Story*. 2005, Boca Raton, FL: CRC Press, Taylor & Francis. 312 p.

[55] Fonseca, D.A., Antunes, P.E. and Cotrim, M.D. Endothelium-dependent vasoactivity of the human internal mammary artery. Coronary Artery Disease, 2014; 25(3): p. 266–274. doi:10.1097/MCA.0000000000000097

[56] Moncada, S. and Vane, J.R. Pharmacology and endogenous roles of prostaglandin endoperoxides, thromboxane A2, and prostacyclin. Pharmacological Reviews, 1978; 30(3): p. 293–331.

[57] Félétou, M. and Vanhoutte, P.M. Endothelium-derived hyperpolarizing factor: where are we now? Arteriosclerosis, Thrombosis, and Vascular Biology, 2006; 26(6): p. 1215–1225. doi:10.1161/01.ATV.0000217611.81085.c5

[58] Koeppen, B.M. and Stanton, B.A. *Berne & Levy Physiology*. 6th edn. 2008, Philadelphia, PA: Mosby.

[59] Sandow, S.L. and Tare, M. C-type natriuretic peptide: a new endothelium-derived hyperpolarizing factor? Trends in Pharmacological Sciences, 2007; 28(2): p. 61–7. doi: 10.1016/j.tips.2006.12.007

[60] Heberlein, K.R., Straub, A.C. and Isakson, B.E. The myoendothelial junction: breaking through the matrix? Microcirculation, 2009; 16(4): p. 307–322. doi: 10.1080/10739680902744404

[61] Kerr, P.M., Tam, R., Ondrusova, K., Mittal, R., Narang, D., Tran, C.H., et al. Endothelial feedback and the myoendothelial projection. Microcirculation, 2012; 19(5): p. 416–422. doi:10.1111/j.1549-8719.2012.00187.x

[62] Thengchaisri, N. and Kuo, L. Hydrogen peroxide induces endothelium-dependent and -independent coronary arteriolar dilation: role of cyclooxygenase and potassium channels. American Journal of Physiology. Heart and Circulatory Physiology, 2003; 285(6): p. H2255–H2263. doi:10.1152/ajpheart.00487.2003

[63] John, L.C. Biomechanics of coronary artery and bypass graft disease: potential new approaches. The Annals of Thoracic Surgery, 2009; 87(1): p. 331–338. doi:10.1016/j.athoracsur.2008.07.023

[64] Vanhoutte, P.M., Shimokawa, H., Tang, E.H. and Feletou, M. Endothelial dysfunction and vascular disease. Acta Physiologica (Oxford), 2009; 196(2): p. 193–222. doi:10.1111/j.1748-1716.2009.01964.x

[65] Michel, T. and Vanhoutte, P.M. Cellular signaling and NO production. Pflugers Archiv, 2010; 459(6): p. 807–816. doi:10.1007/s00424-009-0765-9

[66] Miura, H., Wachtel, R.E., Liu, Y., Loberiza, F.R., Jr., Saito, T., Miura, M., et al. Flow-induced dilation of human coronary arterioles: important role of Ca(2+)-activated K(+) channels. Circulation, 2001; 103(15): p. 1992–1998.

[67] Miura, H., Bosnjak, J.J., Ning, G., Saito, T., Miura, M. and Gutterman, D.D. Role for hydrogen peroxide in flow-induced dilation of human coronary arterioles. Circulation Research, 2003; 92(2): p. e31–e40.

[68] Zinkevich, N.S., Wittenburg, A.L. and Gutterman, D.D. Abstract 15764: role of cyclo-oxygenase in flow-induced dilation of human coronary arterioles depends upon age. Circulation, 2010; 122(Suppl. 21): p. A15764.

[69] Lim, S.L., Lam, C.S., Segers, V.F., Brutsaert, D.L. and De Keulenaer, G.W. Cardiac endothelium-myocyte interaction: clinical opportunities for new heart failure therapies regardless of ejection fraction. European Heart Journal, 2015; 36(31): p. 2050–2060. doi: 10.1093/eurheartj/ehv132

[70] Duncker, D.J., Bache, R.J. and Merkus, D. Regulation of coronary resistance vessel tone in response to exercise. Journal of Molecular and Cellular Cardiology, 2012; 52(4): p. 802–813. doi:10.1016/j.yjmcc.2011.10.007

[71] Dessy, C., Moniotte, S., Ghisdal, P., Havaux, X., Noirhomme, P. and Balligand, J.L. Endothelial beta3-adrenoceptors mediate vasorelaxation of human coronary microarteries through nitric oxide and endothelium-dependent hyperpolarization. Circulation, 2004; 110(8): p. 948–954. doi:10.1161/01.cir.0000139331.85766.af

[72] Margaritis, M., Antonopoulos, A.S., Digby, J., Lee, R., Reilly, S., Coutinho, P., et al. Interactions between vascular wall and perivascular adipose tissue reveal novel roles for adiponectin in the regulation of endothelial nitric oxide synthase function in human vessels. Circulation, 2013; 127(22): p. 2209–2221. doi:10.1161/circulationaha.112.001133

[73] Camici, P.G. and Crea, F. Coronary microvascular dysfunction. New England Journal of Medicine, 2007; 356(8): p. 830–840. doi:10.1056/NEJMra061889

[74] Lanza, G.A. and Crea, F. Primary coronary microvascular dysfunction: clinical presentation, pathophysiology, and management. Circulation, 2010; 121(21): p. 2317–2325. doi:10.1161/CIRCULATIONAHA.109.900191

[75] Seals, D.R., Jablonski, K.L. and Donato, A.J. Aging and vascular endothelial function in humans. Clinical Science (London), 2011; 120(9): p. 357–375. doi:10.1042/cs20100476

[76] LeBlanc, A.J. and Hoying, J.B. Adaptation of the coronary microcirculation in aging. Microcirculation, 2016; 23(2): p. 157–167. doi:10.1111/micc.12264

[77] Muller-Delp, J.M., Gurovich, A.N., Christou, D.D. and Leeuwenburgh, C. Redox balance in the aging microcirculation: new friends, new foes, and new clinical directions. Microcirculation, 2012; 19(1): p. 19–28. doi:10.1111/j.1549-8719.2011.00139.x

[78] Mannacio, V., Di Tommaso, L., Antignano, A., De Amicis, V., Stassano, P., Pinna, G.B., et al. Endothelial nitric oxide synthase expression in postmenopausal women: a sex-specific risk factor in coronary surgery. The Annals of Thoracic Surgery, 2012; 94(6): p. 1934–1939. doi:10.1016/j.athoracsur.2012.06.040

[79] Muir, A.D., McKeown, P.P. and Bayraktutan, U. Role of gender, smoking profile, hypertension, and diabetes on saphenous vein and internal mammary artery endothelial relaxation in patients with coronary artery bypass grafting. Oxidative Medicine and Cellular Longevity, 2010; 3(3): p. 199–205. doi:10.4161/oxim.3.3.11757

[80] Dal Lin, C., Tona, F. and Osto, E. Coronary microvascular function and beyond: the crosstalk between hormones, cytokines, and neurotransmitters. International Journal of Endocrinology, 2015; 2015: p. 312848. doi:10.1155/2015/312848

[81] Bagi, Z., Broskova, Z. and Feher, A. Obesity and coronary microvascular disease – implications for adipose tissue-mediated remote inflammatory response. Current Vascular Pharmacology, 2014; 12(3): p. 453–461.

[82] Houben, A.J., Eringa, E.C., Jonk, A.M., Serne, E.H., Smulders, Y.M. and Stehouwer, C.D. Perivascular fat and the microcirculation: relevance to insulin resistance, diabetes, and cardiovascular disease. Current Cardiovascular Risk Reports, 2012; 6(1): p. 80–90. doi: 10.1007/s12170-011-0214-0

[83] Barua, R.S., Ambrose, J.A., Eales-Reynolds, L.J., DeVoe, M.C., Zervas, J.G. and Saha, D.C. Dysfunctional endothelial nitric oxide biosynthesis in healthy smokers with impaired endothelium-dependent vasodilatation. Circulation, 2001; 104(16): p. 1905–1910.

[84] Celermajer, D.S., Sorensen, K.E., Georgakopoulos, D., Bull, C., Thomas, O., Robinson, J., et al. Cigarette smoking is associated with dose-related and potentially reversible impairment of endothelium-dependent dilation in healthy young adults. Circulation, 1993; 88(5 Pt 1): p. 2149–2155.

[85] Zeiher, A.M., Schachinger, V. and Minners, J. Long-term cigarette smoking impairs endothelium-dependent coronary arterial vasodilator function. Circulation, 1995; 92(5): p. 1094–1100.

[86] Kaufmann, P.A., Gnecchi-Ruscone, T., di Terlizzi, M., Schäfers, K.P., Lüscher, T.F. and Camici, P.G. Coronary heart disease in smokers: vitamin C restores coronary microcirculatory function. Circulation, 2000; 102(11): p. 1233–1238.

[87] Lusis, A.J. Atherosclerosis. Nature, 2000; 407(6801): p. 233–241. doi:10.1038/35025203

[88] Dayanikli, F., Grambow, D., Muzik, O., Mosca, L., Rubenfire, M. and Schwaiger, M. Early detection of abnormal coronary flow reserve in asymptomatic men at high risk for coronary artery disease using positron emission tomography. Circulation, 1994; 90(2): p. 808–817.

[89] Gould, K.L., Martucci, J.P., Goldberg, D.I., Hess, M.J., Edens, R.P., Latifi, R., et al. Short-term cholesterol lowering decreases size and severity of perfusion abnormalities by positron emission tomography after dipyridamole in patients with coronary artery disease. A potential noninvasive marker of healing coronary endothelium. Circulation, 1994; 89(4): p. 1530–1538.

[90] Czernin, J., Barnard, R.J., Sun, K.T., Krivokapich, J., Nitzsche, E., Dorsey, D., et al. Effect of short-term cardiovascular conditioning and low-fat diet on myocardial blood flow and flow reserve. Circulation, 1995; 92(2): p. 197–204.

[91] Kaufmann, P.A., Gnecchi-Ruscone, T., Schafers, K.P., Luscher, T.F. and Camici, P.G. Low density lipoprotein cholesterol and coronary microvascular dysfunction in hypercholesterolemia. Journal of the American College of Cardiology, 2000; 36(1): p. 103–109.

[92] Madonna, R. and De Caterina, R. Cellular and molecular mechanisms of vascular injury in diabetes—part I: pathways of vascular disease in diabetes. Vascular Pharmacology, 2011; 54(3–6): p. 68–74. doi:10.1016/j.vph.2011.03.005

[93] Kannel, W.B. and McGee, D.L. Diabetes and cardiovascular disease. The Framingham study. JAMA, 1979; 241(19): p. 2035–2038.

[94] Di Carli, M.F., Janisse, J., Grunberger, G. and Ager, J. Role of chronic hyperglycemia in the pathogenesis of coronary microvascular dysfunction in diabetes. Journal of the American College of Cardiology, 2003; 41(8): p. 1387–1393.

[95] Chauhan, A., Mullins, P.A., Taylor, G., Petch, M.C. and Schofield, P.M. Both endothelium-dependent and endothelium-independent function is impaired in patients with angina pectoris and normal coronary angiograms. European Heart Journal, 1997; 18(1): p. 60–48.

[96] Epstein, S.E. and Cannon, R.O., 3rd. Site of increased resistance to coronary flow in patients with angina pectoris and normal epicardial coronary arteries. Journal of the American College of Cardiology, 1986; 8(2): p. 459–461.

[97] Buffon, A., Rigattieri, S., Santini, S.A., Ramazzotti, V., Crea, F., Giardina, B., et al. Myocardial ischemia-reperfusion damage after pacing-induced tachycardia in patients with cardiac syndrome X. American Journal of Physiology. Heart and Circulatory Physiology, 2000; 279(6): p. H2627–H2633.

[98] Maseri, A., Crea, F., Kaski, J.C. and Crake, T. Mechanisms of angina pectoris in syndrome X. Journal of the American College of Cardiology, 1991; 17(2): p. 499–506.

[99] Marinescu, M.A., Löffler, A.I., Ouellette, M., Smith, L., Kramer, C.M. and Bourque, J.M. Coronary microvascular dysfunction, microvascular angina, and treatment strategies. JACC: Cardiovascular Imaging, 2015; 8(2): p. 210–220. doi:10.1016/j.jcmg.2014.12.008

[100] Uren, N.G., Crake, T., Lefroy, D.C., de Silva, R., Davies, G.J. and Maseri, A. Delayed recovery of coronary resistive vessel function after coronary angioplasty. Journal of the American College of Cardiology, 1993; 21(3): p. 612–621.

[101] Gregorini, L., Marco, J., Kozakova, M., Palombo, C., Anguissola, G.B., Marco, I., et al. Alpha-adrenergic blockade improves recovery of myocardial perfusion and function after coronary stenting in patients with acute myocardial infarction. Circulation, 1999; 99(4): p. 482–490.

[102] Gregorini, L., Marco, J., Farah, B., Bernies, M., Palombo, C., Kozakova, M., et al. Effects of selective alpha1- and alpha2-adrenergic blockade on coronary flow reserve after coronary stenting. Circulation, 2002; 106(23): p. 2901–2907.

[103] Gregorini, L., Marco, J. and Heusch, G. Peri-interventional coronary vasomotion. Journal of Molecular and Cellular Cardiology, 2012; 52(4): p. 883–889. doi:10.1016/j.yjmcc.2011.09.017

[104] Gregorini, L., Marco, J., Palombo, C., Kozakova, M., Anguissola, G.B., Cassagneau, B., et al. Postischemic left ventricular dysfunction is abolished by alpha-adrenergic blocking agents. Journal of the American College of Cardiology, 1998; 31(5): p. 992–1001.

[105] Kozàkovà, M., Marco, J., Heusch, G., Bernies, M., Bossi, I.M., Palombo, C., et al. The alpha1-adrenergic blocker urapidil improves contractile function in patients 3 months after coronary stenting: a randomized, double-blinded study. American Heart Journal, 2004; 147(2): p. E6. doi:10.1016/j.ahj.2003.08.005

[106] Spyrou, N., Khan, M.A., Rosen, S.D., Foale, R., Davies, D.W., Sogliani, F., et al. Persistent but reversible coronary microvascular dysfunction after bypass grafting. American Journal of Physiology. Heart and Circulatory Physiology, 2000; 279(6): p. H2634–H2640.

[107] Pries, A.R. and Secomb, T.W. Making microvascular networks work: angiogenesis, remodeling, and pruning. Physiology, 2014; 29(6): p. 446–455. doi:10.1152/physiol. 00012.2014

[108] van den Akker, J., Schoorl, M.J., Bakker, E.N. and Vanbavel, E. Small artery remodeling: current concepts and questions. Journal of Vascular Research, 2010; 47(3): p. 183–202. doi:10.1159/000255962

[109] Maron, B.J., Towbin, J.A., Thiene, G., Antzelevitch, C., Corrado, D., Arnett, D., et al. Contemporary definitions and classification of the cardiomyopathies: an American Heart Association Scientific Statement from the Council on Clinical Cardiology, Heart Failure and Transplantation Committee; Quality of Care and Outcomes Research and Functional Genomics and Translational Biology Interdisciplinary Working Groups; and Council on Epidemiology and Prevention. Circulation, 2006; 113(14): p. 1807–1816. doi: 10.1161/circulationaha.106.174287

[110] Elliott, P., Andersson, B., Arbustini, E., Bilinska, Z., Cecchi, F., Charron, P., et al. Classification of the cardiomyopathies: a position statement from the European Society Of Cardiology Working Group on Myocardial and Pericardial Diseases. European Heart Journal, 2008; 29(2): p. 270–276. doi:10.1093/eurheartj/ehm342

[111] Arbustini, E., Narula, N., Tavazzi, L., Serio, A., Grasso, M., Favalli, V., et al. The MOGE(S) classification of cardiomyopathy for clinicians. Journal of the American College of Cardiology, 2014; 64(3): p. 304–318. doi:10.1016/j.jacc.2014.05.027

[112] Neglia, D., Michelassi, C., Trivieri, M.G., Sambuceti, G., Giorgetti, A., Pratali, L., et al. Prognostic role of myocardial blood flow impairment in idiopathic left ventricular dysfunction. Circulation, 2002; 105(2): p. 186–193.

[113] Gil, K.E., Pawlak, A., Frontczak-Baniewicz, M., Gil, R.J. and Nasierowska-Guttmejer, A. The proposed new classification of coronary microcirculation as the predictor of the heart failure progression in idiopathic dilated cardiomyopathy. Cardiovascular Pathology, 2015; 24(6): p. 351–358. doi:10.1016/j.carpath.2015.08.001

[114] Schwartzkopff, B., Frenzel, H., Dieckerhoff, J., Betz, P., Flasshove, M., Schulte, H.D., et al. Morphometric investigation of human myocardium in arterial hypertension and valvular aortic stenosis. European Heart Journal, 1992; 13(Suppl. D): p. 17–23.

[115] Marzilli, M., Sambuceti, G., Testa, R. and Fedele, S. Platelet glycoprotein IIb/IIIa receptor blockade and coronary resistance in unstable angina. Journal of the American College of Cardiology, 2002; 40(12): p. 2102–2109.

[116] Tomai, F., Ribichini, F., Ghini, A.S., Ferrero, V., Ando, G., Vassanelli, C., et al. Elevated C-reactive protein levels and coronary microvascular dysfunction in patients with coronary artery disease. European Heart Journal, 2005; 26(20): p. 2099–2105. doi: 10.1093/eurheartj/ehi356

[117] Teragawa, H., Fukuda, Y., Matsuda, K., Ueda, K., Higashi, Y., Oshima, T., et al. Relation between C reactive protein concentrations and coronary microvascular endothelial function. Heart, 2004; 90(7): p. 750–754. doi:10.1136/hrt.2003.022269

[118] Reffelmann, T. and Kloner, R.A. The no-reflow phenomenon: a basic mechanism of myocardial ischemia and reperfusion. Basic Research in Cardiology, 2006; 101(5): p. 359–372. doi:10.1007/s00395-006-0615-2

[119] Kaul, S. and Ito, H. Microvasculature in acute myocardial ischemia: part II: evolving concepts in pathophysiology, diagnosis, and treatment. Circulation, 2004; 109(3): p. 310–315. doi:10.1161/01.cir.0000111583.89777.f9

[120] Galiuto, L. Optimal therapeutic strategies in the setting of post-infarct no reflow: the need for a pathogenetic classification. Heart, 2004; 90(2): p. 123–125.

[121] Schwartz, B.G. and Kloner, R.A. Coronary no reflow. Journal of Molecular and Cellular Cardiology, 2012; 52(4): p. 873–882. doi:10.1016/j.yjmcc.2011.06.009

[122] Elliott, P.M., Kindler, H., Shah, J.S., Sachdev, B., Rimoldi, O.E., Thaman, R., et al. Coronary microvascular dysfunction in male patients with Anderson-Fabry disease and the effect of treatment with alpha galactosidase A. Heart, 2006; 92(3): p. 357–360. doi:10.1136/hrt.2004.054015

Chapter 3

The Skeletal Muscle Microvasculature and Its Effects on Metabolism

Cathryn M Kolka

Additional information is available at the end of the chapter

http://dx.doi.org/10.5772/63535

Abstract

Skeletal muscle is a major metabolic organ that plays a critical role in regulating glucose homeostasis and lipid utilization. Impaired muscle metabolic response is evident in diseases such as diabetes, obesity and cardiovascular diseases, and is also often associated with microvascular dysfunction. Here, we investigate the changes that can occur in the muscle microvasculature and the profound impact they can have on metabolism.

Under basal conditions, vasoactive compounds are able to affect metabolism in muscle by providing more glucose and oxygen to resting muscle. Insulin and exercise increase the perfusion of muscle, and thus provide more microvascular surface area, increasing the delivery of these metabolites to muscle. Endothelial dysfunction can therefore impair the delivery of oxygen, glucose and hormones to muscle, both through effects on blood flow distribution and the transport of these factors across the endothelium, leading to a decrease in oxygen consumption and glucose metabolism. Obesity and diabetes are associated with endothelial dysfunction and are accompanied by underlying changes in metabolism and reductions in insulin sensitivity.

The muscle is a highly metabolic organ, and the vasculature is essential to maintain appropriate metabolic response; therefore, the muscle microcirculation may be a target for treating metabolic disease.

Keywords: Skeletal muscle, blood flow, capillary, transendothelial transport, diabetes, endothelium, perfusion, exercise, insulin, vasodilation, vasoconstriction

1. Introduction

Skeletal muscle is normally thought of in the context of exercise or posture, and its ability to contract to generate force or motion is an essential part of mobility. It is a highly metabolic organ, responsible for breakdown and storage of glucose and fat in order to provide the energy required for these contractions. In addition, skeletal muscle is the primary tissue responsible for the increased glucose metabolism during hyperinsulinemia and exercise [1]. The vascular system in skeletal muscle is essential in metabolism and exercise, and can directly affect its ability to generate the energy needed for contraction and movement, and to appropriately dispose of glucose. Here, we will discuss the structure and function of the muscle microcirculatory system, and the role that microvascular function plays in muscle metabolism. We will discuss the effects of diet and obesity on vascular function, how these effects may translate to impaired muscle metabolism, and the possibility of targeting the microcirculatory system in order to treat both vascular and metabolic disease.

2. Muscle microcirculatory system

As is common in other tissues, the vascular network in skeletal muscle consists of arteries branching into smaller and smaller vessels. In skeletal muscle, a terminal arteriole gives rise to groups of capillaries that run parallel to muscle fibres, and each muscle fibre can be supplied by several different groups of capillaries from independent terminal arterioles [2]. Vascular casts of the rat hind limb have demonstrated that the muscle capillaries are long and tortuous [3], and thus have a lot of contact with myocytes (**Figure 1**). Original methods to assess the structure and location of the microcirculatory system in skeletal muscle used microscopy to gain 2D images from fixed or frozen tissues. However, the skeletal muscle is particularly sensitive to certain artefacts when freezing [4], and limitations to counting capillaries in 2D include lack of estimation of capillary length, tortuosity or fibre size [5]. More recent advances in 3D visualization *in vivo* supply more spatial information about the relationship between the microcirculation and the muscle tissue, as capillaries are found to be embedded in grooves in the sarcolemma of muscle fibres [6].

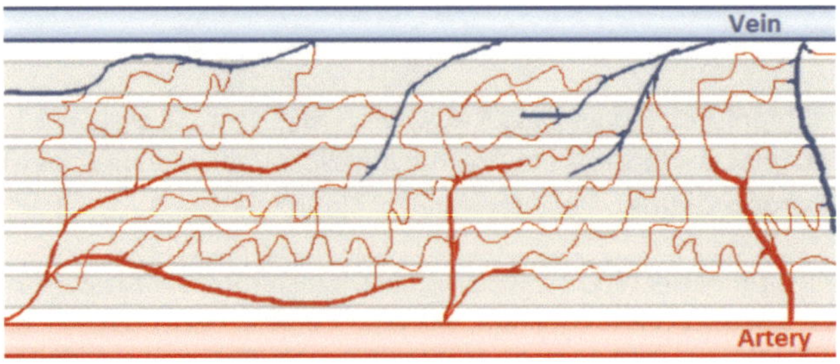

Figure 1. Muscle microcirculatory system. Arteries feed into the muscle, supplying arterioles, each of which controls a capillary network. Blood is then removed from the capillaries through venules and veins. (Grey: muscle fibres. Red: artery, arterioles and capillaries. Blue: venules and vein).

Blood flow through these capillaries can be controlled through dilation or constriction of the blood vessel network. Most of this regulation does not occur at the capillary level, as the capillaries are not associated with an underlying smooth muscle network required for dilation and constriction. While subject to changes in blood flow, as well as being in direct contact with factors in the blood, the capillary itself does not usually regulate blood flow. Instead, the vessels that have smooth muscle surrounding the endothelial wall, such as the arteries, precapillary arterioles, post-capillary venules and veins, are responsible for vasoconstriction and vasodilation. Factors that are vasoactive throughout the body also affect the muscle microvasculature. Nitric oxide (NO), endothelium-derived hyperpolarizing factor and prostacyclin are known vasodilators, and more recently carbon monoxide and hydrogen sulphide have been included in this list [7], and there are a range of hormones that can cause vasoconstriction, including endothelin, angiotensin, serotonin and others. The effects can vary depending on where the vasomotion is taking place. For example, vasoconstriction in the precapillary arteriole will induce low pressure in the capillaries, whereas venular constriction will increase blood pressure in the local capillary environment, and may increase shear stress.

Resting blood flow is low, approximately 5–10 ml/min/100 g [7], but increases rapidly by a factor of up to 20 (up to 80–100 ml/min/100 g) during exercise [8]; however, this can be highly variable depending on the muscle. In resting skeletal muscle, it is estimated that only about 25% of the capillaries are perfused at any time [9], but that this can increase to 100% with exercise; however, some recent publications suggest that no capillaries are unperfused at rest, and instead capillary surface area is recruited by exercise [10]. A coordinated response between the terminal arterioles has been shown, and capillary perfusion can increase through broad regions of a muscle [2]. Early studies by Lindbom and Arfors using intravital microscopy showed that oxygen partial pressure itself in the rabbit tennuisimus muscle could increase perfusion. This is likely mediated through the nervous system [11], which is thought to maintain a low-level vasoconstriction in muscle microvasculature. Thus, the sympathetic nervous system is likely to be important in blood flow regulation [12].

Measurement of functional capillary density in skeletal muscle has been made possible by advances in imaging techniques. Contrast-enhanced ultrasound (CEU) technology is used in perfusion studies in a variety of tissues, and showed that physiologic hyperinsulinemia can increase human skeletal muscle perfusion and microvascular volume [13]. This technique can also detect microvascular complications [14]. However, an *in vitro* study designed to more fully understand the data acquired from CEU has shown that while alterations in the filling rate of the microvascular volume can be detected, CEU cannot discriminate between different flow patterns that reflect changes in capillary perfusion *in vivo* [15]. This may be explained by new developments to the capillary recruitment theory, whereby instead of recruiting previously unperfused capillaries, capillary surface area is recruited by elevating capillary haematocrit and extending the length of the capillary available for exchange [10].

There are several other techniques that have been used to estimate functional capillary density or capillary recruitment. Earlier methods used laser Doppler fluxmetry (LDF) at the muscle surface, and showed effects of different vasoconstrictors to either increase or decrease the capillary surface area [16]. Further studies demonstrated an increase in LDF signal by insulin, but not by adrenaline, which increases bulk flow without effect on capillary recruitment [17], suggesting that LDF does indeed reflect changes in capillary recruitment, and not bulk flow. Skeletal muscle perfusion can also be assessed by nuclear magnetic resonance (NMR) arterial spin labelling, which has been validated as a method with strong spatial and temporal resolution [18], and can be combined with assessments of muscle oxygenation and energy metabolism [8]. Positron emission tomography (PET) utilizes short-lived radioisotopes to measure blood flow and its distribution, and also offers the ability to measure oxygen consumption and extraction. This technique has been used to show that NO is involved in maintaining resting skeletal muscle blood flow [19]. In addition, the PET technique demonstrated that exercise can recruit capillaries [20]. Near-infra red spectroscopy (NIRS) is a non-invasive method that has been used in skeletal muscle to measure blood flow and oxygen consumption [21], and can be used to show differences in oxygen consumption in tissue, which may indicate the distribution of blood flow through skeletal muscle. NIRS has been used to link tissue oxygenation to blood flow in a range of conditions from critically ill patients to athletes [22, 23].

The microvascular endothelium functions as a barrier between the blood and the underlying tissue [24]. In skeletal muscle, there is a continuous endothelial barrier with tight junctions between the endothelial cells, and thus the molecule's ability to reach the muscle is restricted. In comparison, an organ with a discontinuous endothelium or one with large pores in the endothelial barrier, such as liver, has a greater direct contact with molecules in the blood. These differences make the muscle microvasculature highly regulated; thus, the constitution of the plasma is very different to the muscle interstitium. Our own results have shown very different concentrations of insulin and lipid in the muscle interstitium when compared to plasma [25], and the endothelial barrier may account for a lag time of 5 min between plasma and interstitial glucose levels [26], in spite of the fact that glucose is a small molecule thought to easily diffuse across the endothelium. Plasma is therefore substantially different from the interstitial fluid [27, 28]; and as the interstitial environment is largely modified by supply from the blood, or removal through the lymph, the endothelial barrier is an important component of regulating the muscle microenvironment.

In addition to the basic structure of the endothelium, the endothelial glycocalyx is an approximately 1 μm thick layer on the luminal side of the vascular endothelial cells, which consists of a mesh of polysaccharide structures, which provide a layer of protection for the endothelial cells, regulating access of molecules in the plasma based on molecular size, charge and structure [29]. The glycocalyx is a dynamic addition to the endothelial barrier [30–32] and, while perhaps not directly involved in regulating blood flow or metabolism, is a structural and functional barrier that may alter the composition of the muscle interstitium.

Sampling the interstitial environment is difficult, with many techniques inducing inflammation, allowing only small sample sizes, or being unable to provide a dynamic measure of changes in response to certain stimuli [28]. Our own studies use lymph sampling [25, 33–36], which does not induce inflammation at the sampling point, and allows studies of temporal changes. The lymph vessel is highly permeable and has a slow flow rate, allowing equilibration with the interstitial fluid. However, the volume sampled is quite small, restricting this technique to larger animals. In addition, there may be some modification of the lymph fluid, which may alter results [37]. Other techniques can indirectly sample the interstitium, such as microdialysis. For larger molecules, this technique can have a low recovery, providing only a dilute sample, and the insertion of the probe may induce inflammation. However, this technique has been used in many human applications [38–44]. In general, the consensus is that the muscle interstitium is substantially different from plasma, and the muscle microvasculature is an important component of the regulation of the muscle microenvironment.

3. Skeletal muscle metabolism

Metabolism in muscle provides working muscle with energy, and metabolic processes are increased in times of need. Muscle can utilize both glucose and fat for energy, and typically relies on fat oxidation during both increased energy expenditure (exercise) and decreased energy intake (fasting) [45], but is also the primary tissue for insulin-mediated glucose uptake [1]. Plasma free fatty acids typically supply most of the fuel for skeletal muscle under low and moderate levels of exercise [46]; however, rates of glycogen utilization also increase with contraction [47]. The fuel selection is dependent on not only the intensity of exercise but also the type of muscle fibre recruited for exercise and the availability of fuels [48].

Metabolism of both fat and glucose requires mitochondria to generate energy through aerobic respiration. Within the mitochondria, glucose, fats and proteins are broken down through a series of enzymatic reactions, and the products feed into the electron transport chain, causing oxidative phosphorylation and the generation of ATP (energy) (**Figure 2**). Skeletal muscle is heterogenous, and the mitochondrial content of different muscle fibre types is a major component of the metabolic preference of each muscle fibre type. Red muscle contains a high number of mitochondria, thus providing a very high level of oxidative capacity. These red fibres (Type I) are useful in endurance type activities, and are served by an extensive vascular network in order to supply the oxygen required for oxidative phosphorylation and thus efficient production of ATP, which provides the energy for all forms of muscle work [49]. In contrast, Type II muscle fibres, known as white fibres, have lower levels of mitochondria and vessel density. This muscle is typically used for very short maximal intensity activities, such as sprints: it is more glycolytic, such that instead of undergoing full oxidation, glucose is broken down to lactate to give a quick release of energy (**Figure 2**). Recent studies have shown that red fibres have a larger capillary to fibre ratio, a greater capillary density and more tortuous capillary pathways than white [50]. Thus, vascularization is tightly tied to metabolism in skeletal muscle—vascularized muscle is more oxidative, and leads to more complete metabolism of glucose, and less vascularized muscle supplies less oxygen to the myocyte leading to anaerobic respiration and production of lactate [49]. However, studies have shown that capillary density in some muscles has a greater relativity to muscle fibre size, rather than the oxidative capacity of the muscle fibre [5]. Glancy et al. concluded that the embedding of the capillaries in the sarcolemma increased oxygen delivery to the myocyte. Interestingly, the mitochondrial pool was located close to embedded capillaries, though the authors believe that while this increased oxygen delivery to the myocyte, it was not associated with mitochondrial oxygen access [6].

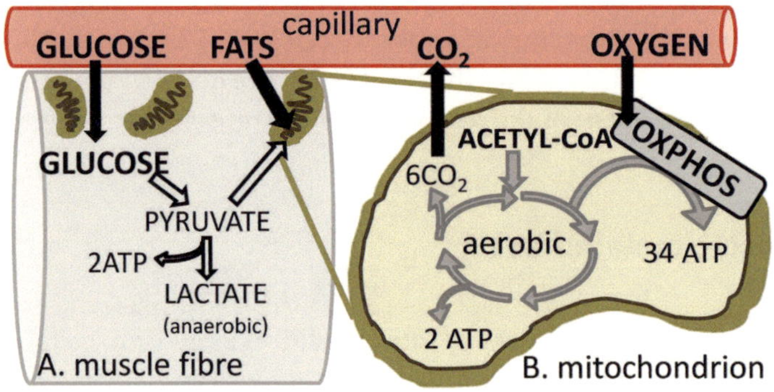

Figure 2. Role of microcirculation in muscle metabolism. Glucose and fats are the main source of energy for muscle fibres (A). Glucose is broken down to pyruvate, which can be metabolized without oxygen to lactate, producing 2ATP, a pathway used preferentially in white muscle fibres. Alternatively, pyruvate can be transported into the mitochondria of the muscle fibre (B), where both pyruvate and fats can be converted to acetyl-CoA. This enters the Krebs cycle and activates oxidative phosphorylation (OXPHOS), requiring the delivery of oxygen from the blood. This method is common in red muscle fibres: it produces much more ATP than anaerobic production of lactate, but also produces carbon dioxide, which must be removed by the blood. Thus, the microcirculation is essential for delivering glucose, fats and oxygen, and removing carbon dioxide from the muscle.

Exercise requires more ATP [49], which can be derived both anaerobically for short-term activity or aerobically using the electron transport chain in mitochondria (**Figure 2**). A model has been generated to predict this transition from rest to work, and has shown the importance of myoglobin in oxygen delivery to working muscle [51]. Exercise causes increases in blood flow primarily to red muscles [52]: muscles consisting of more red fibres showed a quicker increase in blood flow than white, and, interestingly, the red muscles also showed a quicker return to rested blood flow levels than the white [53]. The maximal metabolic rate is related to both mitochondrial size and number as well as capillary volume [54], emphasizing the importance of the microvasculature in metabolism.

Aerobic exercise training has been shown to double skeletal muscle mitochondrial content, yet maximal whole body oxygen uptake only increased approximately 15% [55]. As these effects of exercise on mitochondrial content and oxygen consumption are not proportional, some conclude that the ability to deliver oxygen to mitochondria is in fact limiting to aerobic respiration, rather than mitochondrial content [6, 56]. This contribution of the vasculature may include both the presence of blood vessels and also their function, specifically their ability to redirect blood flow through the muscle.

4. Blood flow distribution affects muscle metabolism

As already discussed, there can be changes in the distribution of blood flow through muscle by altering functional capillary density. This redistribution of flow can directly alter metabolism: some vasoconstrictors and vasodilators can alter oxygen consumption and glucose uptake independently of any direct effects on muscle metabolism [16, 57]. This was demonstrated by showing that the effects of vasoactive substances on metabolism in perfused skeletal muscle were not replicated in incubated skeletal muscle, implicating the essential role of the microvasculature in mediating those changes in metabolism [58, 59]. Vessel surface area, the distance for the factor to travel, and the concentration gradient can all alter the rate of diffusion according to Fick's equation. Vasodilation allows a greater surface area for exchange, and conversely vasoconstriction reduces the surface area for diffusion. However, as discussed above, the areas of the blood vessel responsible for exchange are typically the capillaries, which themselves do not undergo vasomotion, but are controlled by the larger surrounding vessels. Thus, a larger effect on diffusion of oxygen and other metabolites can be induced by vasomotion that alters the distribution of flow through muscle, which will decrease the distance for the factor to travel from the blood vessel to all areas of the muscle, as shown in Fick's equation [60]. When a greater number of capillaries are perfused, as occurs with capillary recruitment, each myocyte is supplied with a great amount of oxygen and glucose, and metabolism is increased. This is independent of extra work being performed by the muscle (such as during exercise), and demonstrates that changes in blood flow even during resting conditions may influence metabolism [60].

4.1. Factors that can induce capillary recruitment

There are several known factors that can increase the number of perfused capillaries. From a physiological perspective, exercise and reactive hyperaemia are both associated with a substantial increase in perfusion. Exercise also induces a major increase in blood flow: while muscle only uses approximately 15% of the cardiac output at rest, this increases to 88% during maximum exercise [49], mainly to muscles consisting predominantly of red fibres [53]. There is also an increase in capillary recruitment with exercise [61–64], and this was associated with an increased perfused capillary density of 1.5- to 3-fold [65]. It is possible that both exercise and reactive hyperaemia induce their blood flow effects through the sympathetic nervous system [11]; however, alternative models of local blood flow regulation have also been postulated [66]. NO does not appear to be involved in exercise-induced capillary recruitment [67], and in fact inhibiting NO during exercise can increase local muscle oxygen uptake, but seems to decrease glucose uptake [19, 67]. As discussed, NO is considered a vasodilator; however, there are some inconsistencies with regards to its effects on metabolism. In resting muscle, inhibition of NO synthesis causes free fatty acid uptake, increased oxygen uptake, but not glucose uptake [68], and the authors proposed a possible contribution of an inhibitory effect of NO on mitochondrial respiration to explain their data; thus, the contribution of NO to basal metabolism may be slight. PET has been used to show that NO is involved in maintaining resting skeletal muscle blood flow, and suppresses resting muscle oxygen uptake, likely because NO competes with oxygen and inhibits mitochondrial respiration [19]; further studies demonstrated that NO may contribute to the regulation of free fatty acid metabolism at rest [68]. Thus, while NO is a known vasodilator, its role in metabolism is unclear. These divergent results may reflect differences depending on the dose of NO inhibitor used, but also may indicate a role of NO in the mitochondrial function of working muscle, as it can inhibit oxidative phosphorylation [69].

While many hormones are themselves vasoactive, including serotonin, epinephrine, norepinephrine and angiotensin, many do not appear to change muscle perfusion. GLP-1 (Glucagon-like peptide-1) increases capillary perfusion, though the involvement of NO in this process is so far controversial [70–73]. GLP-1 receptor agonists have beneficial effects on the vasculature [74–78] and metabolism of glucose [70, 71, 79–81]; though whether this reflects a direct effect on glucose metabolism, an indirect effect through blood flow changes, or a combination of these is not clear. GLP-1 induces angiogenesis, consistent with increasing functional capillary density, though this is a long-term adaptation rather than an acute increase in the perfusion of skeletal muscle [74]. This effect of angiogenesis, or increasing the size and number of capillaries, has been shown to protect against metabolic disease [82].

There are two classes of vasoconstrictors determined based on their general effects on metabolism. Type A vasoconstrictors, including angiotensin, vasopressin, and low doses of norepinephrine and endothelin increase oxygen consumption and perfusion pressure in the constant-flow pump-perfused hindlimb [3, 83, 84]. Type B vasoconstrictors reduce muscle metabolism, such as serotonin (5-hydroxytryptophan) [3, 85]. Studies have shown that vasoconstrictors from these different groups may control different areas of vascular flow in the muscle, as evidenced by both washout of red blood cells that had been trapped in the muscle, and by corrosion casting of the arterial tree [3], a technique which uses a polymer to fill the perfused vascular area, the tissue is then corroded away to form a 3D model. Serotonin was shown to reduce the available capillary surface area, and is associated with a reduction in metabolism measured by oxygen uptake [85].

Angiotensin II (Ang) is often associated with hypertension, and is a vasoconstrictor that can have different effects on metabolism depending on which receptor type it engages. Ang receptor 1 is associated with reduced metabolism, while Ang receptor 2 can recruit the microvasculature [86], and similar effects have been detected in cardiac muscle [87]. In addition, Ang may have effects on blood vessel permeability, which may separately alter the metabolism through increased delivery of oxygen and nutrients [88]. Ang II increases blood flow, but appears to impair insulin-mediated glucose metabolism, without altering the access of insulin to the muscle interstitium [89]. These data on insulin access are not consistent with other published data, indicating that Ang II can reduce the number of insulin receptors on endothelial cells, which may lead to a reduction in receptor-mediated transcytosis [90], if insulin transport is indeed receptor-mediated. Some of these inconsistences may be due to the time of exposure to the vasoconstrictor: one study has shown that short-term Ang II can increase NO production, but long-term can reduce NO bioavailability [91]. Acute Ang receptor blockade has been shown to improve microvascular responses in hypertensive individuals [92], who may have elevated levels of Ang: Ang receptors are therefore considered to be involved in both metabolic and microvascular actions *in vivo* [93].

Endothelin is a vasoconstrictor released in response to insulin [94, 95], and at low doses behaves as a type A vasoconstrictor; increases in glucose uptake and oxygen consumption indicate augmented metabolism in the muscle. However, at high concentrations, this vasoconstriction continues to lead to high blood pressure, and also reduces oxygen consumption and glucose uptake by the muscle [83]. Thus, the concentrations of vasoconstrictors in the system are an important component of their effects on metabolism. However, it is important to realize that, *in vivo*, the plasma does not contain just one vasoconstrictor, but a mix of several vasoactive compounds, and the interactions among these molecules may be complex. Data have shown that adiponectin [96] and insulin [83] can prevent the vasoconstriction induced by endothelin. These results appear to depend on a prior vasodilation before endothelin-mediated vasoconstriction, and yet NO itself is able to prevent the increased pressure after exposure to endothelin [96]. This may perhaps be due to the systemic introduction of NO-donors to the system in comparison to the local action of insulin or adiponectin. The ability of insulin to dilate against endothelin-mediated constriction, and limit effects on pressure and oxygen consumption, has not been observed against any other vasoconstrictor. Thus, there is a very complex balance between a number of hormones and vasoactive molecules that act together to regulate metabolism.

4.2. Insulin's hemodynamic effects also alter metabolism

Insulin is known as a metabolic endocrine hormone; however, amongst its varied effects on nutrient disposal and storage, insulin also has hemodynamic effects and was first noted to increase blood flow at supraphysiological concentrations [97]. Later, physiological concentrations of insulin were found to induce vasodilation of blood vessels [98], and the release of the vasoconstrictor endothelin [94]. It is thought that the combination of the vasodilation by NO and the low dose of endothelin may combine to cause capillary recruitment [94, 95], as many studies have indicated that insulin is capable of inducing capillary recruitment in healthy individuals in skeletal muscle [13, 17, 99–102] and in skin, which is used as a surrogate measure of muscle [103]. Capillary density is directly correlated with insulin sensitivity in human skin [103], reinforcing the idea that capillary recruitment is an important process in insulin-mediated glucose uptake [13, 17, 99–103].

As we show above, altering muscle perfusion is sufficient to change basal metabolism without a direct effect on the myocyte; however, the increased perfusion induced by insulin-mediated capillary recruitment is also hypothesized to assist in the delivery of insulin to the myocyte, thus augmenting insulin's metabolic response. In a study by Miles et al. [104], the half time to maximum response for glucose disposal in dogs exposed to insulin infusion was not significantly different to that of interstitial insulin, yet the effects on arterial insulin were much quicker. This temporal relationship confirms that the time required for insulin to reach the interstitial space is the limiting factor for insulin-mediated glucose uptake, which agrees with results suggesting that insulin rapidly causes glucose uptake in cell culture [105]. Only once insulin is present at the cell surface can it bind to receptors to cause glucose uptake. In fact, the correlation between insulin levels and glucose uptake is strongest when using lymph insulin concentrations to represent the interstitium than the vein or arterial concentrations [33]. The study by Chiu et al. differs from that of Miles et al. because the focus is specifically on the muscle—local glucose uptake across the leg correlates with muscle lymph insulin concentrations, while Miles et al. used thoracic lymph, which is likely to be representative of the whole body, and corresponds well with the whole body glucose disposal rate [104]. Therefore, the concentration of insulin at the cell surface, rather than in the blood, is a better predictor for the rate of insulin-mediated glucose uptake, thus increasing insulin delivery to the muscle is shown to improve insulin's metabolic effects.

As mentioned, insulin can increase the available surface area to augment its access to muscle, but it is possible that there may be other delays in the access of insulin to the interstitial space that are also altered by the microcirculatory system. The effects on metabolism occur during passive diffusion of oxygen, and probably glucose, in muscle. However, there can be regulated steps in transendothelial transport. Transport of insulin across the endothelial barrier is controversial: some studies have shown that transport is saturable, and as such must be receptor-mediated, yet others have shown no saturation, even at high concentrations, claiming that there is no evidence for receptor-mediated transport. The insulin receptors present on endothelial cells are suggested to be an important part of the trafficking of insulin across the endothelial barrier [106, 107]. However, these studies may be of limited relevance as they use a macrovascular cell type rather than a representative cell of a capillary. A knockout mouse model of endothelial IRS-2 is insulin-resistant and showed decreased access of insulin from the blood to the interstitium [108], implicating insulin signalling in transendothelial insulin transport. However, studies of microvascular cells demonstrated that fatty acids impair insulin transcytosis, and interestingly the insulin receptor and insulin signalling pathways did not appear to be involved [109]. There have also been studies showing that insulin itself can increase the accessibility of the glycocalyx in muscle, consistent with reports of insulin effects to increase blood volume [30], and the authors posit that structures within the glycocalyx are involved in insulin transport through the glycocalyx towards the endothelium for subsequent transport to the muscle interstitium. Thus, any defect in endothelial function may have severe implications for metabolism, particularly in the case of insulin and metabolic disease.

5. Vascular dysfunction in metabolic disease

The prevalence of diabetes has been increasing steadily in the United States and in many parts of the world. In 2010, 25.8 million individuals in the United States were diagnosed with diabetes, almost double the rate of ten years earlier [110]. In fact, 11.3% of the adult population was estimated to have diabetes, either diagnosed or undiagnosed. Diabetes is one of the leading causes of death and disease in the world currently, and is linked with a variety of cardiovascular diseases, including heart disease, stroke and hypertension [110]. The links between a metabolic disease such as diabetes and cardiovascular disease are not always readily apparent; however, as we have discussed here, the microcirculation is intrinsically tied to metabolism. Below, we will investigate various aspects of the metabolic syndrome, and how the muscle microvasculature may be affected.

5.1. Hypertension

Hypertension is often characterized by excessive vasoconstriction, which may be driven by dysregulation of the Ang system, excess amounts of endothelin, or changes in the autonomic nervous system. Microvascular dysfunction can occur due to functional issues as discussed here, but also structural impairments of the arterioles or capillaries, which may lead to capillary drop-out: this combined with arteriolar constriction increases peripheral resistance and thus blood pressure [111]. In addition, some forms of hypertension show a decreased capillary permeability, preventing hormone and nutrient access to the underlying tissue [112]. Excessive vasoconstriction by endothelin in hypertension and the metabolic syndrome may prevent appropriate insulin-mediated haemodynamics and also impair basal metabolism [83]. Further, we have shown that high levels of endothelin-1 can also reduce exercise capacity in muscle, likely due to the fact that oxygen and fuel access to the muscle is impaired with excessive vasoconstriction [113].

Some treatments for hypertension also have effects on metabolism. A recent study investigating the use of renal denervation to treat resistant hypertension has demonstrated a simultaneous improvement in metabolic parameters [114]. Recent studies showing negative results of renal denervation on metabolism also did not confirm effects on blood pressure [115, 116], which bring into question the technique of catheter-based renal ablation [117]. Some claim that renal denervation may have beneficial effects on the microvasculature [118], and the original findings posited that the skeletal muscle may be a primary site of improved metabolism [114], but have not yet been confirmed. Further, other studies have found no improvement in endothelial function as measured by peripheral arterial tone (PAT) using Endo-PAT [119], though these studies acknowledge that many of the patients did not have impaired endothelial function initially, thus no improvement may be detectable.

Regardless of the suitability of renal denervation in restoring endothelial function, other hypertensive treatments are known to restore microvascular function, including acute Ang receptor blockade [92]. Hypertension may therefore be linked to metabolic disease, including muscle metabolism, through effects on the microvasculature [111].

5.2. Obesity

Obesity is typically associated with excess caloric intake, or decreased energy expenditure. Our own studies have indicated that a high fat diet can increase both visceral and subcutaneous fat depots and also impair muscle metabolism [120]. Elevated levels of fat can induce inflammation [121] typically through Toll-like receptor 4. This inflammation has been detected in a number of tissues, including the muscle and the vasculature [122], and the type of fats are likely to affect the level of inflammation. Trans fats have been found to be particularly pro-inflammatory [123]. Saturated fatty acids, such as palmitate, activate an inflammatory response in microvascular endothelial cells; however, the related mono-unsaturated fatty acid did not [109]. In one study that used palmitate to induce inflammatory pathways in microvascular endothelial cells, transcytosis of insulin was reduced, and there was increased monocyte migration into the tissue [109]. While these studies were carried out in microvascular endothelial cells from adipose tissue, it is possible that a similar effect occurs in muscle. These *in vitro* studies used palmitate, as it is the most abundant saturated fatty acid in the western diet —whether these effects could also occur *in vivo* must be confirmed. In association with obesity, perivascular fat accumulation in obesity may prevent appropriate vascular function, either through mechanical impairment, vasocrine signalling or the associated inflammation [124, 125].

While there are many studies demonstrating inflammation due to lipid and high fat diet, some show that there may be gender differences, as women do not seem to experience changes in inflammation with lipid infusion, and also experience a lower impairment in insulin sensitivity [126]. Yet, it is still generally accepted that plasma lipid induces endothelial dysfunction [127], and as such, regardless of inflammation, fat may directly alter endothelial function [128] and thus metabolism. Generally, lipids are known to cause endothelial dysfunction [129] and to impair muscle microvascular responses [130], and obesity is associated with blunted microvascular responses in humans [131]. Further, both visceral and subcutaneous adipose tissue are associated with impaired capillary recruitment [132]. A number of adipokines have been associated with effects on muscle metabolism. Adiponectin and leptin improve skeletal muscle metabolism [133], yet perhaps counter-intuitively, levels of adiponectin are inversely related to fat volume. Interestingly, adiponectin can also have beneficial effects on endothelial cells [134]. Leptin can stimulate fatty acid oxidation, and thus protect against fat deposition [135]. However, high levels of leptin with high fat diet [136] can lead to leptin resistance, including in endothelial cells [137]. Proinflammatory cytokines such as TNF-α (tumour necrosis factor-alpha) [138] and C-reactive protein are secreted from adipocytes and may cause insulin resistance at high levels [139]. An effect of TNF-α on endothelial cells is also known [134]. Other proinflammatory cytokines such as interleukin-6 (IL-6) have variable effects on endothelial function and skeletal muscle metabolism [140], and thus overall effects on metabolism are unclear. Alterations in the secretion of adipokines and interleukins from fat depots have been implicated in the progression of both metabolic and vascular disturbances associated with obesity [124], and visceral fat depots have been linked to a pro-inflammatory state and impaired capillary recruitment in skin [132], which may reflect impaired perfusion in skeletal muscle. Thus, obesity is associated with impaired capillary recruitment, which puts endothelial function as a potential link between obesity and metabolic disease.

Obesity is associated with a muscle fibre type switch, promoting a more 'white' muscle [141]. The number of lipid droplets within muscle fibres was twice as abundant in obese compared to lean individuals [142], and intramyocellular lipid is associated with impaired metabolism *in vivo* [143]. This increased fat content may be associated with mitochondrial dysfunction [144]; however, lipid accumulation itself may not alter metabolism [145]. For example, endurance athletes typically have more red muscle fibres, associated with a high capillary density, but also high intramyocellular lipid content. Obese individuals also have high intramyocellular lipid, but less red muscle fibres and a lower capillary density, so it is likely that intramyocellular lipid is only associated with impaired metabolism when the lipid supply is in excess of need. While the energy and lipid oversupply in obesity may impair mitochondrial function [146], the possibility that appropriate blood supply is lacking may also drive the switch to a less efficient muscle fibre type. Obesity as measured by body mass index (BMI) is

http://dx.doi.org/10.5772/63535

associated with a reduced capillary density [147], and both capillary density and muscle fibre type are linked to metabolic disease in humans [148].

Therefore, the exact stimulus for the muscle fibre type switch in obesity is not clear—does a change in the metabolic requirements of white muscle cause capillary drop-out, or does the capillary rarefaction in fact decrease the transport of oxygen and nutrients to the muscle, and thus reduce metabolism? An interesting correlate exists in adipose tissue, where hypoxia due to a low level of blood vessel density was originally thought to be a method to limit adipose tissue expansion [149]. However, recent results have suggested that increased mitochondrial content and angiogenesis in fact alter adipose metabolism to be more energy-efficient [82]. A similar situation may exist in skeletal muscle, such that increased capillary density and function, as well as increases in mitochondria, may prevent an obesity-induced switch to white muscle fibres, and thus assist in preventing metabolic disease.

5.3. Insulin resistance and diabetes

A mixed meal increases flow to muscle capillaries in healthy lean people, and perhaps more importantly increases muscle perfusion, yet this effect is blunted in obese individuals [150]. As the degree of microvascular surface area is related to insulin sensitivity [103, 151], this impaired perfusion is likely to be responsible for impaired glucose disposal after the meal. In fact, in dogs fed a high fat diet, the ability of insulin to increase the dispersion area of insulin is impaired, and is associated with impaired glucose disposal [152]. Impaired insulin-mediated capillary recruitment has been detected in a range of disease models, including inflammation [138, 140], hypertension or excessive vasoconstriction [92, 153], dyslipidemia [129, 132, 154] and obesity in both rodents [138, 155, 156] and humans [147]. In a model of experimental insulin resistance achieved by pancreatic venous diversion in dogs, glucose disposal rate was suppressed, the time for insulin to move into the lymph was delayed and insulin receptor activity was impaired. The authors conclude that transendothelial transport was impaired, and was responsible for one third of the insulin resistance observed in these animals, cellular defects being responsible for the remaining insulin resistance [157].

In general, vascular dysfunction has been observed in prediabetes [158, 159], diabetes [99, 128, 160] and offspring from individuals with type 2 diabetes [161], which may have profound effects on metabolic responses to insulin, as discussed above.

5.4. Complications of diabetes

As mentioned above, many of the leading causes of death associated with diabetes are related to cardiovascular disease. While heart disease and stroke are major macrovascular complications of disease, diabetes has many microvascular co-morbidities, including diabetic retinopathy, peripheral neuropathy and nephropathy. The endothelium has been implicated in diabetic nephropathy [162], and the blood vessels formed in response to reduced perfusion in retinopathy show abnormal structure and function [163]. Because of this association, diabetes is the leading cause of kidney failure, non-traumatic lower-limb amputations and new cases of blindness in adults in the United States [110]. Around 60–70% of people with diabetes have mild to severe nervous system damage, with 30% exhibiting impaired sensation in hands and feet, which can lead to non-traumatic amputation in extreme cases. Impaired blood flow may be one of the early signs of this diabetic neuropathy [164], and denervation of the skeletal muscle can cause muscle atrophy [165]. However, as the nervous system is partly involved in regulating microvascular function [12], through direct or hormonal means, neuropathic changes may also directly alter endothelial function, and therefore muscle metabolism [166]. Targeting endothelial dysfunction is therefore a viable treatment for preventing vascular complications associated with diabetes [167], and may help prevent muscle atrophy.

6. The vascular system as a target for treatment of metabolic disease

Since insulin resistance and its associated pathologies exhibit endothelial dysfunction; it follows that restoring blood flow patterns to normal would ameliorate at least some of the negative outcomes. For example, several studies have suggested that insulin's haemodynamic effects may account for a substantial amount of the metabolic outcome [168], and be impaired in disease and obesity, contributing to the metabolic deficit [97]; therefore, restoring endothelial function could help to improve insulin sensitivity.

Several drugs are also known to have effects on capillary recruitment. As discussed above, Ang can alter metabolism by vasoconstriction, and thus the disruption of the Renin-Angiotensin-Aldosterone system is likely to be a good target for treatment of any associated metabolic disease, whether by using angiotensin receptor blockers or through angiotensin converting enzyme inhibitors [169]. The differential expression of Ang receptors may provide local or tissue specific effects. Irbesartan, an Ang receptor blocker, improves microvascular responses to insulin in hypertensive individuals [92], however does not appear to induce capillary recruitment alone. While angiotensin receptor blockers also have effects in other tissues such as the pancreas [170], it is possible that their measured effects on insulin sensitivity may arise from effects on the muscle microvasculature, leading to alterations in metabolism. In support of this, studies have shown that Ang receptor blockade using losartan increases microvascular perfusion, leading to increased insulin delivery to muscle, and protecting against lipid-induced insulin resistance, thus protecting insulin's metabolic effects [171]. It is also important to note that these effects may not just be driven by plasma levels of vasoconstrictors, but also the receptor expression, as a change in expression of Ang receptor subtypes may alter endothelial function [86], and thus indirectly alter metabolism [93].

Phosphodiesterase (PDE) inhibitors were originally investigated as a possibly microvascular treatment that may increase metabolism. Studies on sildenafil have shown an effect to increase NO and induce arteriolar dilation [172], an effect that is now used in treatment of erectile dysfunction. Tadalafil, a PDE-5 inhibitor, increased capillary recruitment and also increased forearm glucose uptake in women with type 2 diabetes, possibly due to its effects on the microvasculature, though had no effect in healthy women [40]. These microvascular and metabolic effects have led to the proposal that tadalafil may be investigated as a treatment in insulin resistance [173], and this class of drugs have also been investigated in the setting of muscular dystrophy; however, some have shown a direct effect on the myocyte to alter metabolism [174], so studies using this drug to link muscle microvascular function and metabolism are limited.

Some drugs, such as the thiazolidinediones, are known to have effects on blood flow and vasodilation [175, 176]. Some of this class of drugs can increase capillary density through angiogenesis [177], which may contribute to the beneficial metabolic effects of these drugs. However, while improvements in NO bioavailability are seen, this causes only minor effects on skeletal muscle blood flow [178]; and one review has indicated that while the effects of this class of drugs on macrovascular disease are well known, the microvascular effects, particularly to prevent the development of microvascular complications of diabetes, are less impressive [178]. While the thiazolidinediones may be protective in early cardiovascular disease, effects in end-stage atherosclerosis are deleterious [179] and so far data are lacking to indicate any substantial effects on the muscle microvascular to improve metabolism.

The glycocalyx may be considered another target for treatment. This dynamic structure is proposed to be involved in regulating metabolism [30–32], and is impaired by hyperglycemia, ischemia and other aspects of aging and type 2 diabetes [31, 32, 180, 181]. Thus, some have highlighted the glycocalyx as a potential therapeutic target for treatment in the acute care critical situation, long-term vascular health [182], as well as potentially in regulating metabolism; however, specific interventions are so far limited. Methods of protecting or restoring the damaged glycocalyx include synthesis of components or protection against enzymatic degradation, as well as blocking free radical production [182]. Some suggested pharmacological interventions have included infusion of albumin to maintain stability, inhibiting TNF-α, preventing enzymatic attack through use of anti-thrombin, or inhibition of mast-cell degranulation, though these strategies require further investigation [182].

A recent potential target for treatment of metabolic disease and energy excess is brown adipose tissue (BAT), which dissipates excess energy as heat from the body. BAT is scarce in humans, yet browning of white adipose tissue to form beige fat increases energy expenditure. Factors that affect brown adipose tissue, such as exercise, cold exposure and PGC1a (Peroxisome proliferator-activated receptor G coactivator-1 alpha), also can induce changes in skeletal muscle, and some studies have suggested that skeletal muscle may actually play a large role in these increases in energy expenditure [183]. There are several important components to increase the thermogenic capacity of a tissue: there must be an increase in mitochondria to metabolize glucose, uncoupling or proton leak to dissipate the energy, and an adequate supply of oxygen and glucose to cause this aerobic respiration. The angiogenesis that occurs during adipose tissue browning increases oxygen delivery, and we therefore hypothesize that blood vessels are an essential component of increased thermogenesis. This role of angiogenesis has not been completely studied; however, it has been shown that vascular endothelial growth factor-A (VEGF-A) overexpressing transgenic mice have increased vascularization and upregulated uncoupling protein-1 (UCP-1) and PGC-1a in BAT, and improves deleterious effects of high fat diet on metabolism [184]. From a metabolic perspective, overexpression of VEGF in adipose tissue protects against obesity and insulin resistance [82], even in the absence of changes in mitochondrial content and uncoupling, increased functional capillary density by angiogenesis can increase metabolism. Skeletal muscle may undergo a process similar to browning of fat, leading to greater energy expenditure, and thus may be a target for treatment of obesity and its metabolic complications. In general, angiogenesis is likely to be a key player in increased oxidative capacity and energy expenditure in adipose tissue and muscle. If angiogenesis were also linked to increased mitochondrial content, causing a switch to a more 'red' muscle, and with potential effects on uncoupling in muscle, even greater energy consumption would occur.

Thus, there are many drugs and possibly other interventions that may target the muscle microvasculature, but simultaneously impact metabolism in muscle. In addition, factors that can change the basal or stimulated metabolic rate in muscle, by promoting angiogenesis or increased capillary density, may also have the potential for treating diseases associated with obesity and energy excess.

7. Conclusion

Metabolism in skeletal muscle, and in many other tissues, relies on appropriate delivery of oxygen and metabolites by the blood. The microvascular system is a major component in the delivery of any hormone, and should be considered in any endocrine disease. The muscle microvasculature is a dynamic system that can be altered by a wide range of factors, including vasoconstrictors and vasodilators, the nervous system, inflammation, obesity and other disease states. Thus, endothelial function is integral to regulating metabolism, in skeletal muscle and other tissues, and may be a target for treating not just diseases of the vascular system and cardiovascular disorders but also for treatment of metabolic diseases such as diabetes.

Acknowledgements

Many thanks to Dr Richard Bergman, Director of the Diabetes and Obesity Research Institute at Cedars-Sinai Medical Center.

Author details

Cathryn M Kolka

Address all correspondence to: Cathryn.Kolka@cshs.org

Diabetes and Obesity Research Institute, Cedars-Sinai Medical Center, Los Angeles, USA

References

[1] Defronzo RA, Ferrannini E, Sato Y, Felig P, Wahren J. Synergistic interaction between exercise and insulin on peripheral glucose uptake. J Clin Invest 1981; 68(6):1468-1474.

[2] Emerson GG, Segal SS. Alignment of microvascular units along skeletal muscle fibers of hamster retractor. J Appl Physiol (1985) 1997; 82(1):42-48.

[3] Newman JM, Dora KA, Rattigan S, Edwards SJ, Colquhoun EQ, Clark MG. Norepinephrine and serotonin vasoconstriction in rat hindlimb control different vascular flow routes. Am J Physiol 1996; 270(4 Pt 1):E689-E699.

[4] Meng H, Janssen PM, Grange RW, Yang L, Beggs AH, Swanson LC, et al. Tissue triage and freezing for models of skeletal muscle disease. J Vis Exp 2014; (89):10.

[5] Janacek J, Cebasek V, Kubinova L, Ribaric S, Erzen I. 3D visualization and measurement of capillaries supplying metabolically different fiber types in the rat extensor digitorum longus muscle during denervation and reinnervation. J Histochem Cytochem 2009; 57(5):437-447.

[6] Glancy B, Hsu LY, Dao L, Bakalar M, French S, Chess DJ et al. In vivo microscopy reveals extensive embedding of capillaries within the sarcolemma of skeletal muscle fibers. Microcirculation 2014; 21(2):131-147.

[7] Korthuis RJ. Chapter 3: Regulation of Vascular Tone in Skeletal Muscle. Skeletal Muscle Circulation. San Rafael (CA): Morgan and Claypool Life Sciences, 2011.

[8] Carlier PG. Skeletal muscle perfusion and oxygenation assessed by dynamic NMR imaging and spectroscopy. Adv Exp Med Biol 2011; 915:341-6.:341-346.

[9] Korthuis RJ. Exercise hyperemia and regulation of tissue oxygenation during muscular activity. Skeletal Muscle Circulation. San Rafael (CA): Morgan and Claypool Life Sciences, 2011.

[10] Poole DC, Copp SW, Ferguson SK, Musch TI. Skeletal muscle capillary function: contemporary observations and novel hypotheses. Exp Physiol 2013; 98(12):1645-1658.

[11] Thomas GD, Segal SS. Neural control of muscle blood flow during exercise. J Appl Physiol 2004; 97(2):731-738.

[12] Thomas GD. Neural control of the circulation. Adv Physiol Educ 2011; 35(1):28-32.

[13] Coggins M, Lindner J, Rattigan S, Jahn L, Fasy E, Kaul S, et al. Physiologic hyperinsulinemia enhances human skeletal muscle perfusion by capillary recruitment. Diabetes 2001; 50(12):2682-2690.

[14] Song Y, Li Y, Wang PJ, Gao Y. Contrast-enhanced ultrasonography of skeletal muscles for type 2 diabetes mellitus patients with microvascular complications. Int J Clin Exp Med 2014; 7(3):573-579.

[15] Ross RM, Downey K, Newman JM, Richards SM, Clark MG, Rattigan S. Contrast-enhanced ultrasound measurement of microvascular perfusion relevant to nutrient and hormone delivery in skeletal muscle: a model study in vitro. Microvasc Res 2008; 75(3): 323-329.

[16] Clark AD, Youd JM, Rattigan S, Barrett EJ, Clark MG. Heterogeneity of laser Doppler flowmetry in perfused muscle indicative of nutritive and nonnutritive flow. Am J Physiol Heart Circ Physiol 2001; 280(3):H1324-H1333.

[17] Clark AD, Barrett EJ, Rattigan S, Wallis MG, Clark MG. Insulin stimulates laser Doppler signal by rat muscle in vivo, consistent with nutritive flow recruitment. Clin Sci (London) 2001; 100(3):283-290.

[18] Raynaud JS, Duteil S, Vaughan JT, Hennel F, Wary C, Leroy-Willig A, et al. Determination of skeletal muscle perfusion using arterial spin labeling NMRI: validation by comparison with venous occlusion plethysmography. Magn Reson Med 2001; 46(2): 305-311.

[19] Heinonen I, Saltin B, Kemppainen J, Sipila HT, Oikonen V, Nuutila P, et al. Skeletal muscle blood flow and oxygen uptake at rest and during exercise in humans: a pet study with nitric oxide and cyclooxygenase inhibition. Am J Physiol Heart Circ Physiol 2011; 300(4):H1510-17.

[20] Heinonen I, Kemppainen J, Kaskinoro K, Peltonen JE, Borra R, Lindroos MM et al. Comparison of exogenous adenosine and voluntary exercise on human skeletal muscle perfusion and perfusion heterogeneity. J Appl Physiol 2010; 108(2):378-386.

[21] Van Beekvelt MC, Colier WN, Wevers RA, Van Engelen BG. Performance of near-infrared spectroscopy in measuring local O(2) consumption and blood flow in skeletal muscle. J Appl Physiol (1985) 2001; 90(2):511-519.

[22] Mesquida J, Gruartmoner G, Espinal C. Skeletal muscle oxygen saturation (StO2) measured by near-infrared spectroscopy in the critically ill patients. Biomed Res Int 2013; 2013:502194. doi: 10.1155/2013/502194.

[23] Brizendine JT, Ryan TE, Larson RD, McCully KK. Skeletal muscle metabolism in endurance athletes with near-infrared spectroscopy. Med Sci Sports Exerc 2013; 45(5): 869-875.

[24] Kolka CM, Bergman RN. The barrier within: endothelial transport of hormones. Physiology (Bethesda) 2012; 27(4):237-247.

[25] Kolka CM, Richey JM, Castro AV, Broussard JL, Ionut V, Bergman RN. Lipid-induced insulin resistance does not impair insulin access to skeletal muscle. Am J Physiol Endocrinol Metab 2015; 308(11):E1001-E1009.

[26] Kulcu E, Tamada JA, Reach G, Potts RO, Lesho MJ. Physiological differences between interstitial glucose and blood glucose measured in human subjects. Diabetes Care 2003; 26(8):2405-2409.

[27] Aukland K, Reed RK. Interstitial-lymphatic mechanisms in the control of extracellular fluid volume. Physiol Rev 1993; 73(1):1-78.

[28] Wiig H, Swartz MA. Interstitial fluid and lymph formation and transport: physiological regulation and roles in inflammation and cancer. Physiol Rev 2012; 92(3):1005-1060.

[29] Vink H, Duling BR. Capillary endothelial surface layer selectively reduces plasma solute distribution volume. Am J Physiol Heart Circ Physiol 2000; 278(1):H285-H289.

[30] Eskens BJ, Mooij HL, Cleutjens JP, Roos JM, Cobelens JE, Vink H, et al. Rapid insulin-mediated increase in microvascular glycocalyx accessibility in skeletal muscle may contribute to insulin-mediated glucose disposal in rats. PLoS One 2013; 8(1):e55399.

[31] Nieuwdorp M, van Haeften TW, Gouverneur MC, Mooij HL, van Lieshout MH, Levi M, et al. Loss of endothelial glycocalyx during acute hyperglycemia coincides with endothelial dysfunction and coagulation activation in vivo. Diabetes 2006; 55(2):480-486.

[32] Zuurbier CJ, Demirci C, Koeman A, Vink H, Ince C. Short-term hyperglycemia increases endothelial glycocalyx permeability and acutely decreases lineal density of capillaries with flowing red blood cells. J Appl Physiol 2005; 99(4):1471-1476.

[33] Chiu JD, Richey JM, Harrison LN, Zuniga E, Kolka CM, Kirkman EL, et al. Direct administration of insulin into skeletal muscle reveals that the transport of insulin across the capillary endothelium limits the time course of insulin to activate glucose disposal. Diabetes 2008; 57(4):828-835.

[34] Chiu JD, Kolka CM, Richey JM, Harrison LN, Zuniga E, Kirkman EL, et al. Experimental hyperlipidemia dramatically reduces access of insulin to canine skeletal muscle. Obesity (Silver Spring) 2009; 17(8):1486-1492.

[35] Kolka CM, Harrison LN, Lottati M, Chiu JD, Kirkman EL, Bergman RN. Diet-induced obesity prevents interstitial dispersion of insulin in skeletal muscle. Diabetes 2009; 59:619-26.

[36] Kolka CM, Castro AV, Kirkman EL, Bergman RN. Modest hyperglycemia prevents interstitial dispersion of insulin in skeletal muscle. Metabolism 2015; 64(2):330-337.

[37] Scallan JP, Huxley VH. In vivo determination of collecting lymphatic vessel permeability to albumin: a role for lymphatics in exchange. J Physiol 2010; 588(Pt 1):243-254.

[38] Clausen TS, Kaastrup P, Stallknecht B. Proinflammatory tissue response and recovery of adipokines during 4 days of subcutaneous large-pore microdialysis. J Pharmacol Toxicol Methods 2009; 60(3):281-287.

[39] Gudbjornsdottir S, Sjostrand M, Strindberg L, Lonnroth P. Decreased muscle capillary permeability surface area in type 2 diabetic subjects. J Clin Endocrinol Metab 2005; 90(2):1078-1082.

[40] Jansson PA, Murdolo G, Sjogren L, Nystrom B, Sjostrand M, Strindberg L et al. Tadalafil increases muscle capillary recruitment and forearm glucose uptake in women with type 2 diabetes. Diabetologia 2010; 53(10):2205-2208.

[41] Mokshagundam SP, Peiris AN, Stagner JI, Gingerich RL, Samols E. Interstitial insulin during euglycemic-hyperinsulinemic clamp in obese and lean individuals. Metabolism 1996; 45(8):951-956.

[42] Sjostrand M, Holmang A, Strindberg L, Lonnroth P. Estimations of muscle interstitial insulin, glucose, and lactate in type 2 diabetic subjects. Am J Physiol Endocrinol Metab 2000; 279(5):E1097-E1103.

[43] Sjostrand M, Gudbjornsdottir S, Holmang A, Lonn L, Strindberg L, Lonnroth P. Delayed transcapillary transport of insulin to muscle interstitial fluid in obese subjects. Diabetes 2002; 51(9):2742-2748.

[44] Szendroedi J, Frossard M, Klein N, Bieglmayer C, Wagner O, Pacini G, et al. Lipid-induced insulin resistance is not mediated by impaired transcapillary transport of insulin and glucose in humans. Diabetes 2012; 61(12):3176-3180.

[45] Kelley DE. Skeletal muscle fat oxidation: timing and flexibility are everything. J Clin Invest 2005; 115(7):1699-1702.

[46] Romijn JA, Coyle EF, Sidossis LS, Rosenblatt J, Wolfe RR. Substrate metabolism during different exercise intensities in endurance-trained women. J Appl Physiol (1985) 2000; 88(5):1707-1714.

[47] van Loon LJ, Greenhaff PL, Constantin-Teodosiu D, Saris WH, Wagenmakers AJ. The effects of increasing exercise intensity on muscle fuel utilisation in humans. J Physiol 2001; 536(Pt 1):295-304.

[48] Hultman E. Fuel selection, muscle fibre. Proc Nutr Soc 1995; 54(1):107-121.

[49] Atalay M, Hanninen OOP. Muscle Energy Metabolism. In: Hanninen OOP, Atalay M, editors. Physiology and Maintenance, v4. Ramsey, Isle of Man: EOLSS Publishers Co Ltd, 2009.

[50] Murakami S, Fujino H, Takeda I, Momota R, Kumagishi K, Ohtsuka A. Comparison of capillary architecture between slow and fast muscles in rats using a confocal laser scanning microscope. Acta Med Okayama 2010; 64(1):11-18.

[51] Wilson DF. Regulation of metabolism: the work to rest transition in skeletal muscle. Am J Physiol Endocrinol Metab 2016; 309(9):E793-801.

[52] Laughlin MH, Armstrong RB. Muscular blood flow distribution patterns as a function of running speed in rats. Am J Physiol 1982; 243(2):H296-H306.

[53] Armstrong RB, Laughlin MH. Blood flows within and among rat muscles as a function of time during high speed treadmill exercise. J Physiol 1983; 344:189-208.

[54] Weibel ER, Bacigalupe LD, Schmitt B, Hoppeler H. Allometric scaling of maximal metabolic rate in mammals: muscle aerobic capacity as determinant factor. Respir Physiol Neurobiol 2004; 140(2):115-132.

[55] Gollnick PD, Armstrong RB, Saltin B, Saubert CW, Sembrowich WL, Shepherd RE. Effect of training on enzyme activity and fiber composition of human skeletal muscle. J Appl Physiol 1973; 34(1):107-111.

[56] Ingalls CP. Nature vs. nurture: can exercise really alter fiber type composition in human skeletal muscle? J Appl Physiol (1985) 2004; 97(5):1591-1592.

[57] Clark MG, Wallis MG, Barrett EJ, Vincent MA, Richards SM, Clerk LH, et al. Blood flow and muscle metabolism: a focus on insulin action. Am J Physiol Endocrinol Metab 2003; 284(2):E241-E258.

[58] Rattigan S, Dora KA, Colquhoun EQ, Clark MG. Serotonin-mediated acute insulin resistance in the perfused rat hindlimb but not in incubated muscle: a role for the vascular system. Life Sci 1993; 53(20):1545-1555.

[59] Rattigan S, Dora KA, Colquhoun EQ, Clark MG. Inhibition of insulin-mediated glucose uptake in rat hindlimb by an alpha-adrenergic vascular effect. Am J Physiol 1995; 268(2 Pt 1):E305-E311.

[60] Baron AD, Clark MG. Role of blood flow in the regulation of muscle glucose uptake. Annu Rev Nutr 1997; 17:487-99.:487-499.

[61] Rattigan S, Wallis MG, Youd JM, Clark MG. Exercise training improves insulin-mediated capillary recruitment in association with glucose uptake in rat hindlimb. Diabetes 2001; 50(12):2659-2665.

[62] Rattigan S, Wheatley C, Richards SM, Barrett EJ, Clark MG. Exercise and insulin-mediated capillary recruitment in muscle. Exerc Sport Sci Rev 2005; 33(1):43-48.

[63] Wheatley CM, Rattigan S, Richards SM, Barrett EJ, Clark MG. Skeletal muscle contraction stimulates capillary recruitment and glucose uptake in insulin-resistant obese Zucker rats. Am J Physiol Endocrinol Metab 2004; 287(4):E804-E809.

[64] Vincent MA, Clerk LH, Lindner JR, Price WJ, Jahn LA, Leong-Poi H, et al. Mixed meal and light exercise each recruit muscle capillaries in healthy humans. Am J Physiol Endocrinol Metab 2006; 290(6):E1191-E1197.

[65] Honig CR, Odoroff CL, Frierson JL. Capillary recruitment in exercise: rate, extent, uniformity, and relation to blood flow. Am J Physiol 1980; 238(1):H31-H42.

[66] Golub AS, Pittman RN. Bang-bang model for regulation of local blood flow. Microcirculation 2013;20(6):455–83.

[67] Ross RM, Wadley GD, Clark MG, Rattigan S, McConell GK. Local nitric oxide synthase inhibition reduces skeletal muscle glucose uptake but not capillary blood flow during in situ muscle contraction in rats. Diabetes 2007; 56(12):2885-2892.

[68] Heinonen I, Saltin B, Kemppainen J, Nuutila P, Knuuti J, Kalliokoski K, et al. Effect of nitric oxide synthase inhibition on the exchange of glucose and fatty acids in human skeletal muscle. Nutr Metab (Lond) 2013; 10(1):43-10.

[69] Tengan CH, Rodrigues GS, Godinho RO. Nitric oxide in skeletal muscle: role on mitochondrial biogenesis and function. Int J Mol Sci 2012; 13(12):17160-17184.

[70] Chai W, Dong Z, Wang N, Wang W, Tao L, Cao W, et al. Glucagon-like peptide 1 recruits microvasculature and increases glucose use in muscle via a nitric oxide-dependent mechanism. Diabetes 2012; 61(4):888-896.

[71] Chai W, Zhang X, Barrett EJ, Liu Z. Glucagon-like peptide 1 recruits muscle microvasculature and improves insulin's metabolic action in the presence of insulin resistance. Diabetes 2014; 63(8):2788-2799.

[72] Smits MM, Muskiet MH, Tonneijck L, Kramer MH, Diamant M, van Raalte DH et al. GLP-1 Receptor agonist exenatide increases capillary perfusion independent of nitric oxide in healthy overweight men. Arterioscler Thromb Vasc Biol 2015; 35(6):1538-1543.

[73] Sjoberg KA, Holst JJ, Rattigan S, Richter EA, Kiens B. GLP-1 increases microvascular recruitment but not glucose uptake in human and rat skeletal muscle. Am J Physiol Endocrinol Metab 2014; 306(4):E355-E362.

[74] Aronis KN, Chamberland JP, Mantzoros CS. GLP-1 promotes angiogenesis in human endothelial cells in a dose-dependent manner, through the Akt, Src and PKC pathways. Metabolism 2013; 62(9):1279-1286.

[75] Forst T, Weber MM, Pfutzner A. Cardiovascular benefits of GLP-1-based therapies in patients with diabetes mellitus type 2: effects on endothelial and vascular dysfunction beyond glycemic control. Exp Diabetes Res 2012; 2012:635472.

[76] Gurkan E, Tarkun I, Sahin T, Cetinarslan B, Canturk Z. Evaluation of exenatide versus insulin glargine for the impact on endothelial functions and cardiovascular risk markers. Diabetes Res Clin Pract 2014; 106(3):567-575.

[77] Nystrom T, Gutniak MK, Zhang Q, Zhang F, Holst JJ, Ahren B, et al. Effects of glucagon-like peptide-1 on endothelial function in type 2 diabetes patients with stable coronary artery disease. Am J Physiol Endocrinol Metab 2004; 287(6):E1209-E1215.

[78] Yoon JS, Lee HW. Understanding the cardiovascular effects of incretin. Diabetes Metab J 2011; 35(5):437-443.

[79] Gonzalez N, Acitores A, Sancho V, Valverde I, Villanueva-Penacarrillo ML. Effect of GLP-1 on glucose transport and its cell signalling in human myocytes. Regul Pept 2005; 126:203-11.

[80] Ionut V, Hucking K, Liberty IF, Bergman RN. Synergistic effect of portal glucose and glucagon-like peptide-1 to lower systemic glucose and stimulate counter-regulatory hormones. Diabetologia 2005; 48(5):967-975.

[81] Luque MA, Gonzalez N, Marquez L, Acitores A, Redondo A, Morales M, et al. Glucagon-like peptide-1 (GLP-1) and glucose metabolism in human myocytes. J Endocrinol 2002; 173(3):465-473.

[82] Elias I, Franckhauser S, Ferre T, Vila L, Tafuro S, Munoz S, et al. Adipose tissue overexpression of vascular endothelial growth factor protects against diet-induced obesity and insulin resistance. Diabetes 2012; 61(7):1801-1813.

[83] Kolka CM, Rattigan S, Richards S, Clark MG. Metabolic and vascular actions of endothelin-1 are inhibited by insulin-mediated vasodilation in perfused rat hindlimb muscle. Br J Pharmacol 2005; 145(7):992-1000.

[84] Rattigan S, Clark MG, Barrett EJ. Acute vasoconstriction-induced insulin resistance in rat muscle in vivo. Diabetes 1999; 48(3):564-569.

[85] Rattigan S, Appleby GJ, Miller KA, Steen JT, Dora KA, Colquhoun EQ, et al. Serotonin inhibition of 1-methylxanthine metabolism parallels its vasoconstrictor activity and inhibition of oxygen uptake in perfused rat hindlimb. Acta Physiol Scand 1997; 161(2): 161-9.

[86] Muniyappa R, Yavuz S. Metabolic actions of angiotensin II and insulin: a microvascular endothelial balancing act. Mol Cell Endocrinol 2012; 378:59-69.

[87] Zhang C, Hein TW, Wang W, Kuo L. Divergent roles of angiotensin II AT1 and AT2 receptors in modulating coronary microvascular function. Circ Res 2003; 92(3):322-329.

[88] Williams B, Baker AQ, Gallacher B, Lodwick D. Angiotensin II increases vascular permeability factor gene expression by human vascular smooth muscle cells. Hypertension 1995; 25(5):913-917.

[89] Richey JM, Ader M, Moore D, Bergman RN. Angiotensin II induces insulin resistance independent of changes in interstitial insulin. Am J Physiol 1999; 277(5 Pt 1):E920-E926.

[90] Oh SJ, Ha WC, Lee JI, Sohn TS, Kim JH, Lee JM, et al. Angiotensin II inhibits insulin binding to endothelial cells. Diabetes Metab J 2011; 35(3):243-247.

[91] Imanishi T, Kobayashi K, Kuroi A, Mochizuki S, Goto M, Yoshida K, et al. Effects of angiotensin II on NO bioavailability evaluated using a catheter-type NO sensor. Hypertension 2006; 48(6):1058-1065.

[92] Jonk AM, Houben AJ, Schaper NC, de Leeuw PW, Serne EH, Smulders YM, et al. Acute angiotensin II receptor blockade improves insulin-induced microvascular function in hypertensive individuals. Microvasc Res 2011; 82(1):77-83.

[93] Chai W, Wang W, Dong Z, Cao W, Liu Z. Angiotensin II receptors modulate muscle microvascular and metabolic responses to insulin in vivo. Diabetes 2011; 60(11):2939-2946.

[94] Eringa EC, Stehouwer CD, Merlijn T, Westerhof N, Sipkema P. Physiological concentrations of insulin induce endothelin-mediated vasoconstriction during inhibition of NOS or PI3-kinase in skeletal muscle arterioles. Cardiovasc Res 2002; 56(3):464-471.

[95] Verma S, Yao L, Stewart DJ, Dumont AS, Anderson TJ, McNeill JH. Endothelin antagonism uncovers insulin-mediated vasorelaxation in vitro and in vivo. Hypertension 2001; 37(2):328-333.

[96] Bussey CT, Kolka CM, Rattigan S, Richards SM. Adiponectin opposes endothelin-1-mediated vasoconstriction in the perfused rat hindlimb. Am J Physiol Heart Circ Physiol 2011; 301(1):H79-86.

[97] Laakso M, Edelman SV, Brechtel G, Baron AD. Decreased effect of insulin to stimulate skeletal muscle blood flow in obese man. A novel mechanism for insulin resistance. J Clin Invest 1990; 85(6):1844-1852.

[98] Tack CJJ, Schefman AEP, Willems JL, Thien T, Lutterman JA, Smits P. Direct vasodilator effects of physiological hyperinsulin-aemia in human skeletal muscle. European Journal of Clinical Investigation 1996; 26(9):772-778.

[99] Lambadiari V, Triantafyllou K, Dimitriadis GD. Insulin action in muscle and adipose tissue in type 2 diabetes: the significance of blood flow. World J Diabetes 2015; 6(4):626-633.

[100] Rattigan S, Clark MG, Barrett EJ. Hemodynamic actions of insulin in rat skeletal muscle: evidence for capillary recruitment. Diabetes 1997; 46(9):1381-1388.

[101] Vincent MA, Clerk LH, Lindner JR, Klibanov AL, Clark MG, Rattigan S, et al. Microvascular recruitment is an early insulin effect that regulates skeletal muscle glucose uptake in vivo. Diabetes 2004; 53(6):1418-1423.

[102] Zhang L, Vincent MA, Richards SM, Clerk LH, Rattigan S, Clark MG, et al. Insulin sensitivity of muscle capillary recruitment in vivo. Diabetes 2004; 53(2):447-453.

[103] Serne EH, Ijzerman RG, Gans RO, Nijveldt R, de Vries G, Evertz R, et al. Direct evidence for insulin-induced capillary recruitment in skin of healthy subjects during physiological hyperinsulinemia. Diabetes 2002; 51(5):1515-1522.

[104] Miles PD, Levisetti M, Reichart D, Khoursheed M, Moossa AR, Olefsky JM. Kinetics of insulin action in vivo. Identification of rate-limiting steps. Diabetes 1995; 44(8):947-953.

[105] Sasson S, Cerasi E. Substrate regulation of the glucose transport system in rat skeletal muscle. Characterization and kinetic analysis in isolated soleus muscle and skeletal muscle cells in culture. J Biol Chem 1986; 261(36):16827-16833.

[106] Wang H, Liu Z, Li G, Barrett EJ. The vascular endothelial cell mediates insulin transport into skeletal muscle. Am J Physiol Endocrinol Metab 2006; 291(2):E323-E332.

[107] Wang H, Wang AX, Liu Z, Barrett EJ. Insulin signaling stimulates insulin transport by bovine aortic endothelial cells. Diabetes 2008; 57(3):540-547.

[108] Kubota T, Kubota N, Kumagai H, Yamaguchi S, Kozono H, Takahashi T ,et al. Impaired insulin signaling in endothelial cells reduces insulin-induced glucose uptake by skeletal muscle. Cell Metab 2011; 13(3):294-307.

[109] Pillon NJ, Azizi PM, Li YE, Liu J, Wang C, Chan KL, et al. Palmitate-induced inflammatory pathways in human adipose microvascular endothelial cells promote monocyte adhesion and impair insulin transcytosis. Am J Physiol Endocrinol Metab 2015; 309(1):E35-E44.

[110] National Diabetes Fact Sheet: national estimates and general information on diabetes and prediabetes in the United States. Centers for Disease Control and Prevention. 2011.

[111] Karaca U, Schram MT, Houben AJ, Muris DM, Stehouwer CD. Microvascular dysfunction as a link between obesity, insulin resistance and hypertension. Diabetes Res Clin Pract 2014; 103(3):382-387.

[112] Chakir M, Plante GE, Maheux P. Reduction of capillary permeability in the fructose-induced hypertensive rat. Am J Hypertens 1998; 11(5):563-569.

[113] Kolka CM, Rattigan S, Richards SM, Clark MG. Potential for endothelin-1-mediated impairment of contractile activity in hypertension. Clin Exp Pharmacol Physiol 2007; 34(3):217-222.

[114] Mahfoud F, Schlaich M, Kindermann I, Ukena C, Cremers B, Brandt MC et al. Effect of renal sympathetic denervation on glucose metabolism in patients with resistant hypertension: a pilot study. Circulation 2011; 123(18):1940-1946.

[115] Verloop WL, Spiering W, Vink EE, Beeftink MM, Blankestijn PJ, Doevendans PA, et al. Denervation of the renal arteries in metabolic syndrome: the DREAMS-study. Hypertension 2015; 65(4):751-757.

[116] Bhatt DL, Kandzari DE, O'Neill WW, D'Agostino R, Flack JM, Katzen BT, et al. A controlled trial of renal denervation for resistant hypertension. N Engl J Med 2014; 370(15):1393-1401.

[117] Mendelsohn FO. Does complete renal denervation translate into superior clinical outcomes? Lessons learned from denervation of accessory renal arteries. Clin Res Cardiol 2014; 103(9):681-683.

[118] Jiang F, Li H, Zhu F, Zeng L, Wang X, Wang X, et al. Investigation of the mechanism underlying the antihypertensive effect of catheter-based radiofrequency renal sympathetic denervation in hypertensive dogs. Biomed Rep 2015; 3(2):254-260.

[119] Eikelis N, Hering D, Marusic P, Sari C, Walton A, Phillips S, et al. The effect of renal denervation on endothelial function and inflammatory markers in patients with resistant hypertension. Int J Cardiol 2015; 188:96-8. doi: 10.1016/j.ijcard.2015.04.041.

[120] Kim SP, Ellmerer M, Van Citters GW, Bergman RN. Primacy of hepatic insulin resistance in the development of the metabolic syndrome induced by an isocaloric moderate-fat diet in the dog. Diabetes 2003; 52(10):2453-2460.

[121] Holland WL, Bikman BT, Wang LP, Yuguang G, Sargent KM, Bulchand S, et al. Lipid-induced insulin resistance mediated by the proinflammatory receptor TLR4 requires saturated fatty acid-induced ceramide biosynthesis in mice. J Clin Invest 2011; 121:1858-1870.

[122] Krebs M, Roden M. Molecular mechanisms of lipid-induced insulin resistance in muscle, liver and vasculature. Diabetes Obes Metab 2005; 7(6):621-632.

[123] Iwata NG, Pham M, Rizzo NO, Cheng AM, Maloney E, Kim F. Trans fatty acids induce vascular inflammation and reduce vascular nitric oxide production in endothelial cells. PLoS One 2011; 6(12):e29600.

[124] Gu P, Xu A. Interplay between adipose tissue and blood vessels in obesity and vascular dysfunction. Rev Endocr Metab Disord 2013; 14(1):49-58.

[125] Yudkin JS, Eringa E, Stehouwer CD. "Vasocrine" signalling from perivascular fat: a mechanism linking insulin resistance to vascular disease. Lancet 2005; 365(9473):1817-1820.

[126] Hoeg LD, Sjoberg KA, Jeppesen J, Jensen TE, Frosig C, Birk JB, et al. Lipid-induced insulin resistance affects women less than men and is not accompanied by inflammation or impaired proximal insulin signaling. Diabetes 2011; 60(1):64-73.

[127] Symons JD, Abel ED. Lipotoxicity contributes to endothelial dysfunction: a focus on the contribution from ceramide. Rev Endocr Metab Disord 2013; 14(1):59-68.

[128] Okon EB, Chung AW, Zhang H, Laher I, van Breemen C. Hyperglycemia and hyperlipidemia are associated with endothelial dysfunction during the development of type 2 diabetes. Can J Physiol Pharmacol 2007; 85(5):562-567.

[129] de Jongh RT, Serne EH, Ijzerman RG, de Vries G, Stehouwer CD. Free fatty acid levels modulate microvascular function: relevance for obesity-associated insulin resistance, hypertension, and microangiopathy. Diabetes 2004; 53(11):2873-2882.

[130] Liu J, Jahn LA, Fowler DE, Barrett EJ, Cao W, Liu Z. Free fatty acids induce insulin resistance in both cardiac and skeletal muscle microvasculature in humans. J Clin Endocrinol Metab 2011; 96(2):438-446.

[131] Clerk LH, Vincent MA, Jahn LA, Liu Z, Lindner JR, Barrett EJ. Obesity blunts insulin-mediated microvascular recruitment in human forearm muscle. Diabetes 2006; 55:1436-1442.

[132] de Jongh RT, Ijzerman RG, Serne EH, Voordouw JJ, Yudkin JS, de Waal HA, et al. Visceral and truncal subcutaneous adipose tissue are associated with impaired

capillary recruitment in healthy individuals. J Clin Endocrinol Metab 2006; 91(12):5100-5106.

[133] Dyck DJ, Heigenhauser GJ, Bruce CR. The role of adipokines as regulators of skeletal muscle fatty acid metabolism and insulin sensitivity. Acta Physiol (Oxf) 2006; 186(1):5-16.

[134] Xu SQ, Mahadev K, Wu X, Fuchsel L, Donnelly S, Scalia RG, et al. Adiponectin protects against angiotensin II or tumor necrosis factor alpha-induced endothelial cell monolayer hyperpermeability: role of cAMP/PKA signaling. Arterioscler Thromb Vasc Biol 2008; 28(5):899-905.

[135] Solinas G, Summermatter S, Mainieri D, Gubler M, Pirola L, Wymann MP, et al. The direct effect of leptin on skeletal muscle thermogenesis is mediated by substrate cycling between de novo lipogenesis and lipid oxidation. FEBS Lett 2004; 577(3):539-544.

[136] El Akoum S, Cloutier I, Tanguay JF. Vascular smooth muscle cell alterations triggered by mice adipocytes: role of high-fat diet. J Atheroscler Thromb 2012; 19(12):1128-1141.

[137] Singh P, Peterson TE, Sert-Kuniyoshi FH, Jensen MD, Somers VK. Leptin upregulates caveolin-1 expression: implications for development of atherosclerosis. Atherosclerosis 2011; 217(2):499-502.

[138] Youd JM, Rattigan S, Clark MG. Acute impairment of insulin-mediated capillary recruitment and glucose uptake in rat skeletal muscle in vivo by TNF-alpha. Diabetes 2000; 49(11):1904-1909.

[139] Mazzali G, Di F, V, Zoico E, Fantin F, Zamboni G, Benati C, et al. Interrelations between fat distribution, muscle lipid content, adipocytokines, and insulin resistance: effect of moderate weight loss in older women. Am J Clin Nutr 2006; 84(5):1193-1199.

[140] Yuen DY, Dwyer RM, Matthews VB, Zhang L, Drew BG, Neill B, et al. Interleukin-6 attenuates insulin-mediated increases in endothelial cell signaling but augments skeletal muscle insulin action via differential effects on tumor necrosis factor-alpha expression. Diabetes 2009; 58(5):1086-1095.

[141] Kemp JG, Blazev R, Stephenson DG, Stephenson GM. Morphological and biochemical alterations of skeletal muscles from the genetically obese (ob/ob) mouse. Int J Obes (Lond) 2009; 33(8):831-841.

[142] Malenfant P, Joanisse DR, Theriault R, Goodpaster BH, Kelley DE, Simoneau JA. Fat content in individual muscle fibers of lean and obese subjects. Int J Obes Relat Metab Disord 2001; 25(9):1316-1321.

[143] Virkamaki A, Korsheninnikova E, Seppala-Lindroos A, Vehkavaara S, Goto T, Halavaara J, et al. Intramyocellular lipid is associated with resistance to in vivo insulin actions on glucose uptake, antilipolysis, and early insulin signaling pathways in human skeletal muscle. Diabetes 2001; 50(10):2337-2343.

[144] Toledo FG, Goodpaster BH. The role of weight loss and exercise in correcting skeletal muscle mitochondrial abnormalities in obesity, diabetes and aging. Mol Cell Endocrinol 2013; 379:30-34.

[145] Goodpaster BH, He J, Watkins S, Kelley DE. Skeletal muscle lipid content and insulin resistance: evidence for a paradox in endurance-trained athletes. J Clin Endocrinol Metab 2001; 86(12):5755-5761.

[146] Coen PM, Goodpaster BH. Role of intramyocelluar lipids in human health. Trends Endocrinol Metab 2012; 23(8):391-398.

[147] Czernichow S, Greenfield JR, Galan P, Bastard JP, Charnaux N, Samaras K, et al. Microvascular dysfunction in healthy insulin-sensitive overweight individuals. J Hypertens 2010; 28(2):325-332.

[148] Lillioja S, Young AA, Culter CL, Ivy JL, Abbott WG, Zawadzki JK, et al. Skeletal muscle capillary density and fiber type are possible determinants of in vivo insulin resistance in man. J Clin Invest 1987; 80(2):415-424.

[149] Rupnick MA, Panigrahy D, Zhang CY, Dallabrida SM, Lowell BB, Langer R, et al. Adipose tissue mass can be regulated through the vasculature. Proc Natl Acad Sci U S A 2002; 99(16):10730-10735.

[150] Keske MA, Clerk LH, Price WJ, Jahn LA, Barrett EJ. Obesity blunts microvascular recruitment in human forearm muscle after a mixed meal. Diabetes Care 2009; 32:1672-1677.

[151] Ellmerer M, Kim SP, Hamilton-Wessler M, Hucking K, Kirkman E, Bergman RN. Physiological hyperinsulinemia in dogs augments access of macromolecules to insulin-sensitive tissues. Diabetes 2004; 53(11):2741-2747.

[152] Ellmerer M, Hamilton-Wessler M, Kim SP, Huecking K, Kirkman E, Chiu J, et al. Reduced access to insulin-sensitive tissues in dogs with obesity secondary to increased fat intake. Diabetes 2006; 55(6):1769-1775.

[153] Ross RM, Kolka CM, Rattigan S, Clark MG. Acute blockade by endothelin-1 of haemodynamic insulin action in rats. Diabetologia 2007; 50(2):443-451.

[154] Clerk LH, Rattigan S, Clark MG. Lipid infusion impairs physiologic insulin-mediated capillary recruitment and muscle glucose uptake in vivo. Diabetes 2002; 51(4):1138-1145.

[155] St Pierre P, Bouffard L, Papirakis ME, Maheux P. Increased extravasation of macromolecules in skeletal muscles of the Zucker rat model. Obesity (Silver Spring) 2006; 14(5): 787-793.

[156] Wallis MG, Wheatley CM, Rattigan S, Barrett EJ, Clark AD, Clark MG. Insulin-mediated hemodynamic changes are impaired in muscle of Zucker obese rats. Diabetes 2002; 51(12):3492-3498.

[157] Miles PD, Li S, Hart M, Romeo O, Cheng J, Cohen A, et al. Mechanisms of insulin resistance in experimental hyperinsulinemic dogs. J Clin Invest 1998; 101(1):202-211.

[158] Schaefer C, Biermann T, Schroeder M, Fuhrhop I, Niemeier A, Ruther W, et al. Early microvascular complications of prediabetes in mice with impaired glucose tolerance and dyslipidemia. Acta Diabetol 2009; 47(Suppl 1):19-27.

[159] Eringa EC, Serne EH, Meijer RI, Schalkwijk CG, Houben AJ, Stehouwer CD, et al. Endothelial dysfunction in (pre)diabetes: characteristics, causative mechanisms and pathogenic role in type 2 diabetes. Rev Endocr Metab Disord 2013; 14(1):39-48.

[160] Georgescu A. Vascular dysfunction in diabetes: the endothelial progenitor cells as new therapeutic strategy. World J Diabetes 2011; 2(6):92-97.

[161] Goldfine AB, Beckman JA, Betensky RA, Devlin H, Hurley S, Varo N, et al. Family history of diabetes is a major determinant of endothelial function. J Am Coll Cardiol 2006;47(12):2456-2461.

[162] Satchell SC. The glomerular endothelium emerges as a key player in diabetic nephropathy. Kidney Int 2012; 82(9):949-951.

[163] Tremolada G, Del Turco C, Lattanzio R, Maestroni S, Maestroni A, Bandello F, et al. The role of angiogenesis in the development of proliferative diabetic retinopathy: impact of intravitreal anti-VEGF treatment. Exp Diabetes Res 2012; 2012:728325.

[164] Sun PC, Chen CS, Kuo CD, Lin HD, Chan RC, Kao MJ, et al. Impaired microvascular flow motion in subclinical diabetic feet with sudomotor dysfunction. Microvasc Res 2012; 83(2):243-248.

[165] Bongers KS, Fox DK, Ebert SM, Kunkel SD, Dyle MC, Bullard SA, et al. Skeletal muscle denervation causes skeletal muscle atrophy through a pathway that involves both Gadd45a and HDAC4. Am J Physiol Endocrinol Metab 2013; 305(7):E907-E915.

[166] Stirban A. Microvascular dysfunction in the context of diabetic neuropathy. Curr Diab Rep 2014; 14(11):541-0541.

[167] Sharma A, Bernatchez PN, de Haan JB. Targeting endothelial dysfunction in vascular complications associated with diabetes. Int J Vasc Med 2012; 2012:750126.

[168] Vincent MA, Barrett EJ, Lindner JR, Clark MG, Rattigan S. Inhibiting NOS blocks microvascular recruitment and blunts muscle glucose uptake in response to insulin. Am J Physiol Endocrinol Metab 2003; 285(1):E123-E129.

[169] Tocci G, Paneni F, Palano F, Sciarretta S, Ferrucci A, Kurtz T, et al. Angiotensin-converting enzyme inhibitors, angiotensin II receptor blockers and diabetes: a meta-analysis of placebo-controlled clinical trials. Am J Hypertens 2011; 24(5):582-590.

[170] van der Zijl NJ, Moors CC, Goossens GH, Hermans MM, Blaak EE, Diamant M. Valsartan improves {beta}-cell function and insulin sensitivity in subjects with impaired glucose metabolism: a randomized controlled trial. Diabetes Care 2011; 34(4):845-851.

[171] Wang N, Chai W, Zhao L, Tao L, Cao W, Liu Z. Losartan increases muscle insulin delivery and rescues insulin's metabolic action during lipid infusion via microvascular recruitment. Am J Physiol Endocrinol Metab 2013; 304(5):E538-E545.

[172] Yuan Z, Hein TW, Rosa RH, Jr., Kuo L. Sildenafil (Viagra) evokes retinal arteriolar dilation: dual pathways via NOS activation and phosphodiesterase inhibition. Invest Ophthalmol Vis Sci 2008; 49(2):720-725.

[173] Murdolo G, Sjostrand M, Strindberg L, Lonnroth P, Jansson PA. The selective phosphodiesterase-5 inhibitor tadalafil induces microvascular and metabolic effects in type 2 diabetic postmenopausal females. J Clin Endocrinol Metab 2012; 98(1):245-254.

[174] Sabatini S, Sgro P, Duranti G, Ceci R, Di Luigi L. Tadalafil alters energy metabolism in C2C12 skeletal muscle cells. Acta Biochim Pol 2011; 58(2):237-241.

[175] Biscetti F, Straface G, Arena V, Stigliano E, Pecorini G, Rizzo P, et al. Pioglitazone enhances collateral blood flow in ischemic hindlimb of diabetic mice through an Akt-dependent VEGF-mediated mechanism, regardless of PPARgamma stimulation. Cardiovasc Diabetol 2009; 8:49.

[176] Omae T, Nagaoka T, Tanano I, Yoshida A. Pioglitazone, a peroxisome proliferator-activated receptor-gamma agonist, induces dilation of isolated porcine retinal arterioles: role of nitric oxide and potassium channels. Invest Ophthalmol Vis Sci 2011; 52(9): 6749-6756.

[177] Gealekman O, Guseva N, Gurav K, Gusev A, Hartigan C, Thompson M, et al. Effect of rosiglitazone on capillary density and angiogenesis in adipose tissue of normoglycaemic humans in a randomised controlled trial. Diabetologia 2012; 55(10):2794-2799.

[178] Vinik A, Parson H, Ullal J. The role of PPARs in the microvascular dysfunction in diabetes. Vascul Pharmacol 2006; 45(1):54-64.

[179] Sgarra L, Addabbo F, Potenza MA, Montagnani M. Determinants of evolving metabolic and cardiovascular benefit/risk profiles of rosiglitazone therapy during the natural history of diabetes: molecular mechanisms in the context of integrated pathophysiology. Am J Physiol Endocrinol Metab 2012; 302(10):E1171-E1182.

[180] Annecke T, Chappell D, Chen C, Jacob M, Welsch U, Sommerhoff CP, et al. Sevoflurane preserves the endothelial glycocalyx against ischaemia-reperfusion injury. Br J Anaesth 2010; 104(4):414-421.

[181] Groen BB, Hamer HM, Snijders T, van Kranenburg J, Frijns D, Vink H, et al. Skeletal muscle capillary density and microvascular function are compromised with aging and type 2 diabetes. J Appl Physiol (1985) 2014; 116(8):998-1005.

[182] Becker BF, Chappell D, Bruegger D, Annecke T, Jacob M. Therapeutic strategies targeting the endothelial glycocalyx: acute deficits, but great potential. Cardiovasc Res 2010; 87:300-10.

[183] Blondin DP, Labbe SM, Phoenix S, Guerin B, Turcotte EE, Richard D, et al. Contributions of white and brown adipose tissues and skeletal muscles to acute cold-induced metabolic responses in healthy men. J Physiol 2015; 593(3):701-714.

[184] Sun K, Kusminski CM, Luby-Phelps K, Spurgin SB, An YA, Wang QA, et al. Brown adipose tissue derived VEGF-A modulates cold tolerance and energy expenditure. Mol Metab 2014; 3(4):474-483.

Chapter 4

Microcirculation of the Newborn

Ian M.R. Wright and Rebecca M. Dyson

Additional information is available at the end of the chapter

http://dx.doi.org/10.5772/64584

Abstract

Appropriate regulation of microvascular blood flow in the neonate is crucial for cardiorespiratory stability and survival in the period immediately following birth. Inappropriate microvascular dilatation in the first few days of extrauterine life is associated with poor outcomes in preterm neonates. Male very preterm neonates (≤28 weeks completed gestation) have significantly higher flows than females of the same gestational age. This is of clinical importance as preterm males are twice as likely to die as females. Very little is known about the mechanisms underlying microvascular tone regulation in the perinatal period. Previous studies suggest a role for the gasotransmitters nitric oxide and carbon monoxide; however, differences in levels of these molecules do not account for all the variation observed, suggesting another player. In this chapter, the role of the third gasotransmitter—hydrogen sulphide—as a potential mediator of microvascular (dys)function in the preterm is explored.

Keywords: microcirculation, preterm, neonate, gasotransmitters, vasodilatation

1. Introduction

The newborn period represents a time of high mortality and morbidity. In the developed and developing world, perinatal mortality is the major contributor to infant, and thus child mortality [1], with the preterm infant at the greatest risk of poor outcomes. In Western countries, approximately 10% of infants are delivered prematurely (defined as less than 37 completed weeks of gestation) [2]. Both mortality and morbidity increase substantially with decreasing gestation at birth, as does the risk of long-term disability. Thus, the neonatal period, and prematurity in particular, represents a significant burden for the infant, the family and society. There is a marked sex difference in many of these outcomes, with males doing significantly worse, the causes of which are not fully elucidated. Studies of the microcirculation may be important in understanding both the general and sex-specific risks as peripheral blood flow is subject to considerable changes during the first days of postnatal life, a period of marked circulatory vulnerability, especially in preterm infants.

2. Circulatory transition

There is an increasing body of recent work demonstrating the relationship between peripheral microvascular blood flow and measures of neonatal physiological and cardiorespiratory stability during the transitional period. These studies have shown that the evaluation of the peripheral microcirculation is useful for the assessment of cardiovascular changes within the initial extrauterine period [3, 4]. In the newborn, the skin represents a significant microvascular bed, both because of its size and functional perinatal changes. Measurement of cutaneous microvascular behaviour may be more useful at identifying individuals at risk of cardiovascular compromise than traditional blood pressure monitoring, as decreases in peripheral blood flow can be identified before blood pressure drops in states of compensatory peripheral vasoconstriction. Peripheral blood flow may increase early in vasodilatory shock, despite stable systemic blood pressure for some time after onset [5]. This suggests that peripheral microvascular tissue flow evaluation may be useful for early detection of cardiovascular compromise. In addition, the regulatory mechanisms of the peripheral microcirculation contribute to (and may reflect) the underlying neuroendocrine responses to cardiovascular compromise [6, 7]. Finally, the skin allows non-invasive microvascular measurement, a prerequisite for human newborn studies of the microcirculation.

In adults, blood enters the skin through small arterioles, penetrating the subcutaneous tissue toward the skin surface. One artery often branches into several precapillary arterioles (30–80 μm), which pass into the venous plexuses that are organized parallel to the skin surface. Each arteriole can divide into eight to ten capillary loops orientated perpendicular to the skin surface, with one to three loops perfusing each skin papilla [8]. In neonates, however, this is much less organized and the arteriolar-venular anastomoses, and the capillary loops are immature, with a less defined network. Capillary loops are not detectable (outside the nail beds, palms, or soles) until 2 weeks post-partum (and even then, are not distinguishable in all sites until 14 weeks postnatal age or more) [9]. Development and refinement of the vascular network continues until the formation of a more "adult-type" network at approximately 4 months postnatal age. Despite this structural immaturity, the cutaneous microvasculature of both term and preterm infants is capable of responding to external stimuli, such as occlusion or local heating, from shortly after birth [4, 10].

2.1. Preterm infants

Circulatory transition is a period of marked circulatory vulnerability, especially in preterm infants. The preterm heart is structurally and functionally immature and is not capable of adapting to relatively small changes in preload and afterload in order to function effectively and deliver oxygen and nutrients to tissues. Animal studies in neonatal pigs have demonstrated that the preterm heart requires significantly higher levels of preload than term hearts in order to function effectively [11, 12]. Thus, abnormal regulation of vascular resistance, with net effects on preload and/or afterload, may play a major role in the development of cardiovascular compromise in preterm infants [4, 13, 14].

The peripheral microcirculation undergoes rapid and considerable change during the initial extrauterine period [15, 16]. Studies examining microvascular behaviour in the first 3 days of life have reported that peripheral microvascular blood flow is significantly higher in very preterm infants (≤28 weeks gestational age [GA]) as compared to infants born moderately preterm (29–36 weeks GA) [4] or at full term [17]. This increased peripheral blood flow is associated with low blood pressure, physiological instability, and adverse outcome in the initial extrauterine period [4, 18]. Very preterm male infants, those at the greatest risk for poor short- and long-term outcomes [19], have greater baseline microvascular blood flow than female infants of the same gestational age at 24 h age [20], suggesting sex-specific differences in the neonatal ability to control vascular tone.

These studies demonstrate a strong relationship between microvascular flow and mean arterial pressure. Taken together, they suggest that a large proportion of the blood volume is being taken up by the capacitance vessels and the microcirculation in (male) preterm newborns, leading to "functional hypovolaemia" and decreased preload. This may explain why males are more at risk of complications in the first 24–48 h of life [19, 21].

3. Control of microvascular tone in the newborn

During rapid postnatal growth, autoregulatory mechanisms play a major role in maintaining adequate perfusion of developing tissues. Neural and myogenic control of skin blood flow must be rapidly established following birth to allow an effective thermoregulation in the newborn and to ensure that metabolic demands of tissues are met [22]. It is well established that the autonomic nervous system, particularly peripheral sympathetic nervous system activity, plays a central role in the regulation of vascular tone in the transitional circulation of term neonates [23]. The myogenic response contributes to autoregulation of tissue blood flow and is not dependent upon neural innervation or the endothelium in the adult vasculature. However, the myogenic response of juvenile arterioles isolated from Wistar rats is significantly reduced following endothelial removal, suggesting that in juvenile arterioles endothelium-derived factors normally augment myogenic activity over a wide range of pressures [24]. Thus, the endothelium may be more important in the regulation of vascular tone in the transitional circulation compared to the more mature individual. This is likely to be even more important in the preterm infant, where the balance of parasympathetic (vagal) tone to sympathetic drive is relatively increased compared to term infants [25].

Endothelial cells coordinate the release of vasoactive substances which act directly upon vascular smooth muscle cells (VSMCs) and thus elicit constriction or dilation of the blood vessel [26]. How various vascular mediators may interact in the initial extrauterine period is unknown at present, but elucidation of this interplay and the underlying mechanisms may help to understand microvascular dysfunction and cardiorespiratory instability in the early neonatal period.

3.1. Vasoconstriction

Peripheral vascular resistance is known to correlate with the degree of sympathoadrenal activation at birth [27]. This is due to the fact that autonomic nervous system activity is an essential component of circulatory transition and adaptation to extrauterine life. The peripheral sympathetic nervous system plays a central role in regulation of vascular tone during this period largely via the action of norepinephrine, the main sympathetic neurotransmitter regulating the cardiovascular system in the neonate and eliciting vasoconstriction [28]. Its metabolite, normetanephrine, is excreted in the urine and has been used as a measure of total body sympathoadrenal activity [29] with levels shown to be higher in female than male newborns [23]. In that study, normetanephrine was inversely related to both baseline microvascular blood flow and physiological instability immediately following birth in preterm neonates.

Endothelin (ET)-1 is a primary vasoconstrictor in the pulmonary vasculature of the foetus and neonate. ET-1 is produced by endothelial cells in response to a number of stimuli, including shear stress, hypoxia and ischemia [30]. ET-1 binds to one of the three receptors: ET_A, ET_{B1} or ET_{B2} receptors, located in the underlying VSMCs. Studies in neonatal pigs suggest that all three ET receptor subtypes are highly expressed following birth, and play distinct roles in the newborn: in line with previous studies, ET_A andET_{B2} receptors appear to be responsible for the vasoconstrictive action of ET-1, whereas binding of ET-1 to ET_{B1} receptors elicits vasodilatation. Importantly, these receptors follow a distinct expression profile: the pro-constrictive ET_A and ET_{B2} receptors are more abundant in proximal vessels [31], for example, in the pulmonary arteries and veins, respectively [32]; whereas ET_{B1} receptors are more abundant in the distal vasculature, with relatively low expression in arteries [31, 32]. Evidence from newborn piglets suggests that receptor-affinity for ET-1 is higher in veins than arteries, suggesting that in the immediate postnatal period at least, the majority of the ET-1 vasoconstrictive effect is mediated through ET_{B2} receptors [32].

ET-1 can also elicit vasodilatation through endothelium-derived nitric oxide (NO) and prostacyclin, by binding to endothelial ET_{B1} receptors. Endothelial ET_B receptors are expressed more highly in the distal than the proximal vessels [31, 33]. In the pulmonary vasculature, ET_A-mediated contraction decreases and ET_{B1}-mediated NO-dependent relaxation increases with advancing postnatal age [34], suggesting a switch from a constricted to dilated state, which follows the known decrease in pulmonary vascular resistance following birth, allowing for blood oxygenation [35]. In line with this, plasma ET-1 levels peak immediately after birth and then gradually decrease, with concentrations in healthy term newborns more than threefold greater than at 5 or 30 days postnatal age [36–38]. In a recent study of preterm newborns [23], a significant increase of ET-1 after birth was observed in very preterm neonates, but not in more mature neonates. Interestingly, umbilical arterial ET-1 was significantly higher in female preterm neonates, which is of interest given the well characterised sexual dimorphism in the development of respiratory distress [39]. Plasma ET-1, however, did not correlate with peripheral microvascular blood flow or illness severity, suggesting that while ET-1 may play a significant role in the regulation of pulmonary vascular tone, it does not appear to exert a dominant effect over systemic or peripheral microvascular tone [23].

Isoprostanes (prostaglandin-like bioactive molecules generated by free radicals and reactive oxygen species) are also vasoconstrictive in a number of vascular beds in the foetus and neonate. Under normal conditions in the adult, isoprostanes are present at nanomolar concentrations. In the newborn, however, levels are significantly higher due to the oxidative stress of the adaptation to a rapid increase in blood oxygen tension that occurs during the transition from fetal to neonatal life. The isoprostanes elicit vasoconstriction through a number of pathways, including activation of prostanoid and thromboxane receptors, and tyrosine kinase and Rho kinase pathways [40, 41]. As preterm infants are more susceptible to oxidative stress, they have greater isoprostane concentrations, with an inverse correlation between isoprostane levels and gestational age being observed [42]. At term, umbilical cord arterial isoprostane concentrations are higher in male neonates compared to females of the same age [43], which is consistent with the known vulnerability of males to oxidative stress compared to females [44]. Whether this relationship exists at earlier gestational ages is unclear, however, it seems unlikely that this is a major contributor to peripheral vascular tone regulation in the preterm neonate, as it is well documented that these neonates have a loss of peripheral vascular tone (vasodilatation) [20]. Isoprostanes, along with prostaglandins, play a major role in the closure of the ductus arteriosus after birth, suggesting these molecules may play a more significant role in central, rather than microvascular, vasoactive effects during circulatory transition [41].

Overall, the balance of vasoconstrictors to vasodilators in the immediate postnatal period appears to be relatively increased in females and more mature infants and is associated more with the control of central than peripheral vascular tone.

3.2. Vasodilatation

Whilst the above suggests that microvascular dysregulation in the preterm newborn may be associated with impaired vasoconstriction, there is also a potential role for abnormal peripheral vasodilatation leading to the development of cardiovascular compromise and poor outcome [45]. Changes in enzyme expression, receptor density, ion channel activity and intracellular signalling pathways are all likely responsible for the changes in vascular tone regulation observed during circulatory transition. Studies have shown, for example, that the mechanisms mediating endothelium-dependent vasodilatation in the femoral artery of piglets undergo a maturational change during the first weeks of life [46].

Additionally, there are considerable variations in the contribution of vasoactive substances to endothelium-dependent relaxations in different tissues—it appears that nitric oxide (NO) is the principal vasodilator in conduit arteries, whereas other mediators, such as endothelial-derived hyperpolarising factors (EDHF), make a significant contribution at the level of the resistance arteries [47, 48]. Despite this clear role for other mediators, NO is the most extensively studied vasodilator in the preterm newborn [49–53], partly due to its therapeutic use for the treatment of persistent pulmonary hypertension of the newborn.

Vasodilatation of cerebral arterioles in the newborn pig is largely mediated by endothelial prostanoids, with endothelial NO assuming a progressively greater role in vascular tone regulation during subsequent postnatal maturation. Underlying this difference is a twofold to threefold increase in both the expression and activity of endothelial nitric oxide synthase (eNOS) between birth and 3–4 months postnatal age in cerebral microvessels [54–57]. In the cerebral arteries of newborn sheep, NO plays a major role in endothelium-dependent dilatation during the first week of life [58, 59]. Interestingly, it has also been shown that in newborn lambs, the contribution of NO to peripheral vascular tone is relatively low compared to its contribution in the cerebral circulation [60]. This suggests a role for the involvement of other factors regulating systemic vasodilatation, either independently or in concert with NO, during circulatory transition; and that considerable interspecies and regional differences in vasodilator mechanisms exist. Human studies of the perinatal cerebral microvasculature rely on non-invasive measures such as near infrared spectroscopy or minimally invasive techniques such as xenon cerebral blood flow assessment. Neither has been assessed in this age group in relation to the mediators and their interactions described earlier.

3.2.1. Gasotransmitters

As the gasotransmitters, NO, carbon monoxide (CO) and hydrogen sulphide (H_2S) appear to be crucial to the dilatory component in the newborn circulation these will each be dealt with in the following sections.

3.2.1.1. Nitric oxide

NO is known to play a central role in maintaining vascular homeostasis in the transitional circulation [61]. Hypoxic events occurring at birth are known to upregulate eNOS expression leading to increased NO production, eliciting vasodilatation in the systemic microvasculature of the newborn [62, 63]. It has been hypothesised that the overproduction of NO in the perinatal period may lead to poor control of blood flow throughout the peripheral microcirculation of preterm infants, increasing their risk of circulatory compromise [64]. Blood pressure in the preterm neonate is inversely correlated to cGMP levels [61]. A role may exist for NO, it's substrates or second messengers as potential regulators of peripheral blood flow in the preterm infant [61, 65].

Our group, however, has previously shown that changes in human skin microvascular blood flow in the first 3 days of life are not associated with changes in systemic NO production [45]. Additionally, it has been hypothesised that the rate of NO production by eNOS in the endothelium of peripheral microvessels is lower than would be required to activate the downstream sGC pathway in VSMCs responsible for the excessive vasodilatation seen in premature neonates [66, 67]. This has led to the speculation that other mechanisms may be involved in both the production of NO in the microvasculature and its vasoactive effects on VSMCs during the transition from fetal to neonatal circulatory systems, with NO contributing primarily to the maintenance of baseline tone throughout this period, rather than the pathophysiological variations that are seen in microvascular tone.

3.2.1.2. *Carbon monoxide*

Carbon monoxide (CO) is produced endogenously in endothelial cells and VSMCs as a result of catabolism of heme by the enzyme heme oxygenase (HO) [68]. Two functional HO isoforms have been identified in humans and other species—HO-1, the inducible isoform which is upregulated by various stress stimuli (oxidative stress, cytokines, endotoxin and hypoxia) [69] and plays an important role in cellular defence, and HO-2, the constitutive isoform. Vasodilatation by CO is thought to be through similar pathways to NO, with CO inducing VSMC relaxation by the activation of cGMP-dependent pathways [70]; however, evidence of cGMP-independent pathways also exists—with several papers now suggesting that CO-induced vasodilatation is also mediated by large conductance calcium-activated potassium channel (BKCa) activation leading to VSMC hyperpolarisation [71, 72].

HO-1 plays an important role as an antioxidant, anti-inflammatory and anti-apoptotic mediator in prenatal and postnatal development and in the transitional circulation of neonates [69, 71]. HO-2 expression in the cerebral vasculature is developmentally regulated, with significant increases in expression observed with advancing gestational age [73, 74]. HO-2 is highly expressed in cerebral blood vessels in the newborn piglet and in these studies CO was shown to be a potent vasodilator in this microcirculatory bed [71].

CO is thought to play a role in maintaining vascular homeostasis in the fetal circulation, and endogenously produced CO is known to play a role in maintaining the patency of the ductus arteriosus (DA) in utero [75]. We have previously shown that CO is relatively increased in males and younger infants, that is, those who exhibit increased vasodilatation and adverse clinical outcomes [45]. However, the CO findings only explain a proportion of the difference present in early vasodilatation events (r=0.495 at 24 h postnatal age), with differences in NO levels apparently occurring beyond the crucial early period, suggesting at least one other vasodilator is involved.

3.2.1.3. *Hydrogen sulphide*

In adults, interest is increasing in the role of a third gasotransmitter, H_2S, as a vascular mediator important in regulation of microvascular tone. H_2S is produced endogenously in the vasculature in amounts capable of causing vasodilatation and thus may play a role in the regulation of vessel dilatation and control of blood pressure [76–78]. The majority of endogenous H_2S synthesis occurs by two pyridoxal-5′-phosphate (PLP)-dependent enzymes in the transsulphuration pathway: cystathionine-β-synthase (CBS) and cystathionine-γ-lyase (CSE). The substrates for these enzymes include the amino acids cysteine, homocysteine and cystathionine [79]. A third non-PLP-dependent enzyme 3-mercaptopyruvate sulphurtransferase (MST) also contributes to H_2S production by the metabolism of mercaptopyruvate.

In contrast to NO and CO, H_2S is proposed to exert the majority of its vasodilatory effects through the activation and opening of transmembrane ATP-sensitive potassium channels (K_{ATP}) in VSMCs [80]. In VSMCs, opening of K_{ATP} channels leads to hyperpolarisation of the cell membrane, inactivating voltage-dependent calcium channels and resulting in VSMC relaxation [81]. Thus, H_2S has been implicated as a crucial physiological mediator of vascular tone that represents an alternative pathway of vascular tone control to NO and CO. Like all the gasotransmitters, H_2S is lipophilic, ensuring rapid diffusion of the gas throughout the endothelium and VSMCs, despite its intrinsic reactivity with a diverse range of substrates [82, 83]. This diffuse production across the vessel wall and its mechanism of action qualify H_2S as an EDHF [84].

The H_2S producing enzyme CBS is expressed in multiple tissues during development. In the adult, many of these tissues, including the heart and lungs, do not express CBS [85]. In comparison, many studies have suggested that CSE is not expressed during early mammalian development—in human liver, CSE activity is not detectable in fetal liver or in premature or full-term neonatal liver samples and is not detected until several days postnatal age, with levels comparable to that in the adult reached by 3 months postnatal age [86, 87]. Recent studies, however, suggest that this developmental expression pattern may not be consistent across different tissues and vascular networks. Baragatti et al. [82] have recently demonstrated gene expression of CSE, CBS and MST in the ductus arteriosus in fetal mice (MST expression was very low compared with CSE and CBS). The expression of CSE and CBS was localised to the ductus with a specific distribution: CSE staining was more intense in the endothelial layer (45% higher than in the smooth muscle layer). Conversely, CBS staining was 15% higher in the smooth muscle layer compared to the endothelium. This supports an endothelial, CSE-derived source of H_2S in the mammalian foetus. Leffler et al. [88] showed that H_2S may also be important in the transitional cerebral circulation of newborn piglets with endogenous H_2S produced by CSE, but not CBS, in concentrations capable of eliciting pial arteriolar dilatation.

Until recently, very little was known about the role of H_2S in the transitional circulation of the neonate. The above studies demonstrated at least some activity of both CBS and CSE in the transitional circulation of the preterm newborn [89]. CBS expression, and to a lesser extent CSE, is crucial for the survival of newborn animals: CBS-deficient mice ($Cbs^{-/-}$ knockout) display endothelial dysfunction, severe growth retardation and profound lethality at weaning age, as well as the features of homocysteinemia seen in human CBS-deficient patients [90, 91]. CSE may be important in protecting against oxidative stress in the preterm newborn; $Cth^{-/-}$ mice display greater sensitivity to oxidative stress, despite normal serum biochemistry (for example, levels of bilirubin and glutathione) and the absence of histological abnormalities [90, 92].

Studies have now shown evidence of a role for H_2S in physiological microvascular tone regulation during circulatory transition in human infants, with higher production potentially associated with dysregulation in the human preterm male neonate [93, 94]. In preterm neonates (29–36 weeks completed gestation), total body turnover of H_2S (measured as urinary thiosulphate) positively correlates with peripheral microvascular blood flow and negatively correlates with blood pressure, supporting both a role for H_2S in microvascular tone regulation [93]. This increased total body turnover of H_2S was shown to be related independently to all the major risk factors for poor outcome: gestational age, postnatal age and male sex. In these studies, thiosulphate differences were not present in the first few hours immediately after birth, which suggests that very preterm neonates are not born with inherently higher levels of H_2S production, but that this increases significantly following birth [93]. Potential triggers for this could include oxidative stress [95] or inflammation [96], both of which are increased in preterm neonates [97]. The positive relationship of H_2S turnover with microvascular blood flow, and the inverse relationship with blood pressure in more mature neonates, suggests a physiological role of H_2S in this age group, perhaps as a counter to the increased vasoconstrictors (see above) [98], or as a reflection of an organ specific vascular dilatation, such as in the pulmonary circulation [99, 100].

The contribution of H_2S to vasodilatation via different pathways to those of NO and CO, or interactions with these mediators, may represent a crucial role for this gasotransmitter in regulation, or dysregulation of microvascular tone in the neonatal microvasculature.

4. Interactions of the gasotransmitters in the neonate

It is becoming increasingly evident that the complexity of hemodynamic microvascular control is not through the activity of single factors working in isolation, but by the interaction of all these elements [101, 102]. This includes interactions between the three gasotransmitters in the neonatal microcirculation (**Figure 1**).

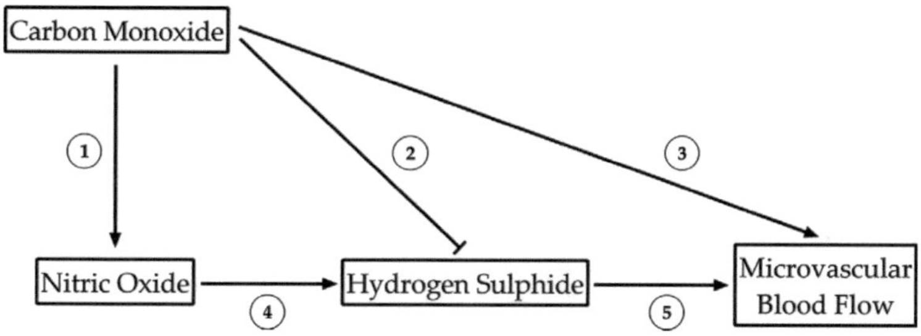

Figure 1. Structural equation modelling of gasotransmitter and microvascular flow interactions in the preterm newborns (males and females combined). NO promotes H_2S production (Interaction 4; overall $p = 0.002$; males $p = 0.06$, females $p < 0.0001$), whilst CO inhibits H_2S only in female infants (Interaction 2; overall $p = 0.18$, males $p = 0.84$, females $p < 0.0001$). The net result is a mild increase in the effect of all vasodilators acting on the microvasculature in males (Interaction 5, $p = 0.006$) compared to the effect of H_2S in isolation (model not shown). In females the model predicted a lower contribution of H_2S on microvascular blood flow when CO and NO were included in the model compared to its effect in isolation. The model predicted covariance in the levels of NO and CO (Interaction 1) but CO had no direct effect on microvascular blood flow (Interaction 3). Inclusion of this pathway, however, improved goodness of fit, most markedly in females (with CO effect $\chi^2 = 0.03$, without $\chi^2 = 0.29$). The inclusion of a direct effect of CO on flow additionally increased the predicted blood flow effect of H_2S in the overall model in both sexes, suggesting a synergistic or permissive action between these molecules. Adapted from Dyson et al. [94].

Knecht et al. [103] found in neonatal pig pial arterioles that CO responses are biphasic: dilatation occurred in response to an acute elevation, such as that produced by inducible HO activity following birth [104], while prolonged or sustained CO exposure caused constriction via NOS inhibition. They speculated that such interaction between CO/HO and NO/NOS could form a negative feedback system for the regulation of cerebrovascular tone. Importantly, the balance of NO and CO systems is different in neonatal and adult cerebrovascular circulations [103]. The role of NO in cerebrovascular control is less in newborn piglets compared to juvenile pigs, consistent with findings in human newborns [45, 55, 57, 61]. In contrast, the pial arteriolar response to CO is greater in newborn piglets compared to older pigs or adult rats. Additionally, they showed that whilst CO-induced dilation in older pigs and rats occurred independently of co-factors, NO and prostacyclin were required for CO-mediated vasodilatation to occur in the newborn [71].

In the mature circulation endogenous production of H_2S appears to be enhanced by NO. H_2S is also known to promote endothelial cell NO release, leading to a threefold increase in vasorelaxation [105, 106]. In adult rats with pulmonary hypertension, the administration of L-arginine (the pre-cursor for NO) increases CSE expression in pulmonary artery VSMCs and also plasma H_2S concentrations [107]. It is unclear whether L-arginine itself or its metabolites induce this upregulation but evidence that NO upregulates CSE expression and H_2S synthesis in VSMCs exists [105]. H_2S can also induce an upregulation of HMOX1—the gene coding for HO-1. By upregulating HO-1 expression, H_2S can thus increase CO production eliciting further vasodilatation. Conversely, administration of an inhibitor of CSE leads to a decrease in CO synthesis [108, 109].

In preterm newborns, a significant positive relationship exists between NO and H_2S [94]. Previous studies have reported that NO inhibits H_2S production via CBS [110, 111] but induces CSE H_2S production [105]. This may suggest that in the human preterm newborn, CSE expression is significantly modulated by NO. Evidence from animal models of prematurity suggest that increases in H_2S associated with microvascular dysregulation are driven by CSE-dependent mechanisms: in preterm animals, H_2S increases during fetal-to-neonatal transition, with significantly higher levels of H_2S produced by tissues collected at 24h postnatal age compared to fetal tissues. Additionally, CSE contribution to total H_2S increases postnatally. H_2S produced by the vasculature (both total H_2S and CSE-derived H_2S) correlates with microvascular blood flow at 24h postnatal age [112]. This suggests that CSE-dependent mechanisms drive the observed increase of H_2S production, and potentially the increased microvascular blood flow and decreased blood pressure, over the first 3 days of life in preterm human neonates [93]. In modelling known interactions of the gasotransmitters in human preterm neonates, a lower contribution of H_2S to microvascular tone regulation in females was predicted when the other gasotransmitters were added into the model [94]. This suggests that the effects of either NO or CO, singly or in combination, negate the effect of H_2S in these female infants to such a degree that there is no net effect on vascular tone. This may be primarily due to CO, which is inversely correlated with H_2S and may reflect an inhibitory action of CO on H_2S [94], in line with published reports [113–115]. Thus in the preterm neonate, because of these dimorphic responses, comparable levels of CO could be associated with microvascular dysregulation and cardiovascular compromise in males but help protect against inappropriate vasodilation in females [45].

4.1. Proposed mechanism of gasotransmitter-regulated microvascular vasodilatation in the newborn

We propose a model of gasotransmitter-dependent vasodilation in the preterm newborn, including a role for oxidative stress in driving dysregulation. It is now evident that all three gasotransmitters may protect against oxidative damage, but may also be cytotoxic via their inhibition of cellular respiration (through inhibition of mitochondrial respiratory chain cytochrome-C-oxidase) and through their marked pro-inflammatory effects [116]. As in the studies performed by Knecht et al., an acute increase in CO, driven in part by the HO-1 response to birth and exposure to high-concentration oxygen during resuscitation [117], drives CO-mediated vasodilatation in the male preterm newborn. Due to lowered antioxidant defences, HO-1 upregulation persists, and the prolonged CO production inhibits NO [103]. This would account for the transient nature of both the CO rise and increased microvascular blood flow observed in the preterm newborn around 24 h postnatal age, which has been shown to not be associated with NO [45]. Additionally, the transsulphuration pathway is upregulated by oxidative stress to produce the antioxidant glutathione. H_2S production is increased by this response, driving aberrant vasodilatation and contributing to hypotension and cardiovascular compromise in the preterm newborn.

We propose varying roles for the three gasotransmitters, allowing for regional and temporal control of blood flow:

- Taking into account gasotransmitter level time course and actions, we propose that NO during circulatory transition is responsible for the maintenance of basal vascular tone—as it is in adults [118, 119]. Levels are relatively stable in the first few days of life, with increases occurring outside the crucial early period of the first 24–48 h following birth [45]. NO in the transitional neonate is not, however, correlated with aberrant peripheral microvascular flow.
- CO has been shown to be a crucial regulator of vascular tone in the cerebral circulation during circulatory transition [71, 120]. It may also explain a proportion of the variance observed in early peripheral vasodilator events [45, 94], both directly and via the sexually dimorphic effects on other vasodilator pathways. The cerebral circulation effects of a CO increase, such as that observed by Stark et al [45], could contribute to the greater incidence of cerebral injury in preterm males.
- Based on our more recent studies, including metabolite measurement, production enzyme assays and interaction modelling, we suggest that H_2S is a key player in the systemic microvasculature in the sick or preterm newborn. Further we propose that H_2S is produced by the peripheral vasculature, particularly via endothelial CSE, and that this closely regulates microvascular tone during this critical period [112].

5. Summary

The microcirculation is structurally and functionally different in the neonate. The ability of the newborn to appropriately distribute blood flow to key vascular beds and to maintain adequate cardiac output is strongly linked to their survival. As cardiac function in the neonate is strongly influenced by both preload and afterload, sex differences in peripheral vascular function in preterm neonates may lead to differences in cardiac function, contributing to physiological instability and thus poor outcomes. In support of this, sexual dimorphism in the functional integrity of the microvasculature, including appropriate control of vasodilatation, is observed in very preterm neonates and is linked to outcome. Gestational age, postnatal age and sex all exert significant effects on peripheral microvascular function, dysregulation of which is associated with clinical illness severity in the neonate; however, the mechanisms by which these factors exert their effects are largely unknown. The gasotransmitters NO, CO and H_2S represent novel mediators which may play a significant role in the regulation of microvascular tone in the newborn: both through their individual roles but also through their potential interactions. The studies outlined above suggest that the gasotransmitters and their interactions could influence the adverse cardiovascular outcomes seen in this population.

6. Conclusions

Cardiovascular compromise is associated with poor outcome in the preterm neonate, with gestational age and male sex as independent risk factors for the development of hypotension and cardiovascular compromise, amongst several other morbidities. A growing body of work has highlighted the importance of the microvasculature in the development of cardiovascular compromise in the preterm newborn, and thus the importance of understanding the contribution of inappropriate peripheral vasodilatation to hypotension, cardiovascular compromise and poor neonatal outcomes.

Potential therapies aimed at either preventing or ameliorating cardiovascular compromise in the preterm neonate must consider the role of microvascular dysfunction, driven by an imbalance in vascular tone mediators, including the gasotransmitters, NO, CO and H_2S. Understanding the aetiology of cardiovascular compromise is crucial for the development of better strategies for monitoring, prevention and treatment of these at risk infants.

Author details

Ian M.R. Wright* and Rebecca M. Dyson

*Address all correspondence to: iwright@uow.edu.au

University of Wollongong and Illawarra Health & Medical Research Institute, Wollongong, NSW, Australia

References

[1] March of Dimes, et al., Born too soon: The global action report on preterm birth, C.P. Howson, M.V. Kinney, and J.E. Lawn, Editors. 2012, World Health Organisation: Geneva.

[2] Blencowe, H., et al., National, regional, and worldwide estimates of preterm birth rates in the year 2010 with time trends since 1990 for selected countries: a systematic analysis and implications. Lancet, 2012. 379(9832): p. 2162–72.

[3] Ishiguro, A., et al., Changes in skin and subcutaneous perfusion in very-low-birth-weight infants during the transitional period. Neonatology, 2011. 100(2): p. 162–8.

[4] Stark, M.J., V.L. Clifton, and I.M. Wright, Microvascular flow, clinical illness severity and cardiovascular function in the preterm infant. Arch Dis Child Fetal Neonatal Ed, 2008. 93(4): p. F271–4.

[5] Ishiguro, A., et al., Peripheral blood flow monitoring in an infant with septic shock. Pediatr Int, 2014. 56(5): p. 787–9.

[6] Ishiguro, A., et al., Skin and subcutaneous blood flows of very low birth weight infants during the first 3 postnatal days. J Matern Fetal Neonatal Med, 2010. 23(6): p. 522–8.

[7] Ishiguro, A., et al., Skin blood flow as a predictor of intraventricular hemorrhage in very-low-birth-weight infants. Pediatr Res, 2014. 75(2): p. 322–7.

[8] Fagrell, B., Peripheral vascular diseases, in Laser Doppler blood flowmetry, A.P. Shepard, P.A. Oberg, and M.A. Norwell, Editors. New York 1990, Kluwer Academic.

[9] Perera, P., A.K. Kurban, and T.J. Ryan, The development of the cutaneous microvascular system in the newborn. Br J Dermatol, 1970. 82: p. 86–91.

[10] Beinder, E., et al., Control of skin blood flow in pre- and full-term infants. Biol Neonate, 1994. 65(1): p. 7–15.

[11] Eiby, Y.A., et al., Left ventricular output and aortic blood flow in response to changes in preload and afterload in the preterm piglet heart. Am J Physiol Regul Integr Comp Physiol, 2012. 303(7): p. R769–77.

[12] Kim, M.Y., et al., Effects of glucocorticoid exposure on growth and structural maturation of the heart of the preterm piglet. PLoS One, 2014. 9(3): p. e93407.

[13] Evans, N., et al., Which to measure, systemic or organ blood flow? Middle cerebral artery and superior vena cava flow in very preterm infants. Arch Dis Child Fetal Neonatal Ed, 2002. 87(3): p. F181–4.

[14] Evans, J.R., et al., Cardiovascular support in preterm infants. Clin Therap, 2006. 28(9): p. 1368-84.

[15] Suichies, H.E., et al., Skin blood flow changes, measured by laser Doppler flowmetry, in the first week after birth. Early Hum Dev, 1990. 23(1): p. 1–8.

[16] Yanowitz, T.D., et al., Postnatal hemodynamic changes in very-low-birthweight infants. J Appl Physiol (1985), 1999. 87(1): p. 370–80.

[17] Dyson, R.M., et al., Early microvascular changes in the preterm neonate: a comparative study of the human and guinea pig. Physiol Rep, 2014. 2(9) e12145.

[18] Schwepcke, A., et al., Microcirculatory mechanisms in postnatal hypotension affecting premature infants. Pediatr Res, 2013. 74(2): p. 186–90.

[19] Kent, A.L., I.M. Wright, and M.E. Abdel-Latif, Mortality and adverse neurologic outcomes are greater in preterm male infants. Pediatrics, 2012. 129(1): p. 124–31.

[20] Stark, M.J., V.L. Clifton, and I.M. Wright, Sex-specific differences in peripheral microvascular blood flow in preterm infants. Pediatr Res, 2008. 63(4): p. 415–9.

[21] Abdel-Latif, M.E., Z. Kecskes, and B. Bajuk, Actuarial day-by-day survival rates of preterm infants admitted to neonatal intensive care in New South Wales and the Australian Capital Territory. Arch Dis Child Fetal Neonatal Ed, 2011 98(3): p. F212–7.

[22] Rutter, N., The dermis. Semin Neonatol, 2000. 5(4): p. 297–302.

[23] Stark, M.J., et al., The influence of sex and antenatal betamethasone exposure on vasoconstrictors and the preterm microvasculature. J Matern Fetal Neonatal Med, 2011. 24(10): p. 1215–20.

[24] Balch-Samora, J., Factors regulating arteriolar tone during microvascular growth. 2007, Ann Arbor: ProQuest. p. 251.

[25] Berry, M., et al., Preterm birth has sex-specific effects on autonomic modulation of heart rate variability in adult sheep. PLoS One, 2013. 8(12): p. e85468.

[26] Stankevicius, E., et al., Role of nitric oxide and other endothelium-derived factors. Medicina (Kaunas), 2003. 39(4): p. 333–41.

[27] Lagercrantz, H., et al., Autonomic reflexes in preterm infants. Acta Paediatr Scand, 1990. 79(8–9): p. 721–8.

[28] Goldstein, D.S., G. Eisenhofer, and I.J. Kopin, Sources and significance of plasma levels of catechols and their metabolites in humans. J Pharmacol Exp Ther, 2003. 305(3): p. 800–11.

[29] Shulman, R.J., et al., Effects of age, feeding regimen, and glucocorticoids on catecholamine and cortisol excretion in preterm infants. JPEN J Parenter Enteral Nutr, 2001. 25(5): p. 254–9.

[30] Gao, Y. and J.U. Raj, Regulation of the pulmonary circulation in the fetus and newborn. Physiol Rev, 2010. 90(4): p. 1291–335.

[31] Soma, S., et al., Localization and distribution of endothelin receptor subtypes in pulmonary vasculature of normal and hypoxia-exposed rats. Am J Respir Cell Mol Biol, 1999. 20(4): p. 620–30.

[32] Perreault, T. and J. Baribeau, Characterization of endothelin receptors in newborn piglet lung. Am J Physiol, 1995. 268(4 Pt 1): p. L607–14.

[33] Yanagisawa, M., et al., A novel potent vasoconstrictor peptide produced by vascular endothelial cells. Nature, 1988. 332(6163): p. 411–5.

[34] Pinheiro, J.M. and A.B. Malik, Mechanisms of endothelin-1-induced pulmonary vasodilatation in neonatal pigs. J Physiol, 1993. 469: p. 739–52.

[35] Emmanouilides, G.C., et al., Pulmonary arterial pressure changes in human newborn infants from birth to 3 days of age. J Pediatr, 1964. 65: p. 327–33.

[36] Nisell, H., et al., Maternal and fetal levels of a novel polypeptide, endothelin: evidence for release during pregnancy and delivery. Gynecol Obstet Invest, 1990. 30(3): p. 129–32.

[37] Radunovic, N., et al., Fetal and maternal plasma endothelin levels during the second half of pregnancy. Am J Obstet Gynecol, 1995. 172(1 Pt 1): p. 28–32.

[38] Endo, A., et al., Nitric oxide and endothelin 1 during postnatal life. Biol Neonate, 1996. 70(1): p. 15–20.

[39] Elsmen, E., I. Hansen Pupp, and L. Hellstrom-Westas, Preterm male infants need more initial respiratory and circulatory support than female infants. Acta Paediatr, 2004. 93(4): p. 529–33.

[40] Belik, J., et al., Isoprostanes in fetal and neonatal health and disease. Free Radic Biol Med, 2010. 48(2): p. 177–88.

[41] Chen, J.X., et al., Isoprostanes as physiological mediators of transition to newborn life: novel mechanisms regulating patency of the term and preterm ductus arteriosus. Pediatr Res, 2012. 72(2): p. 122–8.

[42] Comporti, M., et al., Plasma F2-isoprostanes are elevated in newborns and inversely correlated to gestational age. Free Radic Biol Med, 2004. 37(5): p. 724–32.

[43] Qin, Y., et al., Determinants of umbilical cord arterial 8-iso-prostaglandin F2alpha concentrations. BJOG, 2000. 107(8): p. 973–81.

[44] Minghetti, L., et al., Early-life sex-dependent vulnerability to oxidative stress: the natural twining model. J Matern Fetal Neonatal Med, 2013. 26(3): p. 259–62.

[45] Stark, M.J., V.L. Clifton, and I.M. Wright, Carbon monoxide is a significant mediator of cardiovascular status following preterm birth. Pediatrics, 2009. 124(1): p. 277–84.

[46] Stoen, R., et al., Postnatal changes in mechanisms mediating acetylcholine-induced relaxation in piglet femoral arteries. Pediatr Res, 1997. 41(5): p. 702–7.

[47] Ellinsworth, D.C., et al., Endothelial control of vasodilation: integration of myoendothelial microdomain signalling and modulation by epoxyeicosatrienoic acids. Pflugers Arch, 2014. 466(3): p. 389–405.

[48] Sandow, S.L., Factors, fiction and endothelium-derived hyperpolarizing factor. Clin Exp Pharmacol Physiol, 2004. 31(9): p. 563–70.

[49] Moonen, R.M., et al., Plasma levels of dimethylarginines in preterm very low birth weight neonates: its relation with perinatal factors and short-term outcome. Int J Mol Sci, 2015. 16(1): p. 19–39.

[50] Martin, R.J., M.J. Mhanna, and M.A. Haxhiu, The role of endogenous and exogenous nitric oxide on airway function. Semin Perinatol, 2002. 26(6): p. 432–8.

[51] Nankervis, C.A., P.J. Giannone, and K.M. Reber, The neonatal intestinal vasculature: contributing factors to necrotizing enterocolitis. Semin Perinatol, 2008. 32(2): p. 83–91.

[52] Dani, C. and S. Pratesi, Nitric oxide for the treatment of preterm infants with respiratory distress syndrome. Expert Opin Pharmacother, 2013. 14(1): p. 97–103.

[53] El-Masry, H.M., et al., Nitric oxide and antioxidant enzyme levels in blood of respiratory distress syndrome – Egyptian preterms and their mothers. J Matern Fetal Neonatal Med, 2015. 28(1): p. 41–5.

[54] Armstead, W.M., et al., Different pial arteriolar responses to acetylcholine in the newborn and juvenile pig. J Cereb Blood Flow Metab, 1994. 14(6): p. 1088–95.

[55] Willis, A.P. and C.W. Leffler, Endothelial NO and prostanoid involvement in newborn and juvenile pig pial arteriolar vasomotor responses. Am J Physiol Heart Circ Physiol, 2001. 281(6): p. H2366–77.

[56] Willis, A.P. and C.W. Leffler, NO and prostanoids: age dependence of hypercapniaand histamine-induced dilations of pig pial arterioles. Am J Physiol, 1999. 277(1 Pt 2): p. H299–307.

[57] Zuckerman, S.L., et al., Age dependence of cerebrovascular response mechanisms in domestic pigs. Am J Physiol, 1996. 271(2 Pt 2): p. H535–40.

[58] Williams, J.M. and W.J. Pearce, Age-dependent modulation of endothelium-dependent vasodilatation by chronic hypoxia in ovine cranial arteries. J Appl Physiol (1985), 2006. 100(1): p. 225–32.

[59] Williams, J.M., A.D. Hull, and W.J. Pearce, Maturational modulation of endothelium-dependent vasodilatation in ovine cerebral arteries. Am J Physiol Regul Integr Comp Physiol, 2005. 288(1): p. R149–57.

[60] Hibler, S., H. Toga, and J.U. Raj, Differential role of endothelium-derived nitric oxide in the modulation of the systemic and pulmonary circulation in lambs. Biol Neonate, 1996. 69(2): p. 84–93.

[61] Krediet, T.G., et al., Nitric oxide production and plasma cyclic guanosine monophosphate in premature infants with respiratory distress syndrome. Biol Neonate, 2002. 82(3): p. 150–4.

[62] Li, L., A. Hsu, and P.K. Moore, Actions and interactions of nitric oxide, carbon monoxide and hydrogen sulphide in the cardiovascular system and in inflammation – a tale of three gases! Pharmacol Ther, 2009. 123(3): p. 386–400.

[63] Weindling, M. and F. Paize, Peripheral haemodynamics in newborns: best practice guidelines. Early Hum Dev, 2010. 86(3): p. 159–65.

[64] van Bel, F., et al., Plasma guanosine 3',5'-cyclic monophosphate and severity of peri/intraventricular haemorrhage in the preterm newborn. Acta Paediatr, 2002. 91(4): p. 434–9.

[65] Saugstad, O.D., Update on oxygen radical disease in neonatology. Curr Opin Obstet Gynecol, 2001. 13(2): p. 147–53.

[66] Chen, K. and A.S. Popel, Theoretical analysis of biochemical pathways of nitric oxide release from vascular endothelial cells. Free Radic Biol Med, 2006. 41(4): p. 668–80.

[67] Kavdia, M. and A.S. Popel, Contribution of nNOS- and eNOS-derived NO to microvascular smooth muscle NO exposure. J Appl Physiol, 2004. 97(1): p. 293–301.

[68] Wu, L. and R. Wang, Carbon monoxide: endogenous production, physiological functions, and pharmacological applications. Pharmacol Rev, 2005. 57(4): p. 585–630.

[69] Saukkonen, K., et al., Heme oxygenase 1 polymorphisms and plasma concentrations in critically ill patients. Shock, 2010. 34(6): p. 558–64.

[70] Mustafa, A.K., M.M. Gadalla, and S.H. Snyder, Signaling by gasotransmitters. Sci Signal, 2009. 2(68): p. re2.

[71] Leffler, C.W., et al., Carbon monoxide and cerebral microvascular tone in newborn pigs. Am J Physiol, 1999. 276(5 Pt 2): p. H1641–6.

[72] Naik, J.S., T.L. O'Donaughy, and B.R. Walker, Endogenous carbon monoxide is an endothelial-derived vasodilator factor in the mesenteric circulation. Am J Physiol Heart Circ Physiol, 2003. 284(3): p. H838–45.

[73] Cook, M.N., et al., Ontogeny of heme oxygenase activity in the hippocampus, frontal cerebral cortex, and cerebellum of the guinea pig. Brain Res Dev Brain Res, 1996. 92(1): p. 18–23.

[74] Sun, Y., M.O. Rotenberg, and M.D. Maines, Developmental expression of heme oxygenase isozymes in rat brain. Two HO-2 mRNAs are detected. J Biol Chem, 1990. 265(14): p. 8212–7.

[75] Coceani, F., et al., Carbon monoxide formation in the ductus arteriosus in the lamb: implications for the regulation of muscle tone. Br J Pharmacol, 1997. 120(4): p. 599–608.

[76] Wang, Y.F., et al., Role of gasotransmitters in the pathogenesis of pulmonary hypertension. Beijing Da Xue Xue Bao, 2006. 38(3): p. 326–30.

[77] Pearson, R.J., T. Wilson, and R. Wang, Endogenous hydrogen sulfide and the cardiovascular system-what's the smell all about? Clin Invest Med, 2006. 29(3): p. 146–50.

[78] Zoccali, C., C. Catalano, and S. Rastelli, Blood pressure control: hydrogen sulfide, a new gasotransmitter, takes stage. Nephrol Dial Transplant, 2009. 24(5): p. 1394–6.

[79] Wang, R., Two's company, three's a crowd: can H2S be the third endogenous gaseous transmitter? FASEB J, 2002. 16(13): p. 1792–8.

[80] Beltowski, J., Hydrogen sulfide as a biologically active mediator in the cardiovascular system. Postepy Hig Med Dosw (Online), 2004. 58: p. 285–91.

[81] Giles, T.D., et al., Impaired vasodilation in the pathogenesis of hypertension: focus on nitric oxide, endothelial-derived hyperpolarizing factors, and prostaglandins. J Clin Hypertens (Greenwich), 2012. 14(4): p. 198–205.

[82] Baragatti, B., et al., Hydrogen sulfide in the mouse ductus arteriosus: a naturally occurring relaxant with potential EDHF function. Am J Physiol Heart Circ Physiol, 2013. 304(7): p. H927–34.

[83] Ritter, J.M., Human pharmacology of hydrogen sulfide, putative gaseous mediator. Br J Clin Pharmacol, 2010. 69(6): p. 573–5.

[84] Golding, E.M., et al., Endothelium-derived hyperpolarizing factor in the brain: a new regulator of cerebral blood flow? Stroke, 2002. 33(3): p. 661–3.

[85] Quere, I., et al., Spatial and temporal expression of the cystathionine beta-synthase gene during early human development. Biochem Biophys Res Commun, 1999. 254(1): p. 127–37.

[86] Heinonen, K. and N.C. Raiha, Induction of cystathionase in human fetal liver. Biochem J, 1974. 144(3): p. 607–9.

[87] Levonen, A.L., et al., Human cystathionine gamma-lyase: developmental and in vitro expression of two isoforms. Biochem J, 2000. 347(Pt 1): p. 291–5.

[88] Leffler, C.W., et al., Hydrogen sulfide and cerebral microvascular tone in newborn pigs. Am J Physiol Heart Circ Physiol, 2011. 300(2): p. H440–7.

[89] Hongsprabhas, P., et al., Plasma homocysteine concentrations of preterm infants. Biol Neonate, 1999. 76(2): p. 65–71.

[90] Ishii, I., et al., Cystathionine gamma-Lyase-deficient mice require dietary cysteine to protect against acute lethal myopathy and oxidative injury. J Biol Chem, 2010. 285(34): p. 26358–68.

[91] Walter, J.H., N. Jahnke, and T. Remmington, Newborn screening for homocystinuria. Cochrane Database Syst Rev, 2013. 8: p. CD008840.

[92] Yang, G., et al., H_2S as a physiologic vasorelaxant: hypertension in mice with deletion of cystathionine gamma-lyase. Science, 2008. 322(5901): p. 587–90.

[93] Dyson, R.M., et al., A role for H2S in the microcirculation of newborns: the major metabolite of H2S (thiosulphate) is increased in preterm infants. PLoS One, 2014. 9(8): p. e105085.

[94] Dyson, R.M., et al., Interactions of the gasotransmitters contribute to microvascular tone (dys)regulation in the preterm neonate. PLoS One, 2015. 10(3): p. e0121621.

[95] Wen, Y.D., et al., Hydrogen sulfide protects HUVECs against hydrogen peroxide induced mitochondrial dysfunction and oxidative stress. PLoS One, 2013. 8(2): p. e53147.

[96] Bhatia, M., Role of hydrogen sulfide in the pathology of inflammation. Scientifica (Cairo), 2012. 2012: p. 159680.

[97] Saugstad, O.D., Oxidative stress in the newborn – a 30-year perspective. Biol Neonate, 2005. 88(3): p. 228–36.

[98] Stark, M.J., et al., The influence of sex and antenatal betamethasone exposure on vasoconstrictors and the preterm microvasculature. J Matern Fetal Neonatal Med, 2011. 24(10): p. 1215–20.

[99] Bhutani, V.K., Extrauterine adaptations in the newborn. Semin Neonatol. 1997 2(1): p. 1–12.

[100] Olson, K.R., et al., Hydrogen sulfide as an oxygen sensor/transducer in vertebrate hypoxic vasoconstriction and hypoxic vasodilation. J Exp Biol, 2006. 209(Pt 20): p. 4011–23.

[101] Kubo, S., et al., Direct inhibition of endothelial nitric oxide synthase by hydrogen sulfide: contribution to dual modulation of vascular tension. Toxicology, 2007. 232(1–2): p. 138–46.

[102] Nagpure, B.V. and J.S. Bian, Interaction of hydrogen sulfide with nitric oxide in the cardiovascular system. Oxid Med Cell Longev, 2016. 2016: p. 6904327.

[103] Knecht, K.R., et al., Time-dependent action of carbon monoxide on the newborn cerebrovascular circulation. Am J Physiol Heart Circ Physiol, 2010. 299: p. H70–5.

[104] Maroti, Z., et al., Heme oxygenase-1 expression in premature and mature neonates during the first week of life. Eur J Pediatr, 2007. 166(10): p. 1033–8.

[105] Zhao, W., et al., The vasorelaxant effect of H(2)S as a novel endogenous gaseous K(ATP) channel opener. EMBO J, 2001. 20(21): p. 6008–16.

[106] Szabo, C., Hydrogen sulphide and its therapeutic potential. Nat Rev Drug Discov, 2007. 6(11): p. 917–35.

[107] Wang, Y., et al., Role of hydrogen sulfide in the development of atherosclerotic lesions in apolipoprotein E knockout mice. Arterioscler Thromb Vasc Biol, 2009. 29(2): p. 173–9.

[108] Oh, G.S., et al., Hydrogen sulfide inhibits nitric oxide production and nuclear factor-kappaB via heme oxygenase-1 expression in RAW264.7 macrophages stimulated with lipopolysaccharide. Free Radic Biol Med, 2006. 41(1): p. 106–19.

[109] Qingyou, Z., et al., Impact of hydrogen sulfide on carbon monoxide/heme oxygenase pathway in the pathogenesis of hypoxic pulmonary hypertension. Biochem Biophys Res Commun, 2004. 317(1): p. 30–7.

[110] Taoka, S., et al., Evidence for heme-mediated redox regulation of human cystathionine beta-synthase activity. J Biol Chem, 1998. 273(39): p. 25179–84.

[111] Taoka, S. and R. Banerjee, Characterization of NO binding to human cystathionine beta-synthase: possible implications of the effects of CO and NO binding to the human enzyme. J Inorg Biochem, 2001. 87(4): p. 245–51.

[112] Dyson, R.M., et al., Cystathionine-γ-lyase: a potential target for treatment of microvascular dysregulation following preterm birth? (PS334). J Pediatr Child Health, 2014. 50(Suppl. S1): p. 40–64.

[113] Morikawa, T., et al., Hypoxic regulation of the cerebral microcirculation is mediated by a carbon monoxide-sensitive hydrogen sulfide pathway. Proc Natl Acad Sci U S A, 2012. 109(4): p. 1293–8.

[114] Jin, H.F., et al., Interaction between hydrogen sulfide/cystathionine gamma-lyase and carbon monoxide/heme oxygenase pathways in aortic smooth muscle cells. Acta Pharmacol Sin, 2006. 27(12): p. 1561–6.

[115] Peng, Y.J., et al., H2S mediates O2 sensing in the carotid body. Proc Natl Acad Sci U S A, 2010. 107(23): p. 10719–24.

[116] Baumgart, K., P. Radermacher, and F. Wagner, Applying gases for microcirculatory and cellular oxygenation in sepsis: effects of nitric oxide, carbon monoxide, and hydrogen sulfide. Curr Opin Anaesthesiol, 2009. 22(2): p. 168–76.

[117] Knuppel, R.A., et al., Oxidative stress and antioxidants: preterm birth and preterm infants, in preterm birth – mother and child, J.C. Morrison, Editor. 2012, InTech: Rijeka, Croatia.

[118] Kiely, D.G., et al., Nitric oxide: an important role in the maintenance of systemic and pulmonary vascular tone in man. Br J Clin Pharmacol, 1998. 46(3): p. 263–6.

[119] Stamler, J.S., et al., Nitric oxide regulates basal systemic and pulmonary vascular resistance in healthy humans. Circulation, 1994. 89(5): p. 2035–40.

[120] Knecht, K.R., et al., Time-dependent action of carbon monoxide on the newborn cerebrovascular circulation. Am J Physiol Heart Circ Physiol, 2010. 299(1): p. H70–5.

Chapter 5

The Metabolites of Arachidonic Acid in Microvascular Function

Ines Drenjančević, Ivana Jukić, Zrinka Mihaljević,
Anita Ćosić and Aleksandar Kibel

Additional information is available at the end of the chapter

http://dx.doi.org/10.5772/64676

Abstract

Arachidonic acid (AA) metabolites have an important role in mediating vascular reactivity to various stimuli, affecting tissue perfusion and tissue supply. In addition, they exert proinflammatory or anti-inflammatory effects on vessels. AA is metabolized by cyclooxygenases (COX) 1 and 2 to prostaglandins (PGs) and thromboxane (TX), by lipooxygenase to leukotrienes; by cytochrome P450 (CYP450)-hydroxylase to 20-hydroxyeicosatetraenoic acid (20-HETE) and by CYP450-epoxygenase to epoxyeicosatrienoic acids (EETs). Increased vascular oxidative stress may induce non-enzymatic production of isoprostanes from AA, which, together with vasoconstrictor metabolites of AA underlie endothelial damage and impaired vascular function. The balance among vasodilator and vasoconstrictor metabolites of AA may be disturbed in cardiometabolic diseases. (e.g. hypertension,obesity,diabetes) Dietary habits significantly affect the metabolism of AA, particularly excessive kitchen salt (NaCl) intake. Control of environmental risks factors, good maintenance of the occurring diseases and balanced nutrition with restricted salt intake can significantly improve the metabolism of AA and alleviate microvascular dysfunction and subsequent organ damage. Current research on pharmacological manipulation of certain components of the AA pathways (such as 20-HETE production inhibition or prolongation of the life of epoxyeicoatrienoic acids(EETs) by inhibitors of soluble epoxide hydrolaze (sEH)promises effective therapy of cardiovascular and cerebrovascular diseases in the future.

Keywords: microcirculation, endothelium, arachidonic acid metabolites, 20-HETE, EETs

1. Arachidonic acid metabolites and their receptors

The polyunsaturated omega-6 fatty acid 20:4(ω-6), arachidonic acid (AA), is a major component of cell membranes which is released from the cell membrane phospholipids primarily by phospholipase A_2 (PLA_2). Phospholipases can be activated by stimulation of vascular endothelial cells with various substances, such as acetylcholine (ACh) or shear stress [1]. AA can be metabolized by series of enzymes to numerous biological active metabolites termed "eicosanoids" or be transformed by reactive oxygen species (ROS) in nonenzymatic manner into isoprostanes [2]. The endothelium has a crucial role in maintenance of their circulatory homeostasis by producing and releasing different vasoactive substances, which regulate the tone of the underlying vascular smooth muscle.

Endothelial cells metabolize AA by three enzymatic pathways: cyclooxygenase (COX), lipoxygenase (LOX), or cytochrome P450 (CYP450) pathway, presented in **Figure 1**.

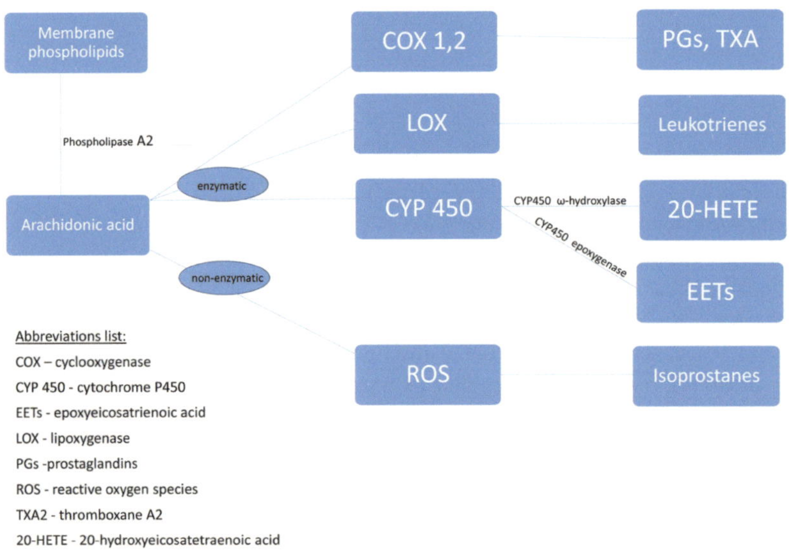

Figure 1. Metabolism of arachidonic acid. COX, cyclooxygenase; CYP 450, cytochrome P450; EETs, epoxyeicosatrienoic acid; LOX, lipoxygenase; PGs, prostaglandins; ROS, reactive oxygen species; TXA2, thromboxane A2; 20-HETE, 20-hydroxyeicosatetraenoic acid.

2. COX pathway

The released AA can be metabolized by COXs into prostanoids, which comprise prostaglandins (PGs) and thromboxanes (TXs). COXs convert AA into endoperoxides (PGH_2), the intermediate of the prostanoid biosynthesis, which can either act as an endothelium-derived contracting factor (EDCF) per se, or be further transformed into prostaglandin PGI_2 (prostacyclin) by prostacyclin synthase, or TXA_2 by thromboxane synthase. It could also be transformed to various other prostaglandins, including PGD_2, PGE_2, and $PGF_2\alpha$ [3]. There are two isoforms of COXs, COX-1 and COX-2, both expressed in physiological and pathological conditions, but their roles, levels of activation, and affinity to AA could be different [2, 4]. In most tissues, COX-1 is constitutively expressed and generates dilator prostaglandins, whereas COX-2 is believed to be primarily an inducible enzyme, activated by pro-inflammatory conditions [2–5]. Oxidative stress can also serve as an initiator of increased COX-2 activity [6].

Numerous studies emphasize the importance of COX-derived metabolites in vascular reactivity regulation: PGs and TXA_2 have a key role in vascular tone expression in both physiological and pathophysiological conditions [2, 7, 8]. The endothelium is the primary source of increased COX activity since endothelial cells contain up to 20 times more COX than vascular smooth muscle cells (VSMC) [9].

3. Prostaglandins and their receptors

Prostanoid receptors, based on their action and signal transduction, can be grouped into three categories: the contractile receptors, the dilatory receptors, and the inhibitory receptors. Prostaglandins and their receptors are presented in **Table 1** [10–13]. The contractile receptors (thromboxane-prostanoid, TP; prostaglandin F, FP; and prostaglandin E_1, EP_1 receptors) mediate Ca^{2+} mobilization and induce smooth muscle contraction. The relaxant receptors (prostacyclin receptor, IP; prostaglandin D_2, DP; prostaglandin E_2, EP_2; and prostaglandin E_4, EP_4) mediate increases in cAMP and induce smooth muscle relaxation. The EP_3 receptor is an inhibitory receptor that mediates decreases in cAMP and inhibits smooth muscle relaxation [14]. Vasodilatory PGs, including PGI_2, PGE_2, and PGD_2 have an important role in regulating renal function; they increase renal blood flow and glomerular filtration rate. PGE_2 is a key regulator of sodium reabsorption in the distal tubules [15]. Therefore, these COX-mediated factors are crucial in the pathogenesis of cardiovascular and kidney diseases.

Prostaglandin I_2 (PGI_2) binds to the prostacyclin receptors (IP) that are located on platelets and vascular smooth muscle cells and mediate inhibition of platelet aggregation and smooth muscle cells relaxation, thus reducing the risk of thrombosis [2, 16, 17]. PGI_2 may represent a compensatory mechanism of vasodilation when the production of nitric oxide (NO) is reduced [18].

The expression of IP receptors was observed by in situ hybridization in various mouse organs showing expression in brain (indicating that IP may be involved in the mediation of pain), in megakaryocytes and the smooth muscles of arteries (consistent with the action of PGI_2 in the cardiovascular system), in afferent arterioles of the glomerulus (indicating its role in regulation of the glomerular filtration rate), and in the thymus and spleen (expressed in mature thymocytes and splenic lymphocytes) [19]. Interaction of PGI_2 with IP receptor plays a central nociceptive role in inflammation. Mice lacking the IP receptor display altered pain perception as well as inflammatory response [20].

AA metabolite	Receptor	Location		Function in health and in the disease
TxA_2	TP-G protein coupled receptor	TPα	Lung, spleen, uterus, placenta, aorta, heart, intestine, liver, eye, thymus, kidney, spinal cord, brain	Thrombosis/hemostasis, modulation of the immune response—*acute myocardial infarction, inflammatory lung disease, hypertension, nephrotic disease*
		TPβ	Human endothelium	
PGD_2	DP_1 DP_2	Blood platelets, VSMC and nervous tissue, including the central nervous system, gastrointestinal SM, uterine SM		Inhibition of platelet aggregation, SM relaxation, possibly inhibition of autonomic neurotransmitter release
PGE_2	EP_1	Human myometrium, kidney, lung		Contraction and relaxation of SM, inhibition and enhancement of neurotransmitter release, inhibition of lipolysis, gastric acid secretion, inflammatory mediator release, Ig expression, immunoregulation, inhibition, and enhancement of nonacid (water) secretion—*inflammation, allergy, parturition, and tumorigenesis (colon cancer), endometriosis*
	EP_2	SM, ileum, thymus, lung, spleen, heart, and uterus		
	EP_3	SM of gastrointestinal, uterine, and vascular origin, gastric mucosa kidney, thymus, spleen, lung, and brain		
	EP_4	SM, endothelium, endometrium		
$PGF_{2\alpha}$	PGF (FP)-G protein coupled receptor—the F prostanoid receptor	FPA FPB	Ovary, myometrium, ocular vasculature, iris sphincter, ocular circular muscles Renal distal convoluted tubule, cortical collecting duct, juxtaglomerular apparatus	Luteolysis, parturition, uterine contraction, aqueous humor homeostasis, water, and electrolyte reabsorption Renin secretion, blood pressure regulation—*pregnancy-induced hypertension, pulmonary and myocardial fibrosis, arrhythmias, myocyte hypertrophy, VSMC hypertrophy, vasoconstriction, atherosclerosis*

AA metabolite	Receptor	Location		Function in health and in the disease
			Lung and cardiac fibroblasts; cardiomyocyte, VSMC	
PGI_2	IP	IP_1 IP_2	Blood platelets, VSMC, sensory afferent nerves, thymus (medulla), spleen, heart/aorta, lung	Local control of vascular tone, platelet aggregation—*hypertension*

TXA2, thromboxane A2; TP, thromboxane receptor; PGD2, prostaglandin D2; DP, prostaglandin D2 receptor; PGE_2, prostaglandin E_2; EP, prostaglandin E_2 receptor; $PGF_{2\alpha}$, prostaglandin F_2alpha; FP, prostaglandin F receptor; PGI_2, prostacyclin; IP, prostacyclin receptor.

Table 1. Eicosanoids and their receptors.

The distribution of EP_1 receptors is restricted to kidney, lung, and stomach. In kidney, they are mainly expressed in collecting duct and can be detected in glomerular mesangial cells, podocytes, and proximal tubule cells. The relationship between EP receptor and blood pressure (BP), indicated by Stock et al. [21] in EP_1 null mice, results from the observed increased concentrations of renin and aldosterone, ongoing activation of the renin-angiotensin system (RAS) and disrupted response to angiotensin II [22].

The EP_2 receptors can be found in vascular and interstitial compartments of the kidney and they are the least abundant among the EP receptors but effectively activate in response to stimuli. PGE_2 evokes contractile and/or relaxant responses of vascular smooth muscles in vitro. Lack of EP_2 receptor and dysfunction of PGE_2 pathway may be involved in elicitation of the salt-sensitive hypertension in EPP/2 mice (mice lacking EP2 receptor). Their results indicate that PGE_2, produced in the body in response to a high-salt (HS) diet, evoked considerable hypertension. It is proposed that the absence of the EP_2 receptor abolishes the ability of the mouse vasculature to vasodilate in response to PGE_2 and unmasks the contractile response via the vasoconstrictor EP receptor(s). EP_2 receptors and EP_4 can also be found in endometrium. The amount and localization of these receptors change during pregnancy, which may correspond to changes in uterine contraction during fertilization and implantation [14].

EP_3 receptors are expressed in smooth muscle layer and kidney. Renal EP_3 is mostly recognized for its pressor effects and its diuretic role opposing vasopressin. It is highly expressed in the distal nephron (mostly in the cortical and medullary collecting duct) [23].

DP is the least expressed receptor found in very low levels in small intestine and brain in humans [24] and moderately expressed in the ileum, lung, stomach, brain, and uterus [25] in mice. FP receptors are mainly expressed in corpus luteum and found to be variable during the estrous cycle indicating a close relationship between FP gene expression and luteolysis. PGF2α is a physiological inducer of luteolysis in pregnancy. Independent of estrous cycle, expression of mouse FP mRNA was found in the kidney, heart, lung, and stomach [26, 27].

Thromboxane A_2 (TXA_2) is a potent vasoconstrictor and a pro-aggregatory substance. The balance between PGI_2 and TXA_2 in the circulation is important for cardiovascular homeostasis [17]. TXA_2 binds to the thromboxane-prostanoid (TP) receptors which are located on platelets and their activation causes platelet aggregation, while in vascular smooth muscle cells, TXA_2 causes vasoconstriction and smooth muscle cells proliferation [4, 5].TP receptors appear to be solely responsible for endothelium-dependent contractions. Endoperoxides (PGH_2) and higher concentrations of prostacyclin (in vascular smooth muscle lacking IP receptor sensitivity) and isoprostanes activate this receptor with a varying range of potency. Role of TP receptors in hypertensive process was shown by Tian et al. on renovascular hypertensive (RVH) rats. They showed that TP receptor hyperresponsiveness to vasoconstrictors and IP receptor insensitivity leads to endothelial dysfunction [6].

4. LOX pathway

The LOX pathways (5, 12, and 15-LOX) of AA metabolism generates eicosanoids (hydroxyeicosatetraenoic acids, HETEs: 12 (S)-HETE, 12 (R)-HETE, and 15 (S)-HETE), lipoxins (LXs), and leukotrienes (LTA_4, LTB_4, LTC_4, LTD_4, and LTE_4) [28]. All of these metabolites have crucial role in pulmonary responses to asthma, inflammation, and atherosclerosis [29–31]. 5-LOX products have been found to be harmful factors in pathological conditions, including cardiovascular and renal diseases [32]. Leukotrienes produced by 12-LOX and 15-LOX cause dilatation, while the 5-LOX generated leukotrienes (LTs), the major LO metabolites associated with vasoconstriction, increased pro-inflammatory cytokines production and also behave as chemotaxins in the blood vessels by recruiting inflammatory cells. LTs are established mediators of pulmonary inflammation and in allergic and pseudoallergic reactions [33] also known as slow-reacting substances of anaphylaxy (SRS-A) which can be produced in basophils and mast cells. Research over the past two decades has established that LTs modulate inflammation in pulmonary arterial hypertension (PAH) [34]. Since LOX pathway does not have much influence on the peripheral vascular function, and pulmonary circulation and pulmonary hypertension are not in the focus of this chapter, the further effects of LOX pathway of AA metabolism will not be discussed here. For comprehensive reading, one may explore many interesting papers, including [35–37].

5. CYP450 pathway

In addition to COX and LOX, CYP450 enzymes (with their numerous isoforms) represent a crucial path in AA metabolism, catalyzing epoxidation reactions (producing EETs) and omega (ω)-hydroxylation reactions (producing 20-HETE) [38]. Two distinct enzymes: CYP-hydroxylase enzymes (CYP4A and CYP4F) generate HETEs (16-, 17-, 18-, 19-, and 20-HETE) while CYP-epoxygenase enzymes generate EETs (5,6-, 8,9-, 11,12-, and 14,15-EET). The CYP epoxygenases, members of CYP2C (predominant in mammals) and CYP2J classes of enzymatic proteins, are primarily located in endoplasmic reticulum of endothelial cells. They convert AA to EETs by adding an epoxide across one of the four double bonds in AA and produce the four mentioned EET regioisomers. CYP epoxygenases demonstrate a very high sequence homology among different species (e.g. human CYP2C8, rat CYP2C23 and mouse CYP2c44) [39–41]. Beside CYP2C8, human arteries and arterioles express CYP2C9, CYP2J2, and soluble epoxide hydrolases (sEH) enzymes [42, 43]. sEH converts EETs to their corresponding diols, dihydroxyeicosatrienoic acids (DHETs), which represent the main EET catabolic pathway. EETs produced by the endothelium hyperpolarize vascular smooth muscle cells VSMCs by opening Ca^{2+}-activated K^+ (K_{Ca}) channels leading to vasodilatation. In contrary, 20-HETE is found to be a vasoconstrictor that inhibits the opening of K_{Ca}.

Key vascular effects of CYP epoxygenase-derived EETs, besides regulating vascular tone and angiogenesis, include autocrine anti-inflammatory actions, limitation of leukocyte adhesion and reducing VSMCs proliferation. They have been found to exhibit protective effects in myocardial and cerebral ischemia and in hypertension-induced renal damage [44].

EETs are also able to modulate vascular responses to other stimuli, such as hormonal and paracrine agents. For instance, vasopressin-induced increase in cytosolic Ca^{2+} in renal mesangial cells is amplified by EETs and reduced when EETs synthesis is inhibited [45]. The responses of afferent arterioles to angiotensin II, endothelin-1, and noradrenaline increase when EETs synthesis is inhibited [45]. In transgenic rats with angiotensin II-dependent hypertension, EETs were shown to be antihypertensive and cardioprotective [46]. Inhibition of EETs synthesis reduces glutamate-induced increase in cerebral blood flow response [47]. Streptozocin-induced diabetes in rats (a model for type 1 diabetes mellitus, DM) reduces the levels of protective EETs, and reduced EETs levels lead to exacerbation of stroke [48]. A similar protective role of EETs was demonstrated in diabetic nephropathy [49], atherosclerosis [50], and cardiac ischemic reperfusion injury in diabetic rats [51]. Reduced CYP activity and EETs production caused by high glucose (through elevated superoxide levels) in coronary endothelial cells has also been implicated in impaired endothelium-dependent vasodilation of coronary arterioles [52]. EETs might constitute a key link between insulin resistance and endothelial dysfunction [53]. Upregulation of the CYP2J group of isoforms in mice (which catalyze EETs formation) leads to attenuation of diabetic nephropathy induced by streptozocin [54].

Both EETs and HETE exert numerous biological signaling effects, including important roles in the vasculature, vessel diameter regulation, and tissue perfusion. EETs function as endothelium-derived hyperpolarizing factor and show mostly vasodilator properties, with their vasodilator effects comparable to that of ACh [46], but some EET subtypes can also mediate vasoconstriction—for example, in kidneys where they can cause constriction of the afferent arterioles [46, 55]. 20-HETE is a potent vasoconstrictor and plays an essential role in the myogenic and tubuloglomerular feedback responses in the afferent arteriole, participating in blood pressure control [56].

Many evidences suggest that alteration in EET pathway contributes to the pathophysiology of hypertension, including BP elevation, endothelial dysfunction, and end-organ damage [44]. Also, EETs have anti-inflammatory and angiogenic function [32]. Imbalance of vasoactive eicosanoids leads to ischemia, thrombosis, coagulopathy, myocardial infarction, and stroke as discussed further in the chapter.

6. Nonenzymatic metabolism of AA

ROS are produced in all layers of the vascular wall by all vascular cell types (endothelium, smooth muscle, and adventitial cells) and by perivascular adipocytes. ROS generated by endothelial cells are superoxide ($O_2\cdot$), hydrogen peroxide (H_2O_2), hydroxyl radicals (HO), and others. Potential sources of endothelial ROS generation include mitochondria, xanthine oxidase (XO), uncoupled NO synthases (NOS), lipoxygenases, cytochrome P450 enzymes, and nicotinamide adenine dinucleotide phosphate (NAD(P)H) oxidases [57]. ROS are formed on sites of inflammation and injury; at low concentrations, ROS can act as a signaling molecule involved in the regulation of fundamental cellular activities such as cell growth and cell adjustments and regulation of endothelial function, while at higher concentrations, ROS can cause cell injury and death. Increased concentration of ROS is associated with changes in endothelial signal transmission and redox-regulated transcription factors in inflammation which may be related to endothelial dysfunction and activation of pathological mechanisms [58]; for example, the development of hypertension. This includes promoting the growth of VSMCs, increased contractility and invasion of monocytes and inflammation, increased permeability of vascular endothelium and enhanced adhesion of leukocytes [58].

ROS can induce peroxidation of AA, which gives rise to the isoprostanes. Several scavenger systems are counteracting the ROS, including enzymes such as superoxide dismutase (SOD), catalase (CAT) and glutathione peroxidase (GPx), and nonenzymatic antioxidants such as vitamin E, vitamin C, β-carotene, and heme-binding proteins, and major of them is SOD [59].

ROS can directly act as endothelium-derived contracting factor (EDCF) [60] or indirectly potentiate EDCF-mediated responses by reducing the bioavailability of NO [61] and activating COX in the VSMCs [3]. Their overproduction leads to increased oxidative stress and development of endothelial dysfunction [62]. Thus, endothelial dysfunction impairs vascular function in various diseases, cardiovascular and endocrine-metabolic disorders. Oxidative stress is characterized by reduced bioavailability of NO and enhanced production of ROS [63] which can exhibit both activating and inhibitory effects on the eicosanoid metabolism, and PGI_2 synthesis is more sensitive then TX and LOX pathways. In blood vessel, production of PGI_2 is selectively inhibited by ROS, whereas TXA_2 synthase is unaffected [64]. ROS can modify vascular tone directly by acting as EDCF or indirectly by reducing the bioavailability of NO which potentiate EDCF-mediated responses.

Urinary isoprostane levels are used as biomarkers of oxidative stress in ischemic-reperfusion injury, atherosclerosis, and hepatic disease. An accumulated body of evidence suggests that there is a cross-talk between 20-HETE and ROS production in response to flow- and pressure-induced stimuli in human and experimental animal microcirculation [65, 66]. Novel data show an association between increased CYP4A activity and oxidative stress in human subjects with hypertension. Increased urinary 20-HETE excretion correlated positively with markers of

http://dx.doi.org/10.5772/64676

oxidative stress and with elevated BP [67]. Similarly, patients recovering from acute ischemic stroke have increased plasma 20-HETE concentrations and elevated plasma oxidative stress markers compared to healthy controls [68].

7. Endothelial dysfunction and metabolites of arachidonic acid

Eicosanoids play an important role in maintenance of vascular reactivity under physiological conditions, but they become deleterious to endothelial function and BP regulation in some conditions with imbalance in the PGI_2/TXA_2 system, in chronic activation of CYP4A and enhanced production of 20-HETE or lack of EETs, as well as in high oxidative stress conditions. At the beginning of the endothelial dysfunction development, there is a compensatory endothelial mechanism of prostacyclin and/or endothelium-derived hyperpolarizing factor (EDHF), which maintains vascular function (**Figure 2**).

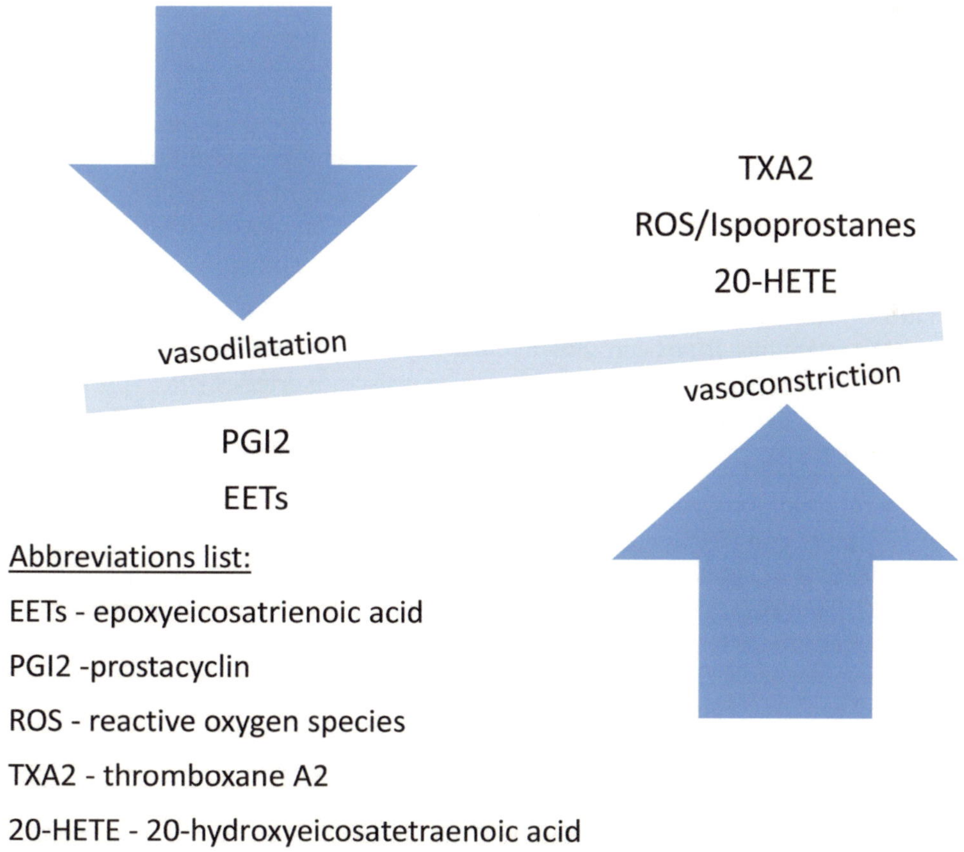

Figure 2. The role of AA metabolites' disbalance in endothelial dysfunction. EETs, epoxyeicosatrienoic acid; PGI2, prostacyclin; ROS, reactive oxygen species; TXA2, thromboxane A2; 20-HETE, 20-hydroxyeicosatetraenoic acid.

Except reduced NO bioavailability and increased ROS production, in some pathological conditions such as hypertension, diabetes, and obesity, there is an overproduction of COX-2-derived prostanoids. Endothelial dysfunction is a hallmark of most cardiovascular and endocrine/metabolic diseases.

8. Obesity

Obesity is associated with microvascular endothelial dysfunction in experimental animal models as well as in obese humans [69, 70]. Human studies have shown that endothelial function of visceral adipose tissue vessels is more damaged compared to subcutaneous adipose tissue vessels [70, 71], and that visceral microenvironment is intrinsically more toxic to the vasculature. Also, COX-derived vasoconstrictors partly contribute to endothelial dysfunction [71, 72]. There is a large body of evidence that endothelial dysfunction precedes and predicts clinical disease [73, 74], suggesting that endothelial dysfunction and impaired vascular reactivity is an initial step in the development of cardiovascular complications caused by obesity. Therefore, endothelial dysfunction in adipose tissue may be a strong prognostic factor for future cardiovascular events [75].

In obesity, chronic exposure of endothelial cells to high levels of circulating fatty acids increases the formation of ROS, which further leads to a disbalance between vasodilation and vasoconstriction leading to net vasoconstriction. Vascular production of PGs can be also altered in obesity because endothelial production of the superoxide anion contributes to enhanced COX expression [76].

Vasodilation in response to flow is reduced in visceral compared to subcutaneous arterioles, and the COX metabolites have been shown to participate in the mechanisms of endothelium-dependent dilation in subcutaneous adipose tissue resistance arteries [70, 71]. Furthermore, ROS (mainly H_2O_2) participate in that response, while the metabolites of the CYP450 partially contribute to dilation of microvessels from both subcutaneous and visceral adipose tissues [70].

In pathological conditions, such as cardiovascular disease and obesity, NO bioavailability is reduced and other endothelium-derived dilator substances compensate for the lack of NO release during flow or agonist activation [70, 77]. The inhibition of NOS augments the contribution of CYP450 metabolites to vasodilation [78], suggesting that EDHF may function as a compensatory mechanism when NO synthesis is impaired in obesity. It is also possible that CYP450 metabolites and COX enzymes are sources of ROS [79], whose production is enhanced in obesity and cardiovascular disease [70, 77].

Taken together, data suggest that endothelium-derived dilator substances other than NO (i.e. H_2O_2 and metabolites of CYP450) may contribute to vasodilation in obesity [70]. Previous studies in the coronary circulation have shown that the P450 component to dilation is present during coronary disease when NO levels are reduced [80]. Therefore, it is possible that the P450 component to dilation in adipose tissue is conserved during disease in the presence and the absence of NO-dependent vasodilation.

9. Arachidonic acid metabolites and hypertension

High BP represents a major risk factor for coronary artery disease, stroke, heart failure, peripheral vascular disease, vision loss, and chronic kidney disease [81, 82]. Reduced releasing of NO and enhanced production of EDCF increase contraction and lead to vascular diseases such as hypertension [83]. Chronically increased arterial BP presumably can cause premature aging of the intima, arterial remodeling, and smooth muscle cells dysfunction. Proper functioning of the endothelium and delayed appearance of vascular complications caused by hypertensive process can be managed by increasing the availability of NO, favoring the EDHF-mediated responses, and preventing the release or action of EDCFs.

Ever since the 1990s when the COX-pathway-independent EDHFs were discovered, substantial number of studies demonstrated CYP450 metabolites of AA to be that other source and these newly discovered EDHFs (EETs and HETEs) were proven to have influence in pathophysiology of many diseases including hypertension. Production of vasoconstrictor cyclooxygenase products, especially ROS, contributes to the development of endothelial dysfunction in hypertension [84, 85]. Until today, wide array of techniques and different types of blood vessels have been comprehensively investigated to discover EET-mediated VSMC signaling mechanisms. Prevailing conclusion of these studies is that EETs activate K^+ channels in vascular smooth muscle cell and in particular the large-conductance K_{Ca} channels causing cell membrane hyperpolarization [86–88]. Another consistent finding has been increase in cAMP in response to EETs, and this signaling pathway has been associated with vasodilation [86–88]. To achieve vasorelaxations, EETs and other EDHFs also require a guanine nucleotide binding protein (protein G) [89, 90]. Capdevila and Falck showed in their study that the EDHF-mediated response (therefore EETs) becomes evident only in the state of reduced NO bioavailability meaning that physiological concentration of NO is adequate to moderate EDHF generation and, under physiological conditions, endothelium-dependent vasodilatation seems to be mainly dependent on NO production [91]. EETs are also contributing to shear stress-dependent hyperpolarization and dilation of skeletal muscle arterioles in mice [92–94]. eNOS-deficient mice have had intact vasorelaxation to shear stress and a reduced vasodilation to ACh also suggesting that EETs can possibly enlarge their contribution to attenuate vascular resistance when NO levels are reduced demonstrating inhibitory interaction between NO and EETs [95]. Another study on essential hypertensive patients showed also connection between impaired NO availability and alternative mechanism of endothelium-dependent vasodilatation, related mainly to compensatory CYP2C9-derived EDHF [96]. Experimental findings in humans have also determined that NO and CYP epoxygenases regulate arterial stiffness in response to flow variations [97]. Early observation on the possible contribution of EETs to BP control and hypertension came from studies on rats treated with an epoxygenase enzyme inhibitor who became hypertensive when fed high salt [98–100]. Study in transgenic mice which expressed human CYP2J2 and CYP2C8 epoxygenases in endothelium and increased endothelial EET biosynthesis has proved that endothelial CYP epoxygenases regulate BP [101]. In fact, these mice exhibit enhanced afferent arteriolar dilation, lower BP, and attenuated hypertension-induced renal injury compared to wild type [101]. These findings suggest the potential therapeutic utility of antihypertensive strategies that may increase CYP-derived

EETs. Recently, a protective role of CYP2J2-derived EETs was found in heart failure [102], suggesting that CYP2J2-derived EETs may be a target for the development of drugs to prevent cardiac hypertrophy and cardiomyocyte apoptosis in heart failure [44]. Sinal et al. showed that mice lacking the sEH gene (epoxide hydrolase 2, Ephx2-/-) have significantly higher circulating EET levels and lower BP compared to wild-type mice. Renal production of DHETs was decreased and EET formation increased in the Ephx2-/-mice, also suggesting an important role for epoxygenase metabolism in the regulation of BP [103]. In addition, the administration of a sEH inhibitor (sEHI) significantly lowers BP in various rodent models of hypertension [103, 104]. The administration of a single dose of an sEHI (*N*,*N*-dicyclohexylurea, DCU) to ANG II-infused rats greatly increased the level of EETs, decreased the urinary DHET excretion, and lowered systolic BP, thus reversing the hypertensive phenotype typical of the spontaneously hypertensive rats (SHR) [105, 106]. However, adverse events may occur in the pulmonary vasculature. EETs, generated in VSMCs of pulmonary blood vessels, increase intracellular Ca^{2+}, thus inducing vasoconstriction and increasing pulmonary artery pressure [107].

10. Role of 20-HETE in hypertension

20-HETE is a CYP450–derived omega-hydroxylation metabolite of arachidonic acid and plays a complex role in blood pressure regulation. 20-HETE biosynthesis is primarily localized to the VSMCs [108], with the exception of endothelium in the pulmonary circulation which may also produce 20-HETE [109]. In physiological conditions, NO, carbon monoxide (CO) and superoxide inhibit the formation of 20-HETE by binding to the heme binding site of the CYP450 pathway enzymes. A role of 20-HETE in NO homeostasis was first suggested by Frisbee et al [110]. They showed that 20-HETE decreases the effect of ACh-induced relaxation in cremasteric arterioles. Studies using endothelial cells demonstrated that 20-HETE stimulates superoxide production by mechanisms that include eNOS uncoupling and activation of NAD(P)H oxidase-dependent and -independent pathways [110–113]. The rate of 20-HETE biosynthesis is inversely proportional to the blood vessel diameter [114]. 20-HETE is not detected in large conduit vessels [115].Therefore, it is largely believed that 20-HETE is an eicosanoid of the microcirculation [116]. In the microvasculature, 20-HETE has been shown to play a pressor role by sensitizing VSMCs to constrictor stimuli and increasing myogenic tone and by acting on the endothelium to further promote endothelial dysfunction and endothelial activation [116].While the formation of 20-HETE in VSMC is stimulated by angiotensin II and endothelin and is inhibited by NO CO, inhibition of 20-HETE synthesis attenuates the vascular responses to angiotensin II, endothelin, noradrenaline, NO, and CO [115]. Other autacoids can also stimulate 20-HETE production, for example, serotonin (5-hydroxytryptamine, 5-HT], and other growth factors [117, 118]. Liu et al. showed that inhibitors of COX-2 increase the levels of 20-HETE [119]. The report by Sacerdoti et al. [120] was the first to implicate 20-HETE in the pathogenesis of hypertension showing that depletion of renal CYP450 normalizes BP in SHR rats. ANG II-mediated hypertension in rats can be decreased by 40% by inhibition of 20-HETE synthesis [116]. Contribution of 20-HETE to blood pressure regulation include diet-, age-, and sex-specific alterations in the expression of CYP enzymes that produce 20-HETE [121]. In pregnancy-induced hypertensive women, the urinary excretion of DHETs is increased compared to healthy pregnant women, which may implicate an increased degradation of EETs [122].

On the contrary, 20-HETE is contributing to antihypertensive mechanisms too; it is involved in the regulation of the pressure-natriuretic response by inhibitory acting on sodium reabsorption and promoting natriuresis in the kidney tubules [123]. HET0016, which is cytochrome P450 ω-hydroxylase inhibitor, attenuates cerebrovascular inflammation, attenuates oxidative stress, and improves vasomotor function in spontaneously hypertensive rats [124].

RAS is the crucial in regulation of body fluid volume and blood pressure [125]. ANG II increases blood pressure by (1) vasoconstriction via AT1R activation, increased sympathetic tone, and the release of arginine-vasopressin and (2) modulation of renal sodium and water reabsorption by stimulating renal AT1R, the production and release of aldosterone, or the sensation of thirst in the central nervous system [116].

ANG II stimulates 20-HETE synthesis in renal microvessels and decreases EET levels by downregulating epoxygenases and increasing their degradation by increasing expression and activity of sEH [117, 126, 127]. In conditions, such as renovascular disease (RVD), there is an increase in the expression of the renin-angiotensin system, associated with enhanced lipid peroxidation related to activation of the renin-angiotensin system [125], elevated levels of ANG II, which parallels an increase in plasma 20-HETE and a decrease in EET plasma levels that supports a pivotal role of EETs in vascular homeostasis [125]. RVD is a relatively rare form of secondary hypertension [128, 129]. The interactions between 20-HETE and the RAS occur at several levels. Increased production of 20-HETE in the peripheral vasculature contributes to the acute vasoconstrictor response to ANG II, whereas acute and chronic inhibition of 20-HETE synthesis attenuates the renal pressor response to ANG II and the development of ANG II-dependent hypertension [116], respectively. The infusion of angiotensin II (ANG II), a potent vessel constrictor, elevates blood pressure in various animal models [106].

In RVD, plasma 20-HETE significantly correlated with plasma renin activity, thus suggesting its role in the elevation of blood pressure through the possible increase of vasomotion and vascular reactivity [130]. All of presented studies suggest that there is a communication network among various eicosanoids. In physiological conditions, eicosanoids are important in the maintenance of vascular tone and reactivity, but in chronic activation of CYP4A/20HETE system or lack of EETs and high oxidative stress, they become deleterious to endothelial function and blood pressure regulation.

11. Arachidonic acid metabolites and high-salt diet

It is well known that increased NaCl intake is an important risk factor for development and progression of hypertension [131, 132], while a reduction in dietary sodium is associated with lowering of BP in many patients with essential hypertension [133]. Furthermore, some studies on normotensive animal models have shown that changes in NaCl intake determined vascular responses to various physiological stimuli, in conduit vessels and resistance arteries, as well as in the microcirculation [134–136].

In contrast to studies which demonstrated deleterious effects of high levels of ANG II and RAS activation on the BP levels [125], there are studies demonstrating that decrease in ANG II circulating levels leads to impaired microvascular endothelial function. This has been recently extensively reported in the paper by Boegehold et al. [137]. One of the most deleterious effects of HS intake is impaired endothelial function [132], and it is crucial to evaluate the altered vascular function in microcirculation because it is a target of the pathological events. In animal models, even a short-term HS diet impairs vascular function by altering the responses to both vasoconstrictor and vasodilator stimuli in different vascular beds [134–136], that is associated with overproduction of vasoconstrictor factors, TXA_2, and PGF2α [134, 136].

In their study, Cavka et al. have shown that one week of HS diet increased plasma levels of potent vasoconstrictor, TXB_2, and that the nonselective COX antagonist indomethacin restored blood flow, whereas the selective COX-2 inhibitor did not cause any change in the impaired hyperemic blood flow in healthy young women [138]. Further, both inhibitors reduce plasma TXA_2 levels, suggesting that some other vasoconstrictor dominantly derived by COX-1 may play important role in impaired microvascular reactivity in subjects on the HS diet. Short-term exposure to a HS diet alter AA metabolism, and COX enzymes (mainly COX-1) play an important role in the development of microvascular endothelial dysfunction [138].

As already mentioned, in vascular pathogenesis, there may be a disbalance where COX-derived constrictors become dominant over the prostacyclin which is usually responsible for vasodilatation under physiological conditions [3, 139]. In endothelial dysfunction, endothelial cells became a source of COX-derived constrictors and enhanced oxidative stress may modify COX-dependent function leading to damaged vascular tone [9] due to decreased NO bioavailability and an increased formation of EDCFs [140]. In animal models, COX-1 metabolites are responsible for endothelium-dependent contractions, but with aging or disease, COX-2 can be induced contributing to EDCF-mediated responses [140, 141].

HS-induced endothelial dysfunction is caused by decreased plasma concentration of ANG II which leads to increased oxidative stress [139, 142, 143], as demonstrated in SS.BN13 consomic rats studies [139], leading to impaired relaxation of middle cerebral artery (MCA) in response to hypoxia and ACh due to decrease in vascular antioxidative capacity [144]. Importance of ANG II is further supported by intravenous infusion of suppressor dose of ANG II during HS diet which restores normal vascular relaxation and restores ROS concentration to normal values [145].

Antioxidative systems are very important in the maintenance of cellular redox homeostasis and prevent excessive accumulation of $O_2^{-}\cdot$ and its reactive metabolites [146]. Reduced activity of antioxidant mechanism, alone or in combination, with increased O_2^{-} production, may contribute to increased vascular $O_2^{-}\cdot$ level associated with a high intake of salt [144]. Several ubiquitous primary antioxidant enzymes such as SOD, catalase, and peroxidase catalyze the conversion of ROS in more stable molecules such as O_2 and water. Until now, research of the influence of high salt intake was based exclusively on changes in the level of SOD isoforms.

Lenda et al. presumed that HS diet decreased the protein expression or activity of the antioxidant enzymes (SOD isoforms) leading to increase oxidative stress, and consequently, reduced dilatation of blood vessels [143, 147]. However, this effect is not uniform at each vascular bed; for example, HS intake has no effect on the expression of CuZn SOD or MnSOD in mesenteric arteries [146] or the expression of CuZn SOD in the arteries of skeletal muscle [141]. Studies on Ren1-BN congenic rats showed that a short-term increase in dietary salt intake reduces the expression of the Cu/Zn SOD and Mn SOD in the cerebral vasculature and that ANG II infusion prevents the reduction of Cu/Zn SOD expression, but not Mn SOD expression, in HS-fed animals [143]. Recent studies showed that, except for reduced protein levels of SOD isoforms, HS intake also significantly reduced the level of mRNA expression of glutathione peroxidase 4 GPx4, very important enzyme in maintaining reduced levels of lipid peroxidation and oxidative stress [142]. Treatment with TEMPOL [136, 148] (which is a SOD mimetic) returns the NO level to the concentrations similar to the ones in the animals on a normal salt diet which indicates that the $O2^{-}\cdot$ is responsible for the oxidation of NO under these conditions. HS diet promotes increased generation of superoxide anion from NOS in spinotrapezius muscle arterioles of C57BL/6J mice, thus impairing endothelium-dependent dilation through reduced NO bioavailability [149].

There are several possible sources of $O_2^{-}\cdot$ in the vascular wall such as mitochondrial respiratory chain, NAD(P)H xanthine oxidase, COX, CYP-450 enzyme, and the NOS [150]. When the bioavailability of NO is greatly reduced, as is the case during HS diet, endothelium activates various compensatory physiological pathways. Impaired endothelium-dependent vasodilation is maintained partially by the production and release of other endothelial vasodilator other than NO, such as prostanoids (prostacyclin) and other endothelium hyperpolarizing factors (EDHFs). In endothelial dysfunction, besides ROS, other harmful metabolites of the arterial wall are formed, that is, TXA_2 and PGH_2 [151]. Endothelial dysfunction is related to pathogenesis of thrombosis and atherosclerosis [151, 152]. mRNA expression of COXs (COX-1 and COX-2) showed a significant reduction of both isoforms in the brain blood vessels after a week of HS intake [153]. New functional studies demonstrated that the flow-mediated dilatation in isolated cerebral arteries of Sprague-Dawley (SD) rats on a high salt is not mediated by COXs neither with EETs [154], which is a further evidence of the abovementioned results of the molecular studies.

Lombard et al. reported that the production of TXA_2 and PGI_2 was altered by HS diet, TXA_2 contributed to impaired vascular response to reduced oxygen partial pressure (PO_2) in animals on HS diet, and that MCA of animals on a HS diet decreased the production of PGI_2 in hypoxic conditions [155].

Taken together, there is a cross-talk between the enzymes producing the vasoactive metabolites and ROS—ROS may be the side-product of impaired activation of COX, NOS, or CYP450 enzymes together with NAD(P)H oxidase activation, and simultaneously, ROS may affect the production of vasoactive metabolites of COX, shifting the production of them from vasodilators to vasoconstrictors and affecting the bioavailability of NO [153, 156, 157] (**Figure 3**).

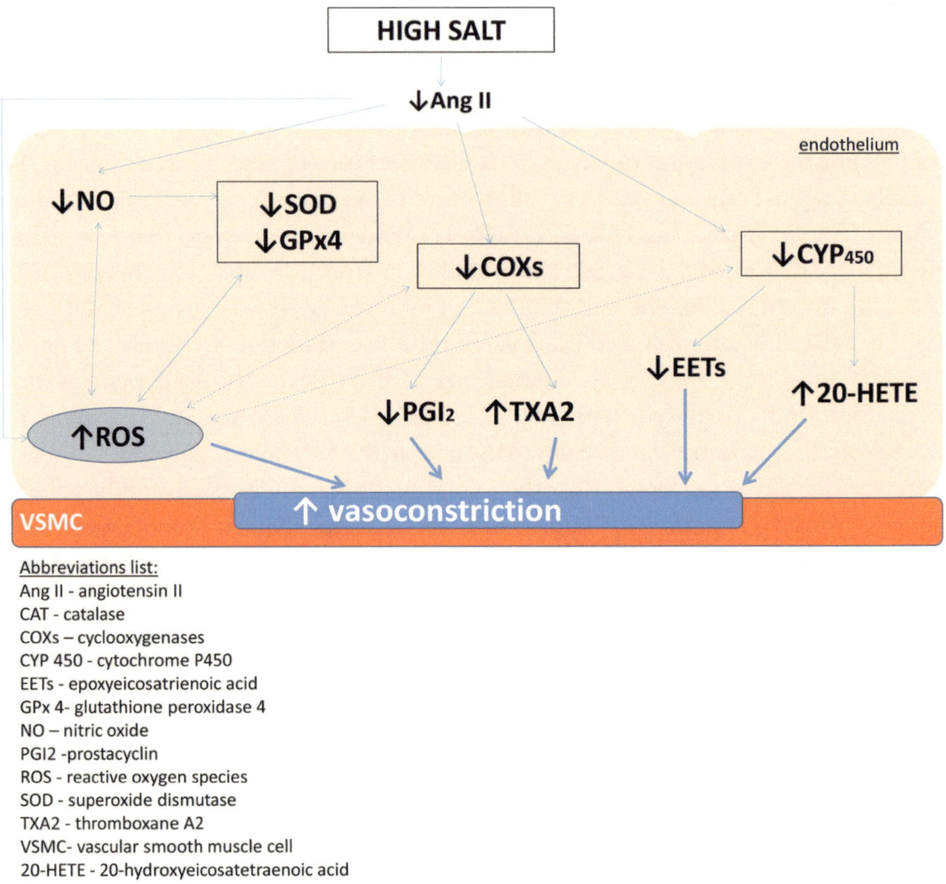

Figure 3. Schematic overview of the influence of high salt intake to increased oxidative stress and reduced vasodilation. Ang II, angiotensin II; CAT, catalase; COXs, cyclooxygenases; CYP 450, cytochrome P450; EETs, epoxyeicosatrienoic acid; GPx 4, glutathione peroxidase 4; NO, nitric oxide; PGI2, prostacyclin; ROS, reactive oxygen species; SOD, superoxide dismutase; TXA2, thromboxane A2; VSMC, vascular smooth muscle cell; 20-HETE, 20-hydroxyeicosatetraenoic acid.

12. Arachidonic acid metabolites and diabetes mellitus

It is clearly recognized that elevated plasma concentration of glucose is responsible for the pathogenesis of vascular complications associated with DM; hyperglycemia can modify vascular function—it compromises the endothelium-dependent relaxation, increases the contractile response of vascular smooth muscle and the development of inflammatory, thrombotic, and atherosclerotic events.

Impaired endothelium-dependent vasodilatation has been shown in various vascular beds of different animal models and in human with DM [62]. In patients with DM type 2 and in diabetic mice, reduced production on NO, increased generation of ROS, and enhanced vasoconstrictor tone were related to impaired endothelium-dependent vasodilation [158]. This attenuated vascular response includes multiple mechanisms, but it seems that increased oxidative stress is the first alteration that triggers more others. Similar to findings in hypertension and high salt diet, endothelial dysfunction in diabetes could also be related to the release of vasoconstrictor mediators, for example, increased production of 20-HETE leading to activation of ROS through an NAD(P)H-dependent pathway. This may have an important therapeutic potential in the treatment of diabetic vascular complications, for example, nephropathy [159].

The impaired endothelium-dependent dilation to ACh in diabetic animals is due to the accompanying release of EDCF and can be attributed to the exposure of the endothelial cells to high blood glucose level, causing increased oxidative stress and overexpression of both COX-1 and COX-2 [160]. Also, as previously mentioned in the paragraph on COXs metabolites and ROS, increased ROS production may determine vasoconstrictor response. Exogenous administration of AA in diabetic dogs induces TXA_2-mediated contraction, while increases the prostacyclin-mediated vasodilation in the arteries of control dogs [161]. ACh-induced vasodilation of diabetic aortas, mesenteric arteries, and femoral arteries is reduced, but COX inhibitors improve that response [162]. Some studies have shown that hyperglycemia increases the expression of COX-2, in large blood vessels and in microcirculation, leading to increased production of vasoconstrictor prostanoids which modify vascular reactivity [162]. Numerous data indicate that there is an increase the release of ROS from endothelial cells in DM, especially superoxide anion, which is thought to be particularly responsible for the increased COX-2 expression [62]. Hyperglycemia increases the release of AA, modifies the formation and function of prostanoids, and thus induces modification of vasomotor tone [62].

Other enzymes, which metabolize AA, are affected by diabetes. Diabetes alters CYP expression and 20-HETE formation, leading to upregulation of CYP4A isoforms and to elevated levels of 20-HETE [115]. The 20-HETE inhibitor HET0016 attenuates the development of diabetes-induced vascular dysfunction, suggesting a contribution of 20-HETE to endothelial dysfunction in diabetes and other insulin-resistant conditions [163]. Recent findings also suggest that 20-HETE impairs insulin-stimulated vasodilator effects that are mediated by the IRS-1/PI3K/AKT/eNOS pathway [163]. Elevated levels of CYP-derived 20-HETE in diabetic patients with cardiac ischemia are associated with dysfunction of circulating endothelial progenitor cells and angiogenic capacity [164]. On the other hand, experiments have indicated that in streptozocin-induced diabetic rats (with impaired endothelial function and contractile responses), the vascular CYP2E1 is significantly increased, leading indirectly to a reduction in the levels of the potent vasoconstrictor 20-HETE (by inhibiting CYP4A enzymes). Preincubation of vessels in vitro with 20-HETE rescued contractile functions, suggesting that the role of 20-HETE in diabetes-induced vascular dysfunction is complex, although those experiments were conducted on aortic vascular models and not in microcirculation [165].

In experiments conducted on two animal models (streptozocin-treated rats) with different levels of glucose metabolism impairment—glucose intolerance model and diabetic model, the expressions of CYP enzymes involved primarily in production of EETs (CYP2J4, CYP2C23) and HETE(CYP4A2 and CYP4A3) were compared, as well as sEH (which degrades EETs) [166]. In the glucose intolerance model, increased degradation of EETs by elevated expression of soluble epoxide hydrolase might contribute to endothelial dysfunction. Findings in the diabetic model suggest a different mechanism, primarily a shift in the balance between EETs and 20-HETE production caused by changes in CYP2J4 and CYP4A3 expression [166–168].

13. Arachidonic acid metabolites and stroke

In recent years, studies suggest that hypertension, a risk factor for stroke, is associated with an increased production of 20-HETE in the wall of cerebral vessels [169]; 20-HETE has a crucial role in cerebral blood flow regulation [170] and is a well-described mediator or neural tissue damage in stroke [169]. 20-HETE increases the production of ROS [171–174], has a role in increasing vasospasm following subarachnoid hemorrhage (SAH), and also affects infarct volume after t-MCAO in rats. Its inhibitors, such as HET0016 [175], reduce vasospasm after SAH and reduce stroke volume and neurological outcome after stroke. Dunn et al. showed that in spontaneously hypertensive rats the CYP4A expression and 20-HETE production were raised in the cerebral vasculature and that inhibition of 20-HETE production noticeably reduced the infarct size and endothelial dysfunction presented in stroke [169]. In humans, excretion of 20-HETE is associated with hypertension and endothelial dysfunction. Ward et al. showed that plasma concentrations of 20-HETE, EETs, and DiHETEs were elevated in patients with acute ischemic stroke and increased oxidative stress was present noticeable by increased plasma F2-isoprostanes [68]. It is considered that free radicals formation that accompanies ischemic brain injury is an acute response [68].

Pretreatment and treatment with 20-HETE inhibitors have been proposed as a new potential approach for stroke treatment [176]. Recently, beside 20-HETE, other metabolites of AA, such as EETs, have been shown to have a potential to alleviate the impairment of tissue perfusion and detrimental outcome of stroke [177–179]. Several studies demonstrated that stabilizing the levels of EETs is important, and that the inhibition of sEH is cerebroprotective against ischemic stroke and SAH [177, 178]. Thus, CYP metabolites could play an important role as new targets for the pharmaceutical industry in managing brain damage that occurs with cerebral ischemia and stroke [180].

14. Conclusion remarks

In conclusion, it is obvious that metabolites of AA play an extremely important role in the mechanisms of microvascular responses and microvascular regulation of tissue blood flow and perfusion. Balance between vasodilator and vasoconstrictor metabolites of AA may be disturbed in various cardiometabolic diseases (such as hypertension, stroke, obesity, diabetes) and underlies endothelial dysfunction which is related to many complications accompanying these diseases. Dietary habits significantly affect the metabolism of AA, particularly excessive NaCl intake or high blood glucose levels lead to endothelial dysfunction, as well. Control of environmental risks factors, good maintenance of the occurring diseases, and balanced nutrition with restricted salt intake can significantly improve metabolism of AA and alleviate possible microvascular dysfunction and subsequent organ damage. Current research on alternative pathways of AA metabolism and pharmacological manipulation with certain components of the AA pathways (such as 20-HETE production inhibition or prolongation of the life of EETs by sEH inhibitors) promises effective therapy of cardiovascular and cerebrovascular diseases in the future.

Author details

Ines Drenjančević[1*], Ivana Jukić[1], Zrinka Mihaljević[1], Anita Ćosić[1] and Aleksandar Kibel[1,2]

*Address all correspondence to: ines.drenjancevic@mefos.hr

1 Department of Physiology and Immunology, Faculty of Medicine University of J.J. Strossmayer Osijek, Osijek, Croatia

2 Department of Heart and Vascular Diseases, Osijek University Hospital, Osijek, Croatia

References

[1] Chawengsub Y, Gauthier KM, Campbell WB. Role of arachidonic acid lipoxygenase metabolites in the regulation of vascular tone. Am J Physiol Heart Circ Physiol. 2009; 297(2):H495–507.

[2] Félétou M, Huang Y, Vanhoutte PM. Endothelium-mediated control of vascular tone: COX-1 and COX-2 products. Br J Pharmacol. 2011; 164:894–912.

[3] Wong MS, Vanhoutte PM. COX-mediated endothelium-dependent contractions: from the past to recent discoveries. Acta Pharmacol Sin. 2010; 31(9):1095–102.

[4] van Hinsbergh WM. Endothelial permeability for macromolecules. Mechanistic aspects of pathophysiological modulation. Arterioscler Thromb Vasc Biol. 1997; 17:1018–23.

[5] FitzGerald GA. Mechanisms of platelet activation: thromboxane A2 as an amplifying signal for other agonists. Am J Cardiol. 1991; 68:11B–15B.

[6] Tian XY, Wong WT, Leung FP, Zhang Y, Wang YX, Lee HK, Ng CF, Chen ZY, Yao X, Au CL, Lau CW, Vanhoutte PM, Cooke JP, Huang Y. Oxidative stress-dependent cyclooxygenase-2-derived prostaglandin f(2α) impairs endothelial function in renovascular hypertensive rats. Antioxid Redox Signal. 2012; 16(4):363–73.

[7] Campbell WB, Falck JR. Arachidonic acid metabolites as endothelium-derived hyperpolarizing factors. Hypertension. 2007; 49:590–6.

[8] Feletou M, Vanhoutte PM. EDHF: an update. ClinSci (Lond). 2009; 117:139–55.

[9] Davidge ST. Prostaglandin H synthase and vascular function. Circ Res. 2001; 89:650–60.

[10] Coleman RA, Smith WL, Narumiya S. International Union of Pharmacology classification of prostanoid receptors: properties, distribution, and structure of the receptors and their subtypes. Pharmacol Rev. 1994; 46(2):205–29.

[11] Zhang J, Gong Y, Yu Y. PG F2α receptor: a promising therapeutic target for cardiovascular disease. Front Pharmacol. 2010; 14(1):116.

[12] Rakhila H, Bourcier N, Akoum A, Pouliot M. Abnormal expression of prostaglandins E2 and F2α receptors and transporters in patients with endometriosis. Biomed Res Int. 2015; 2015:808146.

[13] Pawson AJ, Sharman JL, Benson HE, Faccenda E, Alexander SP, Buneman OP, Davenport AP, McGrath JC, Peters JA, Southan C, Spedding M, Yu W, Harmar AJ; NC-IUPHAR. The IUPHAR/BPS Guide to PHARMACOLOGY: an expert-driven knowledgebase of drug targets and their ligands. Nucleic Acids Res. 2014 Jan;42(Database issue):D1098–106. doi: 10.1093/nar/gkt1143. Epub 2013 Nov 14.

[14] Narumiya S, Sugimoto Y, Ushikubi F. Prostanoid receptors: structures, properties, and functions. Physiol Rev. 1999; 79(4):1193–226.

[15] Harris RC. COX-2 and the kidney. J Cardiovasc Pharmacol. 2006; 47:S37–42.

[16] Mitchell JA, Ali F, Bailey L, Moreno L, Harrington LS. Role of nitric oxide and prostacyclin as vasoactive hormones released by the endothelium. Exp Physiol. 2008; 93(1): 141–7.

[17] Nakayama T. Prostacyclin analogues: prevention of cardiovascular diseases. Cardiovasc Hematol Agents Med Chem. 2006; 4:351–9.

[18] Sandoo A, van Zanten JJ, Metsios GS, Carroll D, Kitas GD. The endothelium and its role in regulating vascular tone. Open Cardiovasc Med J. 2010; 4:302–12.

[19] Oida H, Namba T, Sugimoto Y, Ushikubi F, Ohishi H, Ichikawa A, Narumiya S. In situ hybridization studies of prostacyclin receptor mRNA expression in various mouse organs. Br J Pharmacol. 1995; 116:2828–37.

[20] Sun L, Ye RD. Role of G protein-coupled receptors in inflammation. Acta Pharmacol Sin. 2012; 33:342–50.

[21] Stock JL, Shinjo K, Burkhardt J, Roach M, Taniguchi K, Ishikawa T, Kim HS, Flannery PJ, Coffman TM, McNeish JD, Audoly LP. Theprostaglandin E2 EP1 receptor mediates pain perception and regulates blood pressure. J Clin Invest. 2001; 107:325–31.

[22] Guan Y, Zhang Y, Wu J, Qi Z, Yang G, Dou D, Gao Y, Chen L, Zhang X, Davis LS, Wei M, Fan X, Carmosino M, Hao C, Imig JD, Breyer RM, Breyer MD. Antihypertensive

effects of selective prostaglandinE2 receptor subtype 1 targeting. J Clin Invest. 2007; 117:2496–505.

[23] Nasrallah R, Hassouneh R, Hébert RL. Chronic kidney disease: targeting prostaglandin E2 receptors. Am J Physiol Renal Physiol. 2014; 307:F243–50.

[24] Boie Y, Sawyer N, Slipetz DM, Metters KM, Abramovitz M. Molecular cloning and characterization of the human prostanoid DP receptor. J Biol Chem. 1995; 270:18910–6.

[25] Hirata M, Kakizuka A, Aizawa M, Ushikubi F, Narumiya S. Molecular characterization of a mouse prostaglandin D receptor and functional expression of the cloned gene. Proc Natl Acad Sci USA. 1994; 91:11192–6.

[26] Hasumoto K, Sugimoto Y, Yamasaki A, Morimoto K, Kakizuka A, Negishi M, Ichikawa A. Association of expression of mRNA encoding the PGF2 alpha receptor with luteal cell apoptosis in ovaries of pseudopregnant mice. J Reprod Fertil. 1997; 109(1):45–51.

[27] Hasumoto K, Sugimoto Y, Gotoh M, Segi E, Yamasaki A, Yamaguchi M, Honda H, Hirai H, Negishi M, Kakizuka A, Ichikawa A. Characterization of the mouse prostaglandin F receptor gene: a transgenic mouse study of a regulatory regionthat controls its expression in the stomach and kidney but not in the ovary. Genes Cells. 1997; 2(9):571–80.

[28] Imig JD. Epoxides and soluble epoxide hydrolase in cardiovascular physiology. Physiol Rev. 2012; 92(1):101–30.

[29] Capra V, Thompson MD, Sala A, Cole DE, Folco G, Rovati GE. Cysteinyl-leukotrienes and their receptors in asthma and other inflammatory diseases: critical update and emerging trends. Med Res Rev. 2007; 27:469–527.

[30] Ribeiro JD, Toro AA, Baracat EC. Antileukotrienes in the treatment of asthma and allergic rhinitis. J Pediatr. 2006; 82:S213–21.

[31] Sharma JN, Mohammed LA. The role of leukotrienes in the pathophysiology of inflammatory disorders: is there a case for revisiting leukotrienes as therapeutic targets? Inflammopharmacology. 2006; 14:10–6.

[32] Luo P, Wang MH. Eicosanoids, β-cell function, and diabetes. Prostaglandins Other Lipid Mediat. 2011; 95(1–4):1–10.

[33] Drenjancevic-Peric I, Karner I, Palecek I, Kosovic P, Zuro-Tijardovic I, Soldo I. The cysteinyl-leukotriene-release test in acetylsalicylic acid (ASA) sensitivity. Period Biol. 1999; 101(1):97–100.

[34] Manojlovic D, Drenjancevic I. Molecular mechanisms involved in pulmonary arterial hypertension development. Period Biol. 2011; 113:327–33.

[35] Mashima R, Okuyama T. The role of lipoxygenases in pathophysiology; new insights and future perspectives. Redox Biol. 2015; 6:297–310.

[36] Tian W, Jiang X, Sung YK, Qian J, Yuan K, Nicolls MR. Leukotrienes in pulmonary arterial hypertension. Immunol Res. 2014; 58(2–3):387–93.

[37] Stanke-Labesque F, Pépin JL, Gautier-Veyret E, Lévy P, Bäck M. Leukotrienes as a molecular link between obstructive sleep apnoea and atherosclerosis. Cardiovasc Res. 2014; 101(2):187–93.

[38] Lianos EA. Methods in Molecular Biology, Volume 120. Eicosanoid Protocols. Springer, Humana Press; 1999.

[39] Capdevila JH, Falck JR, Imig JD. Roles of the cytochrome P450 arachidonic acid monooxygenases in the control of systemic blood pressure and experimental hypertension. Kidney Int. 2007; 72:683–9.

[40] Wang H, Lin L, Jiang J, Wang Y, Lu ZY, Bradbury JA, Lih FB, Wang DW, Zeldin DC. Upregulation of endothelial nitric-oxide synthase by endothelium-derived hyperpolarizing factor involves mitogen-activated protein kinase and protein kinase C signaling pathways. J Pharmacol Exp Ther. 2003; 307:753–64.

[41] Karara A, Makita K, Jacobson HR, Falck JR, Guengerich FP, DuBois RN, Capdevila JH. Molecular cloning, expression, and enzymatic characterization of the rat kidney cytochromeP-450 arachidonic acid epoxygenase. J Biol Chem. 1993; 268:13565–70.

[42] Enayetallah AE, French RA, Thibodeau MS, Grant DF. Distribution of soluble epoxide hydrolase and of cytochrome P450 2C8, 2C9, and 2J2 in human tissues. J Histochem Cytochem. 2004; 52:447–54.

[43] Yu Z, Davis BB, Morisseau C, Hammock BD, Olson JL, Kroetz DL, Weiss RH. Vascular localization of soluble epoxide hydrolase in the human kidney. Am J Physiol Renal Physiol. 2004; 286:F720–6.

[44] Tacconelli S, Patrignani P. Inside epoxyeicosatrienoic acids and cardiovascular disease. Front Pharmacol. 2014; 10(5):239.

[45] Zhao X, Imig JD. Kidney CYP450 enzymes: biological actions beyond drug metabolism. Curr Drug Metab. 2003; 4:73–84.

[46] Neckar J, Kopkan L, Huskova Z, Kolar F, Papousek F, Kramer HJ, Hwang SH, Hammock BD, Imig JD, Malý J, Netuka I, Oštádal B, Červenka L. Inhibition of soluble epoxide hydrolase by cis-4-[4-(3-adamantan-1-ylureido)cyclohexyl-oxy]benzoic acid exhibits antihypertensive and cardioprotective actions in transgenic rats with angiotensin II-dependent hypertension. Clin Sci (Lond). 2012; 122:513–25.

[47] Bhardwaj A, Northington FJ, Carhuapoma JR, Falck JR, Harder DR, Traystman RJ, Koehler RC. P-450 epoxygenase and NO synthase inhibitors reduce cerebral blood flow response to N-methyl-D-aspartate. Am J Physiol Heart Circ Physiol. 2000; 279:H1616–24.

[48] Jouihan SA, Zuloaga KL, Zhang W, Shangraw RE, Krasnow SM, Marks DL, Alkayed NJ. Role of soluble epoxide hydrolase in exacerbation of stroke by streptozotocin-induced type 1 diabetes mellitus. J Cereb Blood Flow Metab. 2013; 33:1650–6.

[49] Chen G, Xu R, Wang Y, Wang P, Zhao G, Xu X, Gruzdev A, Zeldin DC, Wang DW. Genetic disruption of soluble epoxide hydrolase is protective against streptozotocin-induced diabetic nephropathy. Am J Physiol Endocrinol Metab. 2012; 303:E563–75.

[50] Theken KN, Schuck RN, Edin ML, Tran B, Ellis K, Bass A, et al. Evaluation of cytochrome P450-derived eicosanoids in humans with stable atherosclerotic cardiovascular disease. Atherosclerosis. 2012; 222:530–6.

[51] Yousif MH, Benter IF, Roman RJ. Cytochrome P450 metabolites of arachidonic acid play a role in the enhanced cardiac dysfunction in diabetic rats following ischaemic reperfusion injury. Auton Autacoid Pharmacol. 2009; 29:33–41.

[52] Tsai SH, Hein TW, Kuo L, Yang VC. High glucose impairs EDHF-mediated dilation of coronary arterioles via reduced cytochrome P450 activity. Microvasc Res. 2011; 82(3): 356–63.

[53] Mustafa S, Sharma V, McNeill JH. Insulin resistance and endothelial dysfunction: are epoxyeicosatrienoic acids the link? Exp Clin Cardiol. 2009; 14:e41–50.

[54] Chen G, Wang P, Zhao G, Xu G, Gruzdev A, Zeldin DC, Wang DW. Cytochrome P450 epoxygenase CYP2J2 attenuates nephropathy in streptozotocin-induced diabetic mice. Prostaglandins Other Lipid Mediat. 2011; 96:63–71.

[55] Wang MH, Brand-Schieber E, Zand BA, Nguyen X, Falck JR, Balu N, Schwartzman ML. Cytochrome P450-derived arachidonic acid metabolism in the rat kidney: characterization of selective inhibitors. J Pharmacol Exp Ther. 1998; 284:966–73.

[56] Fan F, Muroya Y, Roman RJ. Cytochrome P450 eicosanoids in hypertension and renal disease. Curr Opin Nephrol Hypertens. 2015; 24(1):37–46.

[57] Droge W. Free radicals in the physiological control of cell function. Physiol Rev. 2002; 82:47–95.

[58] Lum H, Roebuck KA. Oxidant stress and endothelial cell dysfunction. Am J Physiol Cell Physiol. 2001; 280:C719–41.

[59] Fridovich I. Superoxide anion radical (O2–.), superoxide dismutases and related matters. J Biol Chem. 1997; 272:18515–7.

[60] Katusic ZS, Vanhoutte PM. Superoxide anion is an endothelium-derived contracting factor. Am J Physiol. 1989; 257:H33–7.

[61] Huie RE, Padmaja S. The reaction of NO with superoxide. Free Radic Res Commun. 1993; 18:195–9.

[62] Davel AP, Wenceslau CF, Akamine EH, Xavier FE, Couto GK, Oliveira HT, Rossoni LV. Endothelial dysfunction in cardiovascular and endocrine-metabolic diseases: an update. Braz J Med Biol Res. 2011;44(9):920–32.

[63] Lüscher TF, Vanhoutte PM. The endothelium: modulator of cardiovascular function. CRC Press, Boca Raton; 1990.

[64] Schimke I, Griesmacher A, Weigel G, Holzhutter HG, Muller MM. Effects of reactive oxygen species on eicosanoid metabolism in human endothelial cells. Prostaglandins. 1992; 43(3):281–92.

[65] Tsai IJ, Croft KD, Puddey IB, Beilin LJ, Barden A. 20-Hydroxyeicosatetraenoic acid synthesis is increased in human neutrophils and platelets by angiotensin II and endothelin-1. Am J Physiol Heart Circ Physiol. 2011; 300:H1194–200.

[66] Lukaszewicz KM, Lombard JH. Role of the CYP4A/20-HETE pathway in vascular dysfunction of the Dahl salt-sensitive rat. ClinSci (Lond). 2013; 124(12):695–700.

[67] Ward NC, Puddey IB, Hodgson JM, Beilin LJ, Croft KD. Urinary 20-hydroxyeicosatetraenoic acid excretion is associated with oxidative stress in hypertensive subjects. Free Radic Biol Med. 2005; 38(8):1032–6.

[68] Ward NC, Croft KD, Blacker D, Hankey GJ, Barden A, Mori TA, Puddey IB, Beer CD. Cytochrome P450 metabolites of arachidonic acid are elevated in stroke patients compared with healthy controls. ClinSci (Lond). 2011; 121(11):501–7.

[69] Vanhoutte M. Endothelial dysfunction in obesity. Ann Pharm Fr. 2013; 71:42–50.

[70] Grizelj I, Cavka A, Bian JT, Szczurek M, Robinson A, Shinde S, Nguyen V, Braunschweig C, Wang E, Drenjancevic I, Phillips SA. Reduced flow-and acetylcholine-induced dilations in visceral compared to subcutaneous adipose arterioles in human morbid obesity. Microcirculation. 2015; 22(1):44–53.

[71] Farb MG, Ganley-Leal L, Mott M, Liang Y, Ercan B, Widlansky ME, Bigornia SJ, Fiscale AJ, Apovian CM, Carmine B, Hess DT, Vita JA, Gokce N. Arteriolar function in visceral adipose tissue is impaired in human obesity. Arterioscler Thromb Vasc Biol. 2012; 32:467–73.

[72] Farb MG, Tiwari S, Karki S, Ngo DT, Carmine B, Hess DT, Zuriaga MA, Walsh K, Fetterman JL, Hamburg NM, Vita JA, Apovian CM, Gokce N. Cyclooxygenase inhibition improves endothelial vasomotor dysfunction of visceral adipose arterioles in human obesity. Obesity (Silver Spring). 2014; 22(2):349–55.

[73] Van Gaal LF, Mertens IL, De Block CE. Mechanisms linking obesity with cardiovascular disease. Nature. 2006; 444:875–80.

[74] Despres JP, LemieuxI I. Abdominal obesity and metabolic syndrome. Nature. 2006; 444:881–7.

[75] Nikolopoulou A, Kadoglou NP. Obesity and metabolic syndrome as related to cardiovascular disease. Expert Rev Cardiovasc Ther. 2012; 10:933–9.

[76] Cosentino F, Sill JC, Katusic ZS. Role of superoxide anions in the mediation of endothelium-dependent contractions. Hypertension. 1994; 23:229–35.

[77] Phillips SA, Hatoum OA, Gutterman DD. The mechanism of flow-induced dilation in human adipose arterioles involves hydrogen peroxide during CAD. Am J Physiol Heart Circ Physiol. 2007; 292:H93–100.

[78] Fichtlscherer S, Dimmeler S, Breuer S, Busse R, Zeiher AM, Fleming I. Inhibition of cytochrome P450 2C9 improves endothelium-dependent, nitric oxide-mediated vasodilatation in patients with coronary artery disease. Circulation. 2004; 109:178–83.

[79] Fleming I, Michaelis UR, Bredenkotter D, Fisslthaler B, Dehghani F, Brandes RP, Busse R. Endothelium-derived hyperpolarizing factor synthase (cytochrome P450 2C9) is a functionally significant source of reactive oxygen species in coronary arteries. Circ Res. 2001; 88:44–51.

[80] Miura H, Bosnjak JJ, Ning G, Saito T, Miura M, Gutterman DD. Role for hydrogen peroxide in flow-induced dilation of human coronary arterioles. Circ Res. 2001; 92:e31–40.

[81] Lackland DT, Weber MA. Global burden of cardiovascular disease and stroke: hypertension at the core. Can J Cardiol. 2015; 31(5):569–71.

[82] Mendis S, Puska P, Norrving B. Global atlas on cardiovascular disease prevention and control (1st ed.). World Health Organization in Collaboration with the World Heart Federation and the World Stroke Organization, Geneva; 2011. p. 38. ISBN 9789241564373.

[83] Mattu HS, Randeva HS. Role of adipokines in cardiovascular disease. J Endocrinol. 2013; 216:T17–36.

[84] Pitt B, Pepine C, Willerson JT. Cyclooxygenase-2 inhibition and cardiovascular events. Circulation. 2002; 106:167–9.

[85] Taddei S, Virdis A, Ghiadoni L, Magagna A, Salvetti A. Vitamin C improves endotheliumdependent vasodilation by restoring nitric oxide activity in essential hypertension. Circulation. 1998; 97:2222–9.

[86] Campbell WB, Fleming I. Epoxyeicosatrienoic acids and endothelium-dependent responses. Pflugers Arch. 2010; 459:881–95.

[87] Fleming I. Epoxyeicosatrienoic acids, cell signaling and angiogenesis. Prostaglandins Other Lipid Mediat. 2007; 82:60–7.

[88] Sudhahar V, Shaw S, Imig JD. Epoxyeicosatrienoic acid analogs and vascular function. Curr Med Chem. 2010; 17:1181–90.

[89] Li PL, Campbell WB. Epoxyeicosatrienoic acids activate K+ channels in coronary smooth muscle through a guanine nucleotide binding protein. Circ Res. 1997; 80:877–84.

[90] Li PL, Zhang DX, Ge ZD, Campbell WB. Role of ADP-ribose in 11,12-EET-induced activation of K(Ca) channels in coronary arterial smooth muscle cells. Am J Physiol Heart Circ Physiol. 2002; 282:H1229–36.

[91] Capdevila JH, Falck JR. Biochemical and molecular characteristics of the cytochrome P450 arachidonic acid monooxygenase. Prostaglandins Other Lipid Mediat. 2000; 62:271–92.

[92] Huang A, Sun D, Carroll MA, Jiang H, Smith CJ, Connetta JA, Falck JR, Shesely EG, Koller A, Kaley G. EDHF mediates flow-induced dilation in skeletal muscle arterioles of female eNOS-KO mice. Am J Physiol Heart Circ Physiol. 2001; 280:H2462–9.

[93] Huang A, Sun D, Jacobson A, Carroll MA, Falck JR, Kaley G. Epoxyeicosatrienoic acids are released to mediate shear stress-dependent hyperpolarization of arteriolar smooth muscle. Circ Res. 2005; 96:376–83.

[94] Sun D, Yan C, Jacobson A, Jiang H, Carroll MA, Huang A. Contribution of epoxyeicosatrienoicacids to flow-induced dilation in arteries of male ERalpha knockout mice: role of aromatase. Am J Physiol Regul Integr Comp Physiol. 2007; 293:R1239–46.

[95] Huang A, Sun D, Smith CJ, Connetta JA, Shesely EG, Koller A, Kaley G. In eNOS knockout mice skeletal muscle arteriolar dilation to acetylcholine ACh is mediated by EDHF. Am J Physiol Heart Circ Physiol. 2000; 278:H762–8.

[96] Taddei S, Versari D, Cipriano A, Ghiadoni L, Galetta F, Franzoni F, Magagna A, Virdis A, Salvetti A. Identification of a cytochrome P450 2C9-derived endothelium-derived hyperpolarizing factor in essential hypertensive patients. J Am Coll Cardiol. 2006; 48(3): 508–15.

[97] Bellien J, Favre J, Iacob M, Gao J, Thuillez C, Richard V, Joannides R. Arterial stiffness is regulated by nitric oxide and endothelium-derived hyperpolarizing factor during changes in blood flow in humans. Hypertension. 2010; 55:674–80.

[98] Capdevila JH, Wei S, Yan J, Karara A, Jacobson HR, Falck JR, Guengerich FP, DuBois RN. Cytochrome P-450 arachidonic acid epoxygenase. Regulatory control of the renal epoxygenase bydietary salt loading. J Biol Chem. 1992; 267:21720–6.

[99] Holla VR, Makita K, Zaphiropoulos PG, Capdevila JH. The kidney cytochrome P-450 2C23 arachidonic acid epoxygenase is upregulated during dietary salt loading. J Clin Invest. 1999; 104:751–60.

[100] Makita K, Takahashi K, Karara A, Jacobson HR, Falck JR, Capdevila JH. Experimental and/or genetically controlled alterations of the renal microsomal cytochrome P450 epoxygenase induce hypertension in rats fed a high salt diet. J Clin Invest. 1994; 94:2414–20.

[101] Lee CR, Imig JD, Edin ML, Foley J, DeGraff LM, Bradbury JA, Graves JP, Lih FB, Clark J, Myers P, Perrow AL, Lepp AN, Kannon MA, Ronnekleiv OK, Alkayed NJ, Falck JR, Tomer KB, Zeldin DC. Endothelial expression of human cytochrome P450 epoxygenases lowers blood pressure and attenuates hypertension-induced renal injury in mice. FASEB J. 2010; 24(10):3770–81.

[102] Wang X, Ni L, Yang L, Duan Q, Chen C, Edin ML, Zeldin DC, Wang DW. CYP2J2-derived epoxyeicosatrienoic acids suppress endoplasmic reticulum stress in heart failure. Mol Pharmacol. 2014; 85(1):105–15.

[103] Sinal CJ, Tohkin M, Miyata M, Ward JM, Lambert G, Gonzalez FJ. Targeted disruption of the nuclear receptor FXR/BAR impairs bile acid and lipid homeostasis. Cell. 2000; 102(6):731–44.

[104] Manhiani M, Quigley JE, Knight SF, Tasoobshirazi S, Moore T, Brands MW, Hammock BD, Imig JD. Soluble epoxide hydrolase gene deletion attenuates renal injury and inflammation with DOCA-salt hypertension. Am J Physiol Renal Physiol. 2009; 297(3):F740–8.

[105] Yu Z, Xu F, Huse LM, Morisseau C, Draper AJ, Newman JW, Parker C, Graham L, Engler MM, Hammock BD, Zeldin DC, Kroetz DL. Soluble epoxide hydrolase regulates hydrolysis of vasoactive epoxyeicosatrienoic acids. Circ Res. 2000; 87(11):992–8.

[106] Imig JD, Zhao X, Capdevila JH, Morisseau C, Hammock BD. Soluble epoxide hydrolase inhibition lowers arterial blood pressure in angiotensin II hypertension. Hypertension. 2002; 39(2 Pt 2):690–4.

[107] Bellien J, Joannides R. Epoxyeicosatrienoic acid pathway in human health and diseases. J Cardiovasc Pharmacol. 2013; 61(3):188–96.

[108] Singh H, Cheng J, Deng H, Kemp R, Ishizuka T, Nasjletti A, Schwartzman ML. Vascular cytochrome P450 4A expression and 20-hydroxyeicosatetraenoic acid synthesis contribute to endothelial dysfunction in androgen-induced hypertension. Hypertension. 2007; 50:123–9.

[109] Zhu D, Zhang C, Medhora M, Jacobs ER. CYP4A mRNA, protein, and product in rat lungs: novel localization in vascular endothelium. J Appl Physiol. 2002; 93:330–7.

[110] Frisbee JC, Falck JR, Lombard JH. Contribution of cytochrome P-450 omega-hydroxylase to altered arteriolar reactivity with high-salt diet and hypertension. Am J Physiol Heart Circ Physiol. 2000; 278:H1517–26.

[111] Cheng J, Ou JS, Singh H, Falck JR, Narsimhaswamy D, Pritchard KA Jr, Schwartzman ML. 20-hydroxyeicosatetraenoic acid causes endothelial dysfunction via eNOS uncoupling. Am J Physiol Heart Circ Physiol. 2008; 294:H1018–26.

[112] Guo AM, Scicli G, Sheng J, Falck JC, Edwards PA, Scicli AG. 20-HETE can act as a nonhypoxic regulator of HIF-1alpha in human microvascular endothelial cells. Am J Physiol Heart Circ Physiol. 2009; 297:H602–13.

[113] Medhora M, Chen Y, Gruenloh S, Harland D, Bodiga S, Zielonka J, Gebremedhin D, Gao Y, Falck JR, Anjaiah S, Jacobs ER. 20-HETE increases superoxide production and activates NAPDH oxidase in pulmonary artery endothelial cells. Am J Physiol Lung Cell Mol Physiol. 2008; 294:L902–11.

[114] Marji JS, Wang MH, Laniado-Schwartzman M. Cytochrome P-450 4A isoform expression and 20-HETE synthesis in renal preglomerular arteries. Am J Physiol Renal Physiol. 2002; 283:F60–7.

[115] Roman RJ. P-450 metabolites of arachidonic acid in the control of cardiovascular function. Physiol Rev. 2002; 82(1):131–85.

[116] Alonso-Galicia M, Falck JR, Reddy KM, Roman RJ. 20-HETE agonists and antagonists in the renal circulation. Am J Physiol. 1999; 277(5 pt 2):F790–6.

[117] Croft KD, McGiff JC, Sanchez-Mendoza A, Carroll MA. Angiotensin II releases 20-HETE from rat renal microvessels. Am J Physiol Renal Physiol. 2000; 279:F544–51.

[118] Carroll MA, Balazy M, Huang DD, Rybalova S, Falck JR, McGiff JC. Cytochrome P450-derived renal HETEs: storage and release. Kidney Int. 1997; 51:1696–702.

[119] Liu Y, Webb HK, Fukushima H, Micheli J, Markova S, Olson JL, Kroetz DL. Attenuation of cisplatin-induced renal injury by inhibition of soluble epoxide hydrolase involves nuclear factor kappaB signaling. J Pharmacol ExpTher. 2012; 341:725–34.

[120] Sacerdoti D, Escalante B, Abraham NG, McGiff JC, Levere RD, Schwartzman ML. Treatment with tin prevents the development of hypertension in spontaneously hypertensive rats. Science. 1989; 243:388–90.

[121] Wu CC, GuptaT, Garcia V, Ding Y, Schwartzman ML. 20-HETE and blood pressure regulation: clinical implications. Cardiol Rev. 2014; 22(1):1–12.

[122] Catella F, Lawson JA, Fitzgerald DJ, FitzGerald GA. Endogenous biosynthesis of arachidonic acid epoxides in humans: increased formation in pregnancy-induced hypertension. Proc Natl Acad Sci U S A. 1990; 87(15):5893–7.

[123] Takahashi H, Yoshika M, Komiyama Y, Nishimura M. The central mechanism underlying hypertension: a review of the roles of sodium ions, epithelial sodium channels, the renin-angiotensin-aldosterone system, oxidative stress and endogenous digitalis in the brain. Hypertens Res. 201; 34(11):1147–60.

[124] Toth P, Csiszar A, Sosnowska D, Tucsek Z, Cseplo P, Springo Z, Tarantini S, Sonntag WE, Ungvari Z, Koller A. Treatment with the cytochrome P450 ω-hydroxylase inhibitor HET0016 attenuates cerebrovascular inflammation, oxidative stress and improves vasomotor function in spontaneously hypertensive rats. Br J Pharmacol. 2013; 168(8): 1878–88.

[125] Minuz P, Jiang H, Fava C, Turolo L, Tacconelli S, Ricci M, Patrignani P, Morganti A, Lechi A, McGiff JC. Altered release of cytochrome p450 metabolites of arachidonic acid in renovascular disease. Hypertension. 2008; 51(5):1379–85.

[126] Alonso-Galicia M, Maier KG, Greene AS, Cowley AW Jr, Roman RJ. Role of 20-hydroxyeicosatetraenoic acid in the renal and vasoconstrictor actions of angiotensin II. Am J Physiol Regul Integr Comp Physiol. 2002; 283(1):R60–8.

[127] Ai D, Fu Y, Guo D, Tanaka H, Wang N, Tang C, Hammock BD, Shyy JY, Zhu Y. Angiotensin II up-regulates soluble epoxide hydrolase in vascular endothelium in vitro and in vivo. Proc Natl Acad Sci U S A. 2007; 104(21):9018–23.

[128] Fatica RA, Port FK, Young EW. Incidence trends and mortality in end-stage renal disease attributed to renovascular disease in the United States. Am J Kidney Dis. 2001; 37(6):1184–90.

[129] Kim S, Iwao H. Molecular and cellular mechanisms of angiotensin II-mediated cardiovascular and renal diseases. Pharmacol Rev. 2000; 52(1):11–34.

[130] McGiff JC, Quilley J. 20-HETE and the kidney: resolution of old problems and new beginnings. Am J Physiol. 1999; 277(3 Pt 2):R607–23.

[131] Bragulat E, de la Sierra A. Salt intake, endothelial dysfunction, and salt-sensitive hypertension. J Clin Hypertens (Greenwich). 2002; 4(1):41–6.

[132] Drenjančević-Perić I, Jelaković B, Lombard JH, Kunert MP, Kibel A, Gros M. High-salt diet and hypertension: focus on the renin-angiotensin system. Kidney Blood Press Res. 2011; 34(1):1–11.

[133] Sacks FM, Svetkey LP, VollmerWM, Appel LJ, Bray GA, Harsha D, Obarzanek E, Conlin PR, Miller ER, Simons-Morton DG, Karanja N, Lin PH. For the dash-sodium collaborative researcher group. Effects on blood pressure of reduced dietary sodium and the dietary approaches to stop hypertension (DASH) diet. N Engl J Med. 2001; 344(1):3–10.

[134] Drenjancevic-Peric I, Frisbee JC, Lombard JH. Skeletal muscle arteriolar reactivity in SS.BN13 consomic rats and Dahl salt-sensitive rats. Hypertension. 2003; 41(5):1012–5.

[135] Phillips SA, Drenjancevic-Peric I, Frisbee JC, Lombard JH. Chronic AT(1) receptor blockade alters mechanisms mediating responses to hypoxia in rat skeletal muscle resistance arteries. Am J Physiol Heart Circ Physiol. 2004; 287(2):H545–52.

[136] Zhu J, Mori T, Huang T, Lombard JH. Effect of high-salt diet on NO release and superoxide production in rat aorta. Am J Physiol Heart Circ Physiol. 2004; 286:H575–83.

[137] Boegehold MA, Drenjancevic I, Lombard JH. Salt, angiotensin II, superoxide, and endothelial function. Compr Physiol. 2015; 6(1):215–54.

[138] Cavka A, Cosic A, Jukic I, Jelakovic B, Lombard JH, Phillips SA, Seric V, Mihaljevic I, Drenjancevic I. The role of cyclo-oxygenase-1 in high-salt diet-induced microvascular dysfunction in humans. J Physiol. 2015; 593(24):5313–24.

[139] Drenjancevic-Peric I, Lombard JH. Reduced angiotensin II and oxidative stress contribute to impaired vasodilation in Dahl salt-sensitive rats on low-salt diet. Hypertension. 2005; 45(4):687–91.

[140] Versari D, Daghini E, Virdis A, Ghiadoni L, Taddei S. Endothelium-dependent contractions and endothelial dysfunction in human hypertension. Br J Pharmacol. 2009; 157(4):527–36.

[141] Armstead WM. Cyclooxygenase-2-dependent superoxide generation contributes to age-dependent impairment of G protein-mediated cerebrovasodilation. Anesthesiology. 2003; 98:1378–83.

[142] Ćosić A, Jukić I, Stupin A, Mihalj M, Mihaljević Z, Novak S, Vuković R, Drenjančević I. Attenuated flow-induced dilation of middle cerebral arteries is related to increased vascular oxidative stress in rats on a short-term high salt diet. J Physiol. 2016. DOI: 10.1113/JP272297. [Epub ahead of print]

[143] Lenda DM, Sauls BA, Boegehold MA. Reactive oxygen species may contribute to reduced endothelium-dependent dilation in rats fed high salt. Am J Physiol Heart Circ Physiol. 2000; 279:H7–14.

[144] Durand MJ, Lombard JH. Low-dose angiotensin II infusion restores vascular function in cerebral arteries of high salt-fed rats by increasing copper/zinc superoxide dimutase expression. Am J Hypertens. 2013; 26(6):739–47.

[145] McEwen ST, Schmidt JR, Somber L, de la Cruz L, Lombard JH. Time-course and mechanisms of restored vascular relaxation by reduced salt intake and angiotensin II infusion in rats fed a high-salt diet. Microcirculation. 2009; 16(3):220–34.

[146] Wassmann S, Wassmann K, Nickenig G. Modulation of oxidant and antioxidant enzyme expression and function in vascular cells. Hypertension. 2004; 44:381–6.

[147] Lenda DM, Boegehold MA. Effect of a high salt diet on microvascular antioxidant enzymes. J Vasc Res. 2002; 39:41–50.

[148] Zhu J, Huang T, Lombard JH. Effect of high-salt diet on vascular relaxation and oxidative stress in mesenteric resistance arteries. J Vasc Res. 2007; 44:382–90.

[149] Nurkiewicz TR, Boegehold MA. High salt intake reduces endothelium-dependent dilation of mouse arterioles via superoxide anion generated from nitric oxide synthase. Am J Physiol Regul Integr Comp Physiol. 2007; 292(4):R1550–6.

[150] Li JM, Shah AM. Endothelial cell superoxide generation: regulation and relevance for cardiovascular pathophysiology. Am J Physiol Regul Integr Comp Physiol. 2004; 287:R1014–30.

[151] Taddei S, Ghiadoni L, Virdis A, Versari D, Salvetti A. Mechanisms of endothelial dysfunction: clinical significance and preventive non-pharmacological therapeutic strategies. Curr Pharm Des. 2003; 9:2385–402.

[152] Brunner H, Cockcroft JR, Deanfield J, Donald A, Ferrannini E, Halcox J, et al. Endothelial function and dysfunction. Part II: association with cardiovascular risk factors and diseases. A statement by the Working Group on Endothelins and Endothelial Factors of the European Society of Hypertension. J Hypertens. 2005; 23:233–46.

[153] Ćosić A, Davidović Cvetko E, Jukić I, Drenjančević I. Changes in baseline flow-induced dilation response and interdependence of gene expression caused by the high salt intake in Sprague-Dawley rats. 79th meeting of the Hungarian Physiological Society and the Annual Meeting of the Hungarian Microcirculatory and Vascular Biology Society, Szeged, congress abstract book; 2015. p. 136–37.

[154] Grizelj I, Čavka A, Mihaljević Z, Drenjančević I. The influence of high salt intake on vascular responses of middle cerebral arteries to flow- induced dilation of Sprague-Dawley rats. J Hypertens ESH-ISH Hypertension 2014, Abstract Book. 2014: e217.

[155] Lombard JH, Sylvester FA, Phillips SA, Frisbee JC. High-salt diet impairs vascular relaxation mechanisms in rat middle cerebral arteries. Am J Physiol Heart Circ Physiol. 2003; 284:H1124–33.

[156] Drenjancevic-Peric I, Phillips SA, Falck JR, Lombard JH. Restoration of normal vascular relaxation mechanisms in cerebral arteries by chromosomal substitution in consomic SS.13BN rats. Am J Physiol Heart Circ Physiol. 2005; 289(1):H188–95.

[157] Drenjančević-Perić I, Lombard JH. Introgression of chromosome 13 in Dahl salt-sensitive genetic background restores cerebral vascular relaxation. Am J Physiol Heart Circ Physiol. 2004; 287(2):H957–62.

[158] Okon EB, Chung AWY, Rauniyar P, Padilla E, Tejerina T, McManus BM, Luo H, van Breemen C. Compromised arterial function in human type 2 diabetic patients. Diabetes. 2005; 54:2415–23.

[159] Eid S, Abou-Kheir W, Sabra R, Daoud G, Jaffa A, Ziyadeh FN, Roman L, Eid AA. Involvement of renal cytochromes P450 and arachidonic acid metabolites in diabetic nephropathy. J Biol Regul Homeost Agents. 2013; 27(3):693–703.

[160] Vanhoutte PM, Shimokawa H, Tang EH, Feletou M. Endothelial dysfunction and vascular disease. Acta Physiol (Oxf). 2009; 196(2):193–222.

[161] Gimeno AL, Sterin-Borda L, Borda ES, del Castillo EJ, Gimeno MF. Arachidonate evokes constriction of coronary and mesenteric arteries isolated from diabetic dogs. Adv Prostaglandin Thromboxane Leukot Res. 1983; 12:235–40.

[162] Bagi Z, Erdei N, Papp Z, Edes I, Koller A. Up-regulation of vascular cyclooxygenase-2 in diabetes mellitus. Pharmacol Rep. 2006; 58(Suppl.):52–6.

[163] Li X, Zhao G, Ma B, Li R, Hong J, Liu S, Wang DW. 20-Hydroxyeicosatetraenoic acid impairs endothelial insulin signaling by inducing phosphorylation of the insulin receptor substrate-1 at Ser616. PLoS One. 2014; 9(4):e95841.

[164] Issan Y, Hochhauser E, Guo A, Gotlinger KH, Kornowski R, Leshem-Lev D, Lev E, Porat E, Snir E, Thompson CI, Abraham NG, Laniado-Schwartzman M. Elevated level of pro-inflammatory eicosanoids and EPC dysfunction in diabetic patients with cardiac ischemia. Prostaglandins Other Lipid Mediat. 2013; 100–101:15–21.

[165] Schäfer A, Galuppo P, Fraccarollo D, Vogt C, Widder JD, Pfrang J, Tas P, Barbosa-Sicard E, Ruetten H, Ertl G, Fleming I, Bauersachs J. Increased cytochrome P4502E1 expression and altered hydroxyeicosatetraenoic acid formation mediate diabetic vascular dysfunction: rescue by guanylyl-cyclase activation. Diabetes. 2010; 59(8):2001–9.

[166] Pivackova L, Mensikova L, Gajdacova B, Sotnikova R, Navarova J, Klimas J, Krenek P. 6D.05: endothelial dysfunction in animal models of glucose intolerance and diabetes is accompanied by different expression of key enzymes of epoxyeicosatrienoic acids pathway. J Hypertens. 2015; 33(Suppl. 1):e83–4.

[167] Kibel A, Novak S, Cosic A, Mihaljevic Z, Falck JR, Drenjancevic I. Hyperbaric oxygenation modulates vascular reactivity to angiotensin-(1-7) in diabetic rats: potential role of epoxyeicosatrienoic acids. Diab Vasc Dis Res. 2015;12(1):33–45.

[168] Kibel A, Cavka A, Cosic A, Falck JR, Drenjancevic I. Effects of hyperbaric oxygenation on vascular reactivity to angiotensin II and angiotensin-(1-7) in rats. Undersea Hyperb Med. 2012;39(6):1053–66.

[169] Dunn KM, Renic M, Flasch AK, Harder DR, Falck J, Roman RJ. Elevated production of 20-HETE in the cerebral vasculature contributes to severity of ischemic stroke and oxidative stress in spontaneously hypertensive rats. Am J Physiol Heart Circ Physiol. 2008; 295(6):H2455–65.

[170] Toth P, Rozsa B, Springo Z, Doczi T, Koller A. Isolated human and rat cerebral arteries constrict to increases in flow: role of 20-HETE and TP receptors. J Cereb Blood Flow Metab. 2011; 31:2096–105.

[171] Lange A, Gebremedhin D, Narayanan J, Harder D. 20-Hydroxyeicosatetraenoic acid-induced vasoconstriction and inhibition of potassium current in cerebral vascular smooth muscle is dependent on activation of protein kinase C. J BiolChem. 1997; 272:27345–52.

[172] Harder DR, Gebremedhin D, Narayanan J, Jefcoat C, Falck JR, Campbell WB, Roman R. Formation and action of a P-450 4A metabolite of arachidonic acid in cat cerebral microvessels. Am J Physiol. 1994; 266:H2098–107.

[173] Gebremedhin D, Lange AR, Narayanan J, Aebly MR, Jacobs ER, Harder DR. Cat cerebral arterial smooth muscle cells express cytochrome P450 4A2 enzyme and

produce the vasoconstrictor 20-HETE which enhances L-type Ca2+ current. J Physiol. 1998; 507(Part 3):771–81.

[174] Medhora M, Chen Y, Gruenloh S, Harland D, Bodiga S, Zielonka J, Gebremedhin D, Gao Y, Falck JR, Anjaiah S, Jacobs ER. 20-HETE increases superoxide production and activates NAPDH oxidase in pulmonary artery endothelial cells. Am J Physiol Lung Cell Mol Physiol. 2008; 294:L902–11.

[175] Cambj-Sapunar L, Yu M, Harder DR, Roman RJ. Contribution of 5-hydroxytryptamine1B receptors and 20-hydroxyeiscosatetraenoic acid to fall in cerebral blood flow after subarachnoid hemorrhage. Stroke. 2003;34(5):1269–75.

[176] Renic M, Klaus JA, Omura T, Kawashima N, Onishi M, Miyata N, Koehler RC, Harder DR, Roman RJ. Effect of 20-HETE inhibition on infarct volume and cerebral blood flow after transient middle cerebral artery occlusion. J Cereb Blood Flow Metab. 2009; 29(3): 629.

[177] Qu YY, Yuan MY, Liu Y, Xiao XJ, Zhu YL. The protective effect of epoxyeicosatrienoic acids on cerebral ischemia/reperfusion injury is associated with PI3K/Akt pathway and ATP-sensitive potassium channels. Neurochem Res. 2015; 40(1):1–14.

[178] Zuloaga KL, Krasnow SM, Zhu X, Zhang W, Jouihan SA, Shangraw RE, Alkayed NJ, Marks DL. Mechanism of protection by soluble epoxide hydrolase inhibition in type 2 diabetic stroke. PLoS One. 2014; 9(5):e97529.

[179] Zuloaga KL, Zhang W, Roese NE, Alkayed NJ. Soluble epoxide hydrolase gene deletion improves blood flow and reduces infarct size after cerebral ischemia in reproductively senescent female mice. Front Pharmacol. 2015; 5:290.

[180] Imig JD, Simpkins AN, Renic M, Harder DR. Cytochrome P450 eicosanoids and cerebral vascular function. Expert Rev Mol Med. 2011; 13:e7.

Chapter 6

A Challenged Sympathetic System Is Associated with Retinal Vascular Calibre in a Black Male Cohort: The SABPA Study

Nicolaas T. Malan, Roland von Känel, Wayne Smith, Gavin W. Lambert, Walthard Vilser, Nina Eikelis, Manja Reimann and Leoné Malan

Additional information is available at the end of the chapter

http://dx.doi.org/10.5772/63515

Abstract

Sympathetic system hyperactivity and depression are related to cardiac remodelling in Black men. We investigated whether sympathetic system hyperactivity and depressive symptoms are related to retinal vascular dysregulation. A total of 76 Black and 83 White men (23–68 years of age) from the SABPA study were included. Depressive symptoms, 24h pulse pressure (PP), fasting blood and 24-hour urinary catecholamine data were obtained. Retinal vascular calibre was quantified from digital photographs using standardized protocols. Black men demonstrated increased ($p < 0.05$) hyperpulsatile pressure (PP > 50 mmHg), hypertension (78.9 % vs 48.4%) and depression (34.2% vs. 13.3%) prevalence compared to White men. Despite lower epinephrine levels, epinephrine was associated with arteriolar narrowing and venular widening in the Black men [Adj R2 −0.37 (95% CI: −0.66, −0.09), p=0.013; Adj R2 0.35 (95% CI: 0.13, 0.57), p=0.003]. This might suggest ß-adrenergic hyporesponsivity to epinephrine, which was accompanied by hyperpulsatile blood pressure in the Black group. In the White group, depressive symptoms and norepinephrine were associated with retinal arteriolar narrowing. A profile of ß-adrenergic hyporesponsivity, indicative of a chronically challenged sympathetic system, was associated with retinal vascular remodelling in Black men. ß-adrenergic hyporesponsivity as a result of chronic stress emphasized central control of the brain on the circulatory system irrespective of the vascular bed.

Keywords: Africans, retinal microvascular calibre, 24 h urinary epinephrine, depressive symptoms, ethnicity

INTECH
open science | open minds

1. Introduction

South Africa is facing an epidemic of hypertension (HT) and vascular disease but there still is inadequate information on the physiological factors that are contributing to this process [1, 2]. Microvascular disease seems to play an important role in the development of HT, arterial stiffness and structural remodelling [3]. Currently, HT is regarded as the most important modifiable risk factor for stroke and major macrovascular cerebral complications, but it may also predispose to more subtle cerebral processes based on, amongst others, the microcirculation [4, 5]. Both the ophthalmic artery and the anterior cerebral artery originate from the internal carotid artery and most likely will share common characteristics [6]. Therefore the retinal microvasculature may be an ideal structure to study these abnormalities [7]. Longitudinal studies have shown that an inverse association exists between reduced retinal arteriolar calibre and HT in ageing populations, whilst retinal venular dilation is associated with stroke risk [7, 8]. A higher ratio from either wider retinal arteriolar calibre or narrower retinal venular calibre or both is an index of a better retinal vessel profile [9]. Ref. [8] found racial differences in retinal microvascular calibre of various Asian population groups but whether that is also true for Black and White African men is not clear [8]. In a study using Doppler imagery and iontophoresis of acetylcholine and sodium nitroprusside, it was, however, reported that, after correcting for skin resistance in a Black African group, endothelium-independent microvascular function of Black Africans is attenuated compared to that of White Africans [10]. This might be a contributing factor to the ethnic differences in microvascular disease risk in South Africa.

Enhanced peripheral resistance vascular α-adrenergic responses on exposure to a laboratory stressor, i.e. the handgrip test, were shown in Black Africans during urbanisation when compared to their rural counterparts [11]. Thus overstimulation of the sympathetic nervous system (SNS) and the sympathetic adrenal cortex and medullary stress hormone pathway may explain some of the observed ethnic differences [11–13]. Intense emotional stress may induce sympathetic hyperactivity with persistent increases in catecholamine and cortisol levels, which is detrimental to normal physiological processes [13]. However, during chronic stress this initial hyperactivity may be followed by autonomic exhaustion or depression, receptor hyporesponsivity and decreases in catecholamines and cortisol [14–18]. Phenylethanolamine N-methyltransferase (PNMT) is an enzyme found in the adrenal medulla which converts norepinephrine to epinephrine. PNMT is known to be regulated by glucocorticoids synthesised in the adrenal gland [19]. One-way PNMT expression can be regulated is by corticosterone's positive influence on the maintenance of PNMT mRNA [20]. Chronic depression has been related to attenuated cortisol levels which will lead to a decrease in the synthesis of epinephrine [21]. These alterations in autonomic function are of importance as they have been associated with both depression and cardiovascular pathology [14, 15]. Moreover, chronic psychosocial stress often precedes depression [22] which, in turn, has recently been acknowledged as a risk factor for cardiac remodelling and poor prognosis in patients with coronary heart disease [23]. Indeed, decreased cortisol and catecholamine metabolite responses to a mental stressor were risk factors for the development of vascular diseases in a Black African cohort exhibiting symptoms of depression [24]. There still remains no clear cut or generally accepted model for cortisol responses in depression, as both blunted and increased cortisol activities have previously been noted [21, 25]. Blunted cortisol responses were apparent in individuals with depressive symptoms *after* exposure to the Stroop test [13]. This could imply that the presence of depressive symptoms sensitises the individual to stress and the subsequent development of vascular disease and/or other lifestyle illnesses. Blunted cortisol responses to laboratory and psychosocial stressors have been demonstrated in both clinical and subclinical depression [26, 27]. However, it could be speculated that since depression is a constant state of perceived stress, further exposure to a challenging urban environment or psychosocial stress may result in habituation of the neuroendocrine pathways [28].

The 24 h urinary catecholamines and depressive symptoms might, therefore, indicate a challenged SNS associated with retinal microvascular calibre in an urban-dwelling cohort. Whether sympathetic innervation of the retinal vessels exists, is still being debated although it was recently demonstrated that the choroid of the uvea is densely innervated by the sympathetic system and that both α- and β-adrenergic innervations were demonstrated in the preocular central retinal artery (CRA) in humans [29]. The optic canal is a regular conduit for autonomic nerves of the internal carotid plexus to the eye. However, the possible distribution of α- and β-adrenergic receptors in the arterioles of the CRA is still unknown. Generally, in resistance vessels, vasoconstriction is mediated via $\alpha 1$- and $\alpha 2$-adrenergic receptors whilst β_2-adrenergic receptors mediate vasodilation [2]. It was recently shown that the CRA receives adrenergic and cholinergic innervation supporting autoregulation of intra-retinal vessels [29]. Systemic sympathetic transmitter spillover (epinephrine and norepinephrine) in the carotid and retinal vasculature may thus impact on retinal perfusion. Indeed, Ref. [30] reported associations of psychosocial risk factors and depression with retinopathy signs (microaneurysms, retinal or vitreous haemorrhages, soft or hard exudates or intra-retinal microvascular abnormalities) and suggested the presence of adrenergic receptors in retinal vessels.

They further demonstrated that heterogeneity in psychosocial effects could result from greater vulnerability of subjects with diabetes and HT due to underlying vascular damage associated with these conditions. This appeared to be the case for symptoms of depression, which had a stronger association with retinopathy in subjects with HT compared with those without, 60% versus 30% greater odds of retinopathy [30].

Chronic stress, as presented by depressive symptoms, may thus induce chronic stimulation of the SNS and initial hyperactivity may be followed by autonomic exhaustion, receptor hyporesponsivity and decreases in catecholamines resulting in hyperkinetic blood pressure (BP) values and receptor hyporesponsivity and decreases in catecholamine levels [15, 16, 31]. The main purpose of this study was, therefore, to assess the associations between retinal microvascular calibre, as primary endpoint and systemic adrenergic neurotransmitters and depressive symptoms, in a bi-ethnic cohort of South African men.

2. Main body of paper

2.1. Materials and methods

2.1.1. Design and participants

Urban Black and White African teachers were recruited as part of the prospective Sympathetic activity and Ambulatory Blood Pressure in Africans (SABPA) study [32]. All participants of the first phase of SABPA (2007–2008) were invited to participate in the follow-up. Their ages varied between 23 and 68 years. Of the initial 204 male participants in the first phase, 180 men reported for the second phase where, additionally, retinal blood vessel measurements were obtained. Men are more prone to the development of cardiovascular disease (CVD); therefore, only men were included in order to obtain a homogenous high CVD risk cohort [1, 2].

We excluded one participant with a history of epilepsy and 20 participants who did not have usable retinal microvascular images. Finally we included a total of 76 Black and 83 White Africans in the study. Participants were fully informed about the objectives and procedures of the study prior to their recruitment. All participants provided written, informed consent. The study conformed to the Helsinki Declaration (2007) and was approved by the Ethics Review Board of the North-West University, Potchefstroom Campus (approval number 0003607S6).

2.1.2. Assessment of health behaviour

Participants were in a semi-recumbent position from 07 h15 for at least 2 h during which the 12-lead ECG (NORAV PC 1200) registration was performed followed by blood sampling. Physical activity was assessed with the Actiheart® (GB0/67703, CamNtech Ltd., Cambridgeshire, UK) monitors considering resting metabolic rate. The 12-lead ECG resting heart rate was used to calculate the sleep heart rate required by the Actiheart programme. Quantitative assessment of some markers was done to determine smoking status (cotinine, a nicotine metabolite) and alcohol consumption levels (gamma glutamyl transferase, γ-GT) [33]. All anthropometric measurements were performed in triplicate by registered level II anthropometrists according to standardised procedures. The body mass index (BMI) as well as body surface area (BSA) was calculated. BSA was based on the Mosteller formula [34]. Intra- and inter-variability was less than 5%.

2.1.3. Depressive symptoms

The Patient Health Questionnaire (PHQ-9) was used to determine the depressive symptom score of the participants [35]. The PHQ-9 is a measure of depressive symptom severity and has been validated in various ethnic groups including sub-Saharan Africans [36]. The questionnaire is designed for use in primary health-care settings adapting diagnostic criteria from the DSM-IV (Diagnostic and Statistical Manual of Mental Disorders, Fourth Edition). Each item of the PHQ-9 evaluates the presence of one of the nine DSM-IV criteria of major depression [35]. In the current study, the Cronbach alpha-reliability index for the total PHQ-9 score was 0.80. Items on the questionnaire are scored to reflect the frequency of symptom occurrence during

http://dx.doi.org/10.5772/63515

the prior two weeks on a scale of zero to three, with zero reflecting "not at all" and three "nearly every day," thus providing continuous score between 0 and 27 [35]. Examples of questions are: "Feeling down/depressed/hopeless; feeling bad about yourself *OR* that you are a failure/that you have let yourself or your family down, thoughts that you would be better off dead/of hurting yourself in some way" [35]. The recommended and established PHQ-9 cut-off point of ≥10 was used to indicate the presence of depressive symptoms [35].

2.1.4. Cardiovascular measurements

On the morning of the first clinical assessment day, ABPM and 2-lead electrocardiograph monitors were attached to participants on the non-dominant arm at their workplace between 07 h00 and 07 h30 (Meditech CE120 CardioTens®; Meditech, Budapest, Hungary). The ABPM was programmed to measure BP at time intervals shown for assessing sympathetic activity at 30-min intervals during the day (07 h00–22 h00) and every hour during night time (22 h00–06 h00) [37]. The successful inflation rate over this period was 85.8% (±9.14) in Africans and 90.4% (±8.61) in Whites. Hypertensive status and CVD risk were classified from 24 h ABPM as systolic blood pressure (SBP) ≥ 130 mmHg and/or diastolic blood pressure (DBP) ≥ 80 mmHg [38]. Hyperpulsatile pulse pressure (PP) was defined as 24 h SBP–24 h DBP > 50 mmHg [39]. The apparatus was removed after the last BP measurement at 07 h30 the next day.

2.1.5. Measurement of retinal vascular calibre

Static retinal microvascular measurements were performed in a well-controlled light and temperature regulated laboratory using an Imedos Retinal Vessel Analyser (Germany) with a Zeiss FF450^{Plus} camera and the VesselMap 1 Version 3.10 software. No intake of food or caffeine containing beverages, alcohol, smoking or exercise was allowed one hour prior to retinal vessel measurements. Participants were introduced to the procedure and screened for Acute angle-closure glaucoma risk with a small light source by a trained registered nurse. Mydriasis was induced in the right eye of the participant by means of a drop containing tropicamide 1% and benzalkonium chloride 0.01% (m/v). In the event of previous injury to the right eye, the left eye was used (Black men N = 3; White men N = 1). Retinal vascular calibre was measured in the monochrome images by manually selecting first-order vessel branches in a measuring zone located between 0.5 and 1.0 optic disc diameters from the margin or the optic disc. Upon selection of the vessel, the VesselMap 2, Version 3.02 software, automatically delineated the vessels' measuring area. The colour photograph was used as a reference to ascertain correct identification of venules and arterioles. Identification of vessels was done by two experienced scientists who had to agree on the vessel type before selection. Automated software calculations, based on the Knudtson revision of the Parr-Hubbard formulas, determined estimates from the six largest arterioles and venules and were summarised as the central retinal arterial equivalent (CRAE) and central retinal venular equivalent (CRVE), respectively [40]. AVR was also calculated (CRAE/CRVE). Arterio-venular nicking was defined when a small arteriole crossed a small venule and resulted in the compression of the vein with bulging on either side of the crossing. A higher ratio from either wider retinal arteriolar calibre or narrower retinal venular calibre or both is an index of a better retinal vessel profile [9]. As the image scale of each eye was unknown, the values of CRAE and CRVE were expressed as measuring units (MU). 1 MU is equivalent to 1 μm when the dimensions of the eye being examined correspond to those of the normal Gullstrand eye. Reproducibility was computed for a randomly selected cohort with a correlation coefficient of 0.84. The ICC analysis involved a mixed-model framework, whereby random effects were assumed for subjects and fixed effects were assumed for the graders. The Cronbach's alpha-reliability index for the AVR was 0.91 for this randomised cohort. Retinal pathology as seen in hypertensive/diabetic retinopathy and including optic nerve cup/disc ratio and arterio-venular nicking was diagnosed by a registered ophthalmologist.

2.1.6. 24 h urinary catecholamines

A three-litre container, washed with 9 ml of 20% HCl, ensured preservation of urinary metanephrines and an accurately 24 h timed specimen (Sarstedt®, Nümbrecht, Germany). Sampling began and ended with an empty bladder and participants were instructed to complete a 24 h diary to indicate voiding time, volume and fluid intake.

2.1.7. Biochemical analyses

Sodium fluoride blood samples, serum and whole blood EDTA samples were analysed for glucose, lipids, C-reactive protein (CRP), cotinine, γ-GT and glycated haemoglobin (HbA_{1c}), using Unicel DXC 800 (Beckman and Coulter, USA), Modular ROCHE Automized (Switzerland) and the Konelab™ 20I Sequential Multiple Analyzer Computer (ThermoScientific, Vantaa, Finland), respectively. An acidified sample from the 24 h urine collection was stored at −80°C until analysis within one year after collection [41]. Urinary epinephrine and norepinephrine values were determined using the 3-Cat Urine ELISA Fast Track kit (LDN, Nordhorn, Germany). Intra- and inter-assay coefficients for epinephrine were 5.50% and 9.62%, respectively, and for norepinephrine 2.70% and 8.59%.

2.1.8. Statistical methods

Data were analysed using Statistica® software version 12.0 (Statsoft Inc., Tulsa, USA, 2012). Skewness of data was tested and γ-GT and CRP values were logarithmically transformed. Independent T-tests determined participant characteristic differences. A priori covariates which are implicated in higher sympathetic activity and CVD risk included age, BSA, physical activity, log γ-GT, log CRP and cholesterol [33, 38]. Chi-square (χ^2) statistics compared proportions. General linear model analyses, independent of a priori covariates, were computed to test interactions with race for depressive symptoms, norepinephrine-to-creatinine ratio (NECR), epinephrine-to-creatinine ratio (ECR) and potential cardiovascular risk markers (i.e. PP) and retinal vasculature markers, and, as a result of the high correlation between CRAE and CRVE, CRAE was adjusted for CRVE and vice versa [42]. ANCOVA's determined significant differences by comparing ethnic male groups from least square means analyses whilst adjusting for covariates (age, BSA, physical activity, log γ-GT, log CRP, cholesterol).

Multiple linear regression analyses were computed in the total male cohort and in separate race groups. Unadjusted associations between retinal vessel calibre markers, depressive symptoms and catecholamines were computed in the male cohorts. Forward stepwise multiple regression analyses were performed in various models based on significant interactions for race. Dependent variables were AVR, CRVE and CRAE. Independent covariates included age, BSA, physical activity, log γ-GT, log CRP, cholesterol 24 h PP, depressive symptoms, NECR and ECR. As a result of the high correlation between CRAE and CRVE, CRAE was added as covariate for CRVE and vice versa.

Sensitivity analyses: Forward stepwise regression analyses with similar dependent and independent covariates were repeated in several models in both ethnic male groups, by (a) excluding HIV-positive status participants (N = 16) (b) including only 24 h hypertensive participants and (c) adding HT medication users, cotinine and/or serum glucose as independent covariates. Significance was noted as $p \leq 0.05$.

2.2. Results

General linear model analyses showed ethnic differences for principal variables investigated, NECR and ECR ($F_{1.151} = 20.66$, $p < 0.0001$), depressive symptoms ($F_{1.165} = 4.45$, $p = 0.04$) as well as AVR ($F_{1.150} = 9.09$, $p = 0.003$), independent of a priori covariates.

Table 1 shows unadjusted baseline characteristics of the Black and White men. The Black men displayed lower waist circumference, BSA, BMI and physical activity but a larger metabolic risk with higher glucose, HbA_{1c}, cholesterol, CRP and γ-GT than their White counterparts. They also had a higher depressive symptom score with 34.2% of the Black men above the cut-off point for modestly severe depressive symptoms [36] compared to 13.3% of the White men. Despite their higher depressive symptom score, the Black men had lower 24 h urine NECR and 24 h urine ECR ratios than the White men. The Black group had higher BP, PP, arterio-venular nicking, optic nerve cup/disc ratio and CRVE values, whilst their retinal AVR was smaller compared to that of the White group.

	Black men (N = 76)	White men (N = 83)	P
Lifestyle and biochemical variables			
Age (years)	45.4 ± 6.9	48.8 ± 10.2	0.016
BMI (kg/m^2)	28.4 ± 5.77	30.4 ± 5.24	0.026
BSA (m^2)	1.99 ± 0.22	2.24 ± 0.21	<0.0011
Waist circumference (cm)	98.3 ± 14.8	106.2 ± 13.2	<0.001
Physical activity (kcal/24 h)	3464.2 ± 1284.5	4101.2 ± 1859.2	0.015
Cholesterol (mmol/L)	4.63 ± 1.02	4.22 ± 1.00	0.012
HDL cholesterol (mmol/L)	0.93 ± 0.35	0.84 ± 0.22	0.054

	Black men (N = 76)	White men (N = 83)	P
Glucose (mmol/L)	5.75 ± 1.71	4.65 ± 1.30	<0.001
Glycated haemoglobin (%)	6.18 ± 1.40	5.70 ± 0.88	0.010
γ-Glutamyl transferase (U/L)	71.7 ± 61.9	36.7 ± 41.2	<0.001
C-reactive protein (mg/L)	5.91 ± 12.2	2.84 ± 10.0	0.084
Cotinine (ng/mL)	48.3 ± 97.8	29.5 ± 98.7	0.232
Depressive symptoms score	7.59 ± 4.51	4.86 ± 4.23	<0.0011
Depressive symptoms (PHQ-9 ≥ 10) N (%))	26 (34.2)	11 (13.3)	<0.001
24 h endocrine variables			
24 h urine norepinephrine/creatinine ratio (nmol/mmol)	15.3 ± 10.7	28.4 ± 20.5	<0.001
24 h urine epinephrine/creatinine ratio (nmol/mmol)	2.61 ± 1.70	4.71 ± 3.17	<0.001
Cardiovascular variables			
24 h SBP (mmHg)	137 ± 15	128 ± 11	<0.001
24 h DBP (mmHg)	87 ± 10	80 ± 7	<0.001
24 h PP (mmHg)	51 ± 8	48 ± 6	0.034
24 h heart rate (beats/min)	78 ± 9	72 ± 10	<0.001
Central retinal arterial equivalent (MU)	147.9 ± 13.2	150.4 ± 11.9	0.218
Central retinal venular equivalent (MU)	251.4 ± 19.2	237.9 ± 18.6	<0.001
Retinal arteriolar-to-venular ratio	0.59 ± 0.06	0.63 ± 0.04	<0.001
Optic nerve cup/disc ratio (right eye)	0.37 ± 0.19	0.28 ± 0.24	0.011
Hypertensive/diabetic retinopathy (%)	75.0	36.3	<0.001
Arterio-venular nicking (N (%))	59 (77.6)	20 (24.1)	<0.001
HT (SBP > 130 and/or DBP > 80 mmHg) (N (%))	60 (78.9)	40 (48.4)	0.001
HT medication (% of hypertensives)	36.6	34.1	0.274

Data presented as unadjusted means with standard deviation or percentages. Where BMI, body mass index; BSA, body surface area; PHQ, Patient Health Questionnaire; 24 h SBP, 24 h systolic blood pressure; 24 h DBP, 24 h diastolic blood pressure; 24 h PP, 24 h pulse pressure; HT, hypertension; MU, measuring units, equal to μm in the normal Gullstrand eye.

Table 1. Comparing unadjusted mean (±SD) baseline characteristics of Black and White men.

In **Table 2**, principal variables were compared considering a priori covariates. In the Black male cohort, a similar trend was revealed with increased hyperpulsatile PP (>50 mmHg) accompanied by more depressive symptoms, lower AVR and also lower urine NECR and ECR values compared to their White counterparts. However, only the AVR was smaller in the Blacks whilst neither CRAE nor CRVE was different between the race groups.

	Black men (N = 76)	White men (N = 83)	P
24 h SBP (mmHg)	140 (137, 144)	126 (123, 130)	<0.001
24 h DBP (mmHg)	88 (86, 90)	79 (77, 81)	<0.001
24 h PP (mmHg)	52 (50, 54)	47 (45, 50)	<0.001
Central retinal arterial equivalent (MU)	147.4 (144.0, 150.8)	150.9 (147.6, 154.1)	0.21
Central retinal venular equivalent (MU)	248.0 (242.9, 253.1)	241.2 (236.4, 246.1)	0.11
Retinal arteriolar-to-venular ratio	0.60 (0.58, 0.61)	0.63 (0.61, 0.64)	0.01
24 h urine ECR (nmol/mmol)	14.3 (9.76, 18.9)	30.0 (25.7, 34.3)	<0.001
24 h urine NECR (nmol/mmol)	2.08 (1.14, 3.02)	5.82 (4.94, 6.69)	<0.001
Depressive symptom score	7.11 (6.02, 8.21)	4.71 (3.84, 5.79)	0.006

Comparing adjusted mean (± SD) pulse pressure, retinal vessel calibre, depressive symptoms and 24 h urinary catecholamines in a cohort of Black and White men. Values were adjusted for age, body surface area, physical activity, log γ-glutamyl transferase, log C-reactive protein and cholesterol. Where 24 h SBP, 24 h systolic blood pressure; 24 h DBP, 24 h diastolic blood pressure; 24 h PP, 24 h pulse pressure; MU, measuring units, equal to μm in the normal Gullstrand eye; 24 h NECR ratio, 24 h urinary norepinephrine-to-creatinine ratio; 24 h ECR ratio, 24 h urinary epinephrine-to-creatinine ratio.

Table 2. Comparing adjusted mean (±95% CI) baseline characteristics of Black and White men.

Forward stepwise linear regression analyses (**Table 3**) revealed expected patterns of associations between the dependent retinal microvascular calibre variables (AVR, CRAE and CRVE) and independent variable, PP, in the total group (Model 1). AVR and CRAE were negatively associated with PP, whilst CRVE showed a positive association with PP. In the total group, negative associations were found between AVR, CRAE and depressive symptoms, whilst no associations were found between any of the retinal microvascular variables and NECR or ECR. In the separate ethnic groups, AVR was negatively associated with PP in both racial groups. CRAE was negatively associated with PP in the White men whilst positively associated with CRVE in the Black men. In the White group, AVR and CRAE were negatively associated with depressive symptoms, whilst AVR was, rather unexpectedly, positively associated with NECR. In the Black group, AVR and CRAE were negatively associated with ECR, whilst a positive association existed with CRVE. No unadjusted or adjusted associations between depressive symptoms and the catecholamines were revealed (data not shown).

No changes in the outcome of the data occurred with sensitivity analyses after excluding HIV-positive status participants or including 24 h hypertensive participants. Adding HT medication users, cotinine and serum glucose as independent covariates also did not alter any of the associations.

Model 1: Total group (N = 159)			
	AVR	CRAE	CRVE
Adjusted R^2	0.28	0.36	0.39
β (95% CI)			
Race	0.16 (0.002, 0.32), p = 0.049	–	−0.20 (−0.36,−0.04), p = 0.017
24 h PP (mmHg)	−0.24 (−0.38,−0.10), p = 0.001	−0.24 (−0.38,−0.11), p = 0.001	0.17 (0.04, 0.31), p = 0.014
Depressive symptoms	−0.19 (−0.34,−0.05), p = 0.014	−0.23 (−0.30,−0.15), p = 0.001	–
24 h urine ECR	–	–	NS
24 h urine NECR	–	NS	–

Model 2: Separate ethnic groups						
	Black men (N = 76)			White men (N = 83)		
	AVR	CRAE	CRVE	AVR	CRAE	CRVE
Adjusted R^2	0.24	0.15	0.29	0.27	0.59	0.52
β (95% CI)						
24 h PP (mmHg)	−0.24 (−0.46,−0.01), p = 0.048	–	0.23 (0.01, 0.45), p = 0.045	−0.30 (−0.48,−0.11), p = 0.003	−0.22 (−0.36,−0.08), p = 0.003	–
Depressive symptoms	–	–	–	−0.27 (−0.46,−0.08), p = 0.007	−0.18 (−0.32,−0.04), p = 0.014	–
24 h urine ECR (nmol/mmol)	−0.35 (−0.57,−0.12), p = 0.004	−0.37 (−0.66,−0.09), p = 0.013	0.35 (0.13, 0.57), p = 0.003	–		–
24 h urine NECR (nmol/mmol)	–	NS	–	0.19 (0.0, 0.38), p = 0.050		–

Covariates included age, body surface area, physical activity, log γ-glutamyl transferase, log C-reactive protein and cholesterol. In models with CRAE as a dependent variable, adjustment for CRVE was made and vice versa. Where AVR, arteriolar-to-venular ratio; CRAE, central retinal arterial equivalent; CRVE, central retinal venular equivalent; 24 h PP, 24 h pulse pressure; ECR, epinephrine-to-creatinine ratio; NECR, norepinephrine-to-creatinine ratio; NECR, norepinephrine-to-creatinine ratio.

Table 3. Forward stepwise regression analyses predicting relationships between the 24 h urinary catecholamine levels, depressive symptoms and retinal vessel parameters.

2.3. Discussion

The aim of this study was to evaluate the association between the retinal microvascular calibre as primary endpoint and systemic adrenergic transmitters and depressive symptoms as independent variables, comparing a Black and White male cohort from South Africa.

The main novel finding suggests a cardiometabolic vulnerable profile in terms of more depressive symptoms, PP, arterio-venular nicking, optic nerve cup/disc ratio and CRVE values, whilst their retinal AVR was smaller in the Black men. Despite lower catecholamine levels, epinephrine was positively associated with arteriolar narrowing, venular widening and hyperpulsatile BP (indicative of arterial stiffness) in the Black men.

2.3.1. *Ethnicity and retinopathy*

Although cultural differences exist between the Black and White groups, all the participants were teachers with the same educational background, income and working conditions. Despite these similarities, the Black group clearly exhibited a poorer health profile than their White counterparts with regard to cardiometabolic and mental health characteristics. They presented with increased cardiometabolic risk markers such as hyperglycaemia, cholesterol, inflammation, alcohol consumption and depressive symptoms. The Black group's mean BP values were above the cut-off point for HT (ABPM ≥ 130/80) [38], which reflect in the HT prevalence of nearly 80% in this group. Elevated BP and PP are associated with structural microvascular changes and our findings are in line with those references [43, 44]. Indeed, elevated BP and PP were associated with attenuated retinal arteriolar and increased venular diameter values and consequently also the AVR. This may impact on vascular wall remodelling as is evident from the presence of arteriolar narrowing, AV nicking, retinopathy [45] and possibly progression towards subclinical atherosclerosis. If the effect of elevated glucose as well as HbA_{1c} levels is added which, in the case of the Black men, are both, according to the American Diabetes Association, above the cut-off point indicative of a prediabetic state, changes in the retinal vessels comparable to those in diabetic subjects could be expected. The prevalence of AV nicking and hypertensive/diabetic retinopathy is a clear indication.. that the retinal vasculature is showing signs of structural changes and reduced microvascular health in both groups but especially in the Black group.

2.3.2. *Retinal vessel calibre and depressive symptoms*

Depression has recently been acknowledged as a major risk factor for poorer prognosis in patients with coronary heart disease by the American Heart Association [23]. The depressive symptom score of the Black men was significantly higher than that of the White men with 34 % of the group exceeding the cut-off point for moderately severe depression, thereby worsening their CVD risk. Although underlying stress levels, as assessed using the depressive symptoms risk score, were elevated in the Black men, both their 24 h ECR and NECR levels were lower compared to their White counterparts. During chronic stress the initial hyperactivity may be followed by autonomic exhaustion, receptor hyporesponsivity and decreases in catecholamines and cortisol [14–18]. PNMT converts norepinephrine to epinephrine and is regulated by glucocorticoids synthesised in the adrenal gland [19]. One way that it can regulate PNMT expression is by corticosterone's positive influence on the maintenance of PNMT mRNA [20]. Therefore a reduction in cortisol will lead to a decrease in the synthesis of epinephrine. These alterations in autonomic function are of importance as they have been associated with both depression and cardiovascular pathology [14, 15]. It is known that depression is often preceded by psychosocial stress [22] which might, therefore, also be associated with the risk for cardiac remodelling as well as a poor prognosis in individuals with coronary heart disease [23]. This notion is enhanced by the finding that in a Black cohort with symptoms of depression, attenuated cortisol and catecholamine metabolites were identified as risk factors for the development of vascular diseases [24]. Even though depression [46], diabetes and HT are associated with activation of the SNS [31], we could not replicate these findings.

Our results, therefore, oppose the findings from Ref. [47], showing a positive association between NECR excretion and moderate depressive symptoms. As more depressive symptoms and a hypertensive state are evident in the Black men, the SNS and adrenal medulla may present neural fatigue or "burnout." Our findings could, therefore, indicate a possible down-regulation of norepinephrine and epinephrine secretion as a consequence of long-term overstimulation of the SNS and possible β-adrenergic hyporesponsivity in the Black men. In support of this notion, depressed heart rate variability (HRV) was associated with increased parasympathetic dominance albeit cardiac contractility (24-h heart rate and SBP) in the current African men at baseline, rather suggesting β-adrenergic receptor activation [1, 48]. Conversely, increased SNS activity and a possible vagal-impaired HR profile may however contribute to disturbed endothelial function, possibly because of activation of β-adrenergic receptors [49]. When α-adrenergic responsiveness though prevails [48], dysregulation or desensitisation of β-adrenergic receptors may occur. This was evident in the clustering of increased 24-h heart rate, SBP and depressed HRV values which indicated a possible diminished β-adrenergic responsiveness and vagal-impaired response [1]. A plausible explanation may be that depressed HRV as a reflection of α-adrenergic sympathetic overdrive could also be due to poor ventricular performance as was observed in another study [50].

It supports previous findings in these SABPA Black men, where blunted neuroendocrine responses were associated with vascular wall remodelling concurring with a profile of autonomic exhaustion and emotional distress [14, 16]. Our subsample of White men showed a 13% prevalence of depressive symptoms which were inversely associated with the retinal vessel calibre. Findings from the ARIC study compare favourably with the White group where the depressive symptom score was associated with retinal arteriolar narrowing. In contrast, we could not replicate these findings in the Black group. Clearly prospective studies are needed to determine causality [30].

2.3.3. Retinal microvascular calibre and catecholamines

SNS activation is present in both diabetes and HT [31] and may be associated with microvascular calibre. Increased perfusion pressure enforces.... contraction in the ocular arteries, which are resistance vessels and regulated by myogenic mechanisms (Bayliss effect) [51]. Retinal microvascular calibre associations with the adrenergic transmitters revealed different profiles in the two ethnic groups. Chronic SNS activation will desensitise the baroreceptors with compensatory increases in BP and PP as was shown in the Black group [1]. In the Black group, the smaller CRAE and a larger CRVE are both associated with epinephrine but not with norepinephrine levels. This may imply that epinephrine will reduce blood flow to the retina by stimulating arteriolar contraction but also increasing the draining of blood away from the retina by stimulating venular dilation. Myogenic tone may however be impaired in Blacks and increase retinal venular widening especially during chronic pressure overload with increased hyperpulsatility. An overactive sympathetic system and/or chronic depression symptoms might therefore explain part of the mechanism. Presently, instead of epinephrine's normal arterial vasodilatory response [52], it induces vasoconstriction, which may suggest hyporesponsivity or down-regulation of the β_2-adrenergic receptors as was also shown previously [1].

Therefore, this hyporesponsivity may be a homeostatic reaction to protect the retina from SNS-stimulated increases in hyperpulsatile pressure in a cohort who has more depressive symptoms. This may be true for both the retina and the brain as emotional stress can also provoke reversible cerebral vasoconstriction similar to retinal vasoconstriction [53].

Both a smaller AVR and a larger CRVE are associated with a greater risk for stroke mortality [7]. This also suggests that β-adrenoceptor hyporesponsivity due to SNS hyperactivity as reflected in lower catecholamine levels might constitute an increased risk for vascular hypertrophy and eventually stroke in the Black male cohort. The same associations were not seen in the White men, maybe as result of their lower depressive symptom scores as well as their lower BP and PP levels. The prevalence of depressive symptoms and possible down-regulated catecholamine profile presuming chronic distress in the Black men compared to their White counterparts, therefore, may explain the differences or lack of association between the catecholamine levels and AVR in the Whites.

2.3.4. Retinal microvascular calibre and local or systemic sympathetic activation

Whether local or systemic catecholamine levels are associated with retinopathy is hotly debated [29, 30]. Recently, both α- and β-adrenergic innervation was demonstrated in the preocular CRA in humans [29]. It seems clear that some aspects of sympathetic transmission regulate choroidal and CRA blood flow by way of changes in vascular smooth muscle tone [54]. The inverse association between AVR and ECR may support a vasodilatory (venular) or vasoconstrictive (arteriolar) tone in the retinal vessels. A notion for vasoconstriction is suggested as a hypertensive state increases peripheral vascular resistance in the retinal arterioles [7]. Therefore, increased or hyperpulsatile PP exerting mechanical stress on the vessel walls may contribute to a diminished β-adrenergic albeit an augmented α-adrenergic responsiveness in Black men [1, 33] and subsequent risk of vascular hypertrophy [1] and possibly arteriolar narrowing. The profile of β-adrenergic hyporesponsivity in Black men emphasises central control of the brain on the circulatory system irrespective of the vascular bed.

Several limitations should be noted. The cross-sectional design of the current study prevents us from being able to infer causality. Studies showing direct evidence of sympathetic tone and retinal vascular remodelling in human models could greatly contribute to our knowledge in this field. Larger sample sizes and more diverse data on autonomic and endothelial function are needed to delineate possible physiological mechanisms and the role of the ageing process. Only an indirect measure of SNS activity via 24 h catecholamine concentrations was measured and more direct measurements should be implemented, along with the determination of the corticosteroid profile. A more representative sample of the whole population is necessary to draw generalised conclusions.

2.4. Conclusions

A profile of β-adrenergic hyporesponsivity was evident in Black men. They revealed more depressive symptoms, indicative of a chronically challenged SNS, which were associated with retinal vascular remodelling and possible vascular hypertrophy. Whether these changes precede or result from hyperpulsatile pressure impacting on retinal autoregulation is still debatable.

Acknowledgements

The present work was partially supported by the North-West Department of Education, South African Medical Research Council, National Research Foundation, North-West University, ROCHE Diagnostics, South Africa, and Metabolic Syndrome Institute, France. We gratefully acknowledge the voluntary collaboration of the participants. The SABPA study would not have been possible without the valuable contributions of co-investigators and technical staff.

Sources of funding

The present work was partially supported by the North-West Department of Education, South African Medical Research Council, National Research Foundation, North-West University, ROCHE Diagnostics, South Africa, and the Metabolic Syndrome Institute, France. None of the funding sources had any other involvement in the study design, data collection, analysis or interpretation or in the writing of the manuscript.

Compliance with ethical standards: The ethics on publishing scientific articles were followed. The authors report no relationships that could be construed as a conflict of interest. Any opinion, findings and conclusions or recommendations expressed in this material are those of the author(s) and therefore the NRFs do not accept any liability in regard thereto.

Abbreviations

ambulatory blood pressure measurement (ABPM)

arteriolar-to-venular ratio (AVR)

blood pressure (BP)

body surface area (BSA)

body mass index (BMI)

cardiovascular disease (CVD)

central retinal arterial equivalent (CRAE)

central retinal artery (CRA)

central retinal venular equivalent (CRVE)

C-reactive protein (CRP)

diastolic blood pressure (DBP)

electrocardiogram (ECG)

http://dx.doi.org/10.5772/63515

epinephrine-to-creatinine ratio (ECR)

gamma glutamyl transferase (γ-GT)

glycated haemoglobin (HbA_{1c})

heart rate variability (HRV)

hypertension (HT)

measuring units, equal to µm in the normal Gullstrand eye (MU)

norepinephrine-to-creatinine ratio (NECR)

Patient Health Questionnaire (PHQ-9)

phenylethanolamine N-methyltransferase (PNMT)

pulse pressure (PP)

Sympathetic activity and **A**mbulatory **B**lood **P**ressure in **A**fricans (**SABPA**) study

sympathetic nervous system (SNS)

systolic blood pressure (SBP)

Author details

Nicolaas T. Malan[1*], Roland von Känel[1,2], Wayne Smith[1], Gavin W. Lambert[3], Walthard Vilser[4], Nina Eikelis[3], Manja Reimann[5] and Leoné Malan[1]

*Address all correspondence to: nico.malan@nwu.ac.za

1 Hypertension in Africa Research Team (HART), Faculty of Health Sciences, North West University, Potchefstroom, South Africa

2 Department of Psychosomatic Medicine, Clinic Barmelweid, Barmelweid, Switzerland

3 Laboratory of Human Neurotransmitters, Baker IDI Heart and Diabetes Institute, Melbourne, Victoria, Australia

4 Imedos GmbH, Jena, Germany

5 Autonomic and Neuroendocrinological Laboratory Dresden, Department of Neurology, University Hospital Carl Gustav Carus, Dresden University of Technology, Dresden, Germany

References

[1] Malan L, Hamer M, Schlaich MP, et al. Defensive coping facilitates higher blood pressure and early sub-clinical structural vascular disease via alterations in heart rate variability: the SABPA study. Atherosclerosis 2013;227:391–97.

[2] Opie LH, Seedat YK. Hypertension in Sub-Saharan populations. Circulation 2005;112:3562–68.

[3] Rizzoni D, Porteri E, Castellano M, et al. Vascular hypertrophy and remodelling in secondary hypertension. Hypertrophy 1996;28:785–90.

[4] Sierra C. Cerebral small vessel disease, cognitive impairment and vascular dementia. Panminerva Med 2012;54:179–188.

[5] Malan L, Hamer M, von Känel R, et al. Chronic depression symptoms and salivary NOx associated with retinal vascular dysregulation: the SABPA study. Nitric Oxide 2016;55–56:11–17. doi: 1016/j.niox.2016.02.008.

[6] Patton N, Aslam T, MacGillivray A, et al. Retinal vascular image analysis a potential screening tool for cerebrovascualr disease: a rationale based on homology between cerebral and retinal microvasculatures. J Anat 2005;206:319–48.

[7] Cheung CY, Ikram K, Sabanayagam C, Wong TY. Retinal microvasculature as a model to study the manifestations of hypertension. Hypertension 2012;60:1094–103.

[8] Li X, Wong LL, Cheung CY, et al. Racial differences in retinal vessel geometric characteristics: a multiethnic study in healthy Asians. Invest Ophthalmol Vis Sci 2013;54:3650–56.

[9] Henderson AD, Bruce BB, Newman NJ, Biousse V. Hypertension-related eye abnormalities and the risk of stroke. Rev Neurol Dis 2011;8:1–9.

[10] Pienaar PR, Micklesfield LK, Gill JMR, et al. Ethnic differences in microvascular function in apparently healthy South African men and women. Exp Physiol 2014;99:985–94.

[11] Malan L, Schutte AE, Malan NT, et al. Specific coping strategies of Africans during urbanization: comparing cardiovascular responses and perception of health data. Biol Psychol 2006;72:305–10.

[12] Hamer M, Malan L. Psychophysiological risk markers of cardiovascular disease. In: Psychophysiological Biomarkers of Health. Special Edition. Neurosci Biobehav Rev 2010;35:76–83.

[13] De Kock A, Malan L, Hamer M, Cockeran M, Malan NT. Defensive coping and renovascular disease risk—adrenal fatigue in a cohort of Africans and Caucasians: the SABPA study. Phys Behav 2015;147:213–19.

[14] de Kock A, Malan L, Hamer M, Malan NT. Defensive coping and subclinical vascular disease risk—associations with autonomic exhaustion in Africans and Caucasians: the SABPA study. Atherosclerosis 2012;225:438–43.

[15] Hamer M, Malan L, Schutte AE, et al. Conventional and behavioral risk factors explain differences in sub-clinical vascular disease between black and Caucasian South Africans: the SABPA study. Atherosclerosis 2011;215:237–42.

[16] Mashele N, Malan L, van Rooyen JM. et al. Blunted neuro-endocrine responses linking depressive symptoms and ECG left ventricular hypertrophy in black Africans: the SABPA study. Cardiovasc Endocrinol 2014;3:59–65.

[17] Armario A, Vallès A, Dal-Zotto S, et al. A single exposure to severe stressors causes long-term desensitisation of the physiological response to the homotypic stressor. Stress 2004;7:157–72.

[18] Petrowski K, Herold U, Joraschky P, Wittchen H, Kirschbaum C. A striking pattern of cortisol non-responsiveness to psychosocial stress in patients with panic disorder with concurrent normal cortisol awakening responses. Psychoneuroendocrinology 2010;35:414–21.

[19] Betito K, Diorio J, Meaney MJ, Boksa P. Adrenal phenylethanolamine N-methyltransferase induction in relation to glucocorticoid receptor dynamics: evidence that acute exposure to high cortisol levels is sufficient to induce the enzyme. J Neurochem 1992;58:1853–62.

[20] Ciaranello RD. Regulation of phenylethanolamine N-methyltransferase. Biochem Pharmacol 1978;27:1895–97.

[21] Hellhammer DH, Wüst S, Kudielka BM. Salivary cortisol as a marker in stress research. Psychoneuroendocrinology 2009;34:163–71.

[22] Young EA, Altemus M. Puberty, ovarian steroids, and stress. Ann N Y Acad Sci 2004;1021:124–33.

[23] Lichtman J, Froelicher ES, Blumenthal JA. et al. Depression as a risk factor for poor prognosis among patients with acute coronary syndrome: Systematic review and recommendations. A Scientific Statement from the American Heart Association. Circulation 2014;129:1350–69.

[24] Mashele N, Malan L, Van Rooyen JM, et al. Depression, cardiometabolic function and left ventricular hypertrophy in African men and women: the SABPA study. J Clin Exp Hypertens 2013;35:213–19.

[25] Burke HM, Fernald LC, Gertler PJ, Adler NE. Depressive symptoms are associated with blunted cortisol stress responses in very low-income women. Psychosom Med 2005;67:211–16.

[26] Burke HM, Davis MC, Otte C, Mohr DC. Depression and cortisol stress response: a meta-analysis. Psychoneuroendocrinology 2005;30:846–56.

[27] Peeters F, Nicholson NA, Berkhof J. Cortisol responses to daily events in major depressive disorder. Psychosom Med 2003;65:836–41.

[28] Gerra G, Zaimovic A, Mascetti GG, et al. Neuroendocrine responses to experimentally induced psychological stress in healthy humans. Psychoneuroendocrinology 2001;26:97–107.

[29] Bergua M, Kapsreiter WL, Neuhuber HA et al. Innervation pattern of the preocular human central retinal artery. Exp Eye Res 2013;110:142–47.

[30] Jensen RA, Shea S, Ranjit N. et al. Psychosocial risk factors and retinal microvascular signs. The Multi-Ethnic Study of Atherosclerosis. Am J Epidemiol 2010;171:522–31.

[31] Schlaich MP, Kaye DM, Lambert E, et al. Relation between cardiac sympathetic activity and hypertensive left ventricular hypertrophy. Circulation 2003;108:560–65.

[32] Malan L, Hamer, M, Frasure-Smith N. et al. COHORT PROFILE: Sympathetic activity and Ambulatory Blood Pressure in Africans (SABPA) Prospective Cohort Study. Int J Epidemiol 2015;44:1814–1822.

[33] Malan NT, Stadler T, Schlaich MP, et al. Chronic distress and acute vascular responses associated with ambulatory blood pressure in low-testosterone African men: the SABPA study. J Hum Hypertens 2014;28:393–98.

[34] Mosteller RD. Simplified calculation of body-surface area. N Eng J Med 1987;317:1098.

[35] Kroenke K, Spitzer RL. The PHQ-9: a new depression diagnostic and severity measure. Psychiatr Ann 2002;32:1–7.

[36] Monahan PO, Shacham E, Reece M, et al. Validity/reliability of PHQ-9 and PHQ-2 depression scales among adults living with HIV/AIDS in Western Kenya. J Gen Intern Med 2009;24:189–97.

[37] Kohara K, Nishida W, Maguchi M, Hiwida K. Autonomic nervous function in non-dipper essential hypertensive participants: evaluation by power spectral analysis of heart rate variability. Hypertension 1995;26:808–14.

[38] Mancia G, Fagard R, Narkiewicz K, et al. ESH/ESC guidelines for the management of arterial hypertension. The Task Force for the management of arterial hypertension of the European Society of Hypertension (ESH) and of the European Society of Cardiology (ESC). J Hypertens 2013;31:1281–357.

[39] Hayman DM, Xiao Y, Yao Q, et al. Alterations in pulse pressure affect artery function. Cell Mol Bioeng 2012;5:474484.

[40] Knudtson MD, Lee KE, Hubbard LD, et al. Revised formulas for summarizing retinal vessel diameters. Curr Eye Res 2003;27:143–49.

[41] Boomsma F, Alberts G, van Eijk L, et al. Optimum collection and storage conditions for catecholamine measurements in human plasma and urine. Clin Chem 1993;39:2503–08.

[42] Nguyen TT, Wang JJ, Sharrett AR. et al. Relationship of retinal vascular caliber with diabetes and retinopathy. Diabetes Care 2008;31:544–49.

[43] Ikram MK, Ong YT, Cheung CY, Wong TY. Retinal vascular caliber measurements: clinical significance, current knowledge and future perspectives. Ophthalmologia 2013; 229: 125–36.

[44] Schram MT, Chaturvedi N, Fuller JH, Stehouwer CD, EURODIAB Prospective Complications Study Group. Pulse pressure is associated with age and cardiovascular disease in type 1 diabetes: the Eurodiab Prospective Complications Study. J Hypertens 2003;21:2035–044.

[45] Liew G, Campbell S, Klein R, et al. Ten-year longitudinal changes in retinal microvascular lesions. The Atherosclerosis Risk in Communities Study. Ophthalmology 2011;118:1612–18.

[46] Grippo A, Johnson AK. Stress, depression and cardiovascular dysregulation: a review of neurobiological mechanisms and the integration of research from preclinical disease models. Stress 2009;12:1–21.

[47] Otte C, Neylan TC, Pipkin SS. et al. Depressive symptoms and 24-hour urinary norepinephrine excretion levels in patients with coronary disease: findings from the Heart and Soul Study. Am J Psychiatry 2005;162:2139–45.

[48] Malan L, Hamer M, Schlaich MP, et al. Facilitated defensive coping, silent ischemia and ECG left ventricular hypertrophy: the SABPA Study. J Hypertens 2012;30:543–50.

[49] Yeung AC, Ganz P, Selwyn AP. Interactions between mental stress and coronary endothelial dysfunction. Homeostasis 1993;34:244–51.

[50] Van Lill AS, Malan L, van Rooyen JM, et al. Baroreceptor sensitivity and left ventricular hypertrophy in urban South African men: the SABPA study. Blood Pressure 2011;20:355–61.

[51] Feihl F, Liaudet L, Waeber B, Levy BI. Hypertension: a disease of the microcirculation. Hypertension 2006;48:1012–17.

[52] Opie LH. Heart Physiology—From Cell to Circulation, 4th ed. Philadelphia: Lippincott Williams & Wilkins, 2004: 421 p.

[53] Flammer J. Psychophysical mechanisms and treatment of vasospastic disorders in normal-tension glaucoma. Bull Soc Belge Opthalmol 1992;244:129–34.

[54] Steinle JJ, Smith PG. Role of adrenergic receptors in vascular remodelling of the rat choroid. Brit J Pharmacol 2002;136:730–34.

Chapter 7

Pathogenesis of Leukoaraiosis: A Review

Matija Zupan

Additional information is available at the end of the chapter

http://dx.doi.org/10.5772/63655

Abstract

Leukoaraiosis (LA) represents the most common phenotype of cerebral small vessel disease. It is of undoubted significance regarding its vast prevalence and neuropsychiatric consequences, such as cognitive impairment, higher risk for ischaemic stroke and death. It has been associated with increasing age and conventional vascular risk factors (VRF). Despite huge efforts, LA pathogenesis is still incompletely understood. The hypotheses of ischaemia and malfunctioning blood-brain barrier seem to oppose each other. Hence, the focus has turned to endothelial dysfunction, through which both aforementioned mechanisms could be coupled. The VRF, which are almost universally present in patients with LA, have a detrimental impact on endothelium on their own. However, in LA there may be an additional or even primary endothelial dysfunction at play. This seems to be at the core of LA pathogenesis, leading to chronic ischaemia in cerebral white matter and blood-brain barrier dysfunction culminating in LA. The genetic susceptibility to harmful effects of VRF on endothelial function seems to play an important role. Regarding the burden of LA, interventional approaches should be aimed at decelerating or even halting the progression of the disease. These should focus on strict management of VRF and strategies to enhance endothelial function.

Keywords: cerebral small vessel disease, endothelial dysfunction, leukoaraiosis, pathogenesis, L-arginine

1. Introduction

Leukoaraiosis (LA) represents the most common phenotype of cerebral small vessel disease (CSWD) [1]. It is of undoubted clinical significance regarding its vast prevalence (10–27% in otherwise healthy subjects between 50 and 75 years of age) and neuropsychiatric consequences, such as cognitive impairment, higher risk for ischaemic stroke and death [2]. It has been associated with increasing age and conventional vascular risk factors (VRF), such as arterial hypertension

(AH). Despite huge efforts, LA pathogenesis is still incompletely understood. The hypotheses of ischaemia [3] and malfunctioning blood-brain barrier (BBB) [4] seem to oppose each other. Hence, the focus has turned to endothelial dysfunction, which may explain both aforementioned mechanisms [5]. The VRF, which are almost universally present in patients with LA, have a detrimental impact on endothelium on their own. LA pathogenesis mirrors the interplay between various factors. Endothelial dysfunction seems to be at the core of LA pathogenesis, leading to chronic ischaemia in cerebral white matter (WM) and BBB dysfunction culminating in LA. The genetic susceptibility to harmful effects of VRF on endothelial function seems to play an important role besides the presence and the extent of VRF [6]. Endothelial dysfunction could even be the primary event in LA pathogenesis [7]. Regarding the clinical and socioeconomic burden of LA, interventional approaches should aim at decelerating or even halting the progression of the disease. In the author's view, these should focus on strict management of VRF and strategies to enhance endothelial function in patients with LA.

This chapter outlines the different concepts of LA pathogenesis. The LA pathophysiology will be thoroughly presented, covering basic principles, such as cerebral microcirculation, autoregulation and blood pressure regulation, the interplay between VRF and LA, the role of endothelial function, various functions of nitric oxide (NO) and L-arginine. The differences in LA pathogenesis in different WM regions will be presented. The alternative hypotheses of LA pathogenesis will also be covered. The proposed genetic mechanisms putatively involved in LA pathogenesis will also be mentioned. To conclude, the interventional approaches with the aim of actively influencing the natural path of the disease will be outlined.

2. Definition of cerebral small vessel disease

2.1. Leukoaraiosis

Cerebral small vessel disease is a frequent finding on neuroradiological imaging in elderly population. Leukoaraiosis is a common term denoting diffuse confluent changes of WM with often irregular margins in elderly population with VRF [8]. The changes are hypodense on computer tomographic images (CT) and hyperintensive on T2-weighted and flow-attenuated inversion recovery (FLAIR) magnetic resonance images (MRI). Their appearance directly reflects a higher proton density and water content in the affected WM. The term was used for the first time in 1987 to describe changes in subcortical WM on CT [9]. The WM changes were bilateral, symmetric, diffuse and restricted to periventricular regions extending to semioval centre. The first recognition of CSWD dates back to the late nineteenth century (Binswanger and Alzheimer), but from today's perspective their patients probably had diseased cerebral vessels due to neurosyphilis [10]. With the advent of modern imaging techniques in the 1970s, it was possible for the first time to show WM lesions *in vivo*. The scientific community had thought for a long time that LA is merely a coincidental finding without any significant clinical consequences. Especially during the recent years, we have seen many new discoveries showing that LA is associated with cognitive impairment and higher risk for stroke and death [2]. It is known that LA is a risk factor for dementia and myocardial infarction [11]. In patients older than 60 years, one-sixth of the population develops dementia and another sixth stroke. Taken together, one-third of the population is affected. Leukoaraiosis is more prevalent in patients who have already sustained a stroke. It is also known that the presence of LA represents a risk factor for the first and consequent strokes. The association between LA and stroke can be regarded in two different ways. Stroke and LA share the same VRF. In LA there is a chronic WM perfusion impairment, which is more prone to the development of a frank ischaemic infarction. There is a strong association between LA and lacunar infarctions (LI), which are both part of the wide spectrum of CSWD and frequently coexist in the same patient. Leukoaraiosis is also associated with cerebral atrophy. The progression of LA is associated with declining WM and cerebral grey matter (GM) mass; consequentially, the cerebral ventricles enlarge. Atrophy of GM could be regarded as the consequence of deafferentation, because the loss of subcortical WM leads to the interruption of corticosubcortical connections.

2.2. Other manifestations of cerebral small vessel disease

Lacunar infarctions develop due to the occlusion of small perforate arteries and represent the second manifestation of CSWD, albeit with different pathophysiology. Enlarged Virchow-Robin perivascular spaces are a frequent finding in CSWD and normally appear in the vicinity of the affected vessels. On CT they can easily be confused with LI, but one can definitely distinguish them from LI on MRI. Cerebral microbleeds are small intraparenchymal bleeds in perivascular spaces and represent the leakage of blood constituents through the affected vessel wall and can frequently be encountered in LA, especially in cerebral amyloid angiopathy and also in patients with untreated AH. They may harbour a greater risk for frank cerebral intraparenchymal bleed, especially if patients are prescribed anticoagulants.

3. Risk factors for developing leukoaraiosis

Although some studies have not revealed the association between LA and VRF, the former is more frequently found in patients with a history of stroke and putative vascular cognitive impairment. The most significant risk factors for LA are cerebrovascular and cardiovascular diseases [12]. The prevalence of LA typically rises with age. There is a close, albeit not exclusive, association with AH and antihypertensive therapy. A very significant risk factor for LA is advancing age. Although LA should be regarded as a pathological entity, it could at least partly be a process of normal ageing. It is not clear at what age LA begins to develop. There are no conclusive data on the "normal" extent of LA for any given age. According to the majority of studies, at least scant WM changes could be expected in subjects older than 50 or 65 years. Systematic review of studies has not revealed significant differences in LA prevalence among sexes. Possibly, LA is more prevalent in blacks compared to Caucasians mainly due to higher prevalence of AH in blacks, whereby it is usually also less well treated with resultant higher absolute values of arterial blood pressure (ABP). Blacks could even be more prone to the harmful effects of AH. Arterial hypertension is the strongest modifiable risk factor for LA [12]. According to different studies, it is present in 24.6 to 54.9% of LA patients [13]. Both higher systolic and diastolic pressures contribute. There is no threshold level of ABP above which LA starts to emerge, but merely the association represents a continuum. Diurnal swaying of ABP is also important. Recently published data from the United States revealed that higher pulse pressure has a significant influence on progression of cognitive impairment in people over 45 years of age [14].

Diabetes mellitus (DM) has been implicated especially in the formation of periventricular LA. Higher blood glucose fasting levels are associated with LA. The finding that higher levels of insulin were found in patients with DM and LA may suggest that insulin resistance could be a risk factor for developing LA. However, the pathophysiological mechanisms are presently unknown. On the other hand, many studies have not found a significant correlation between LA and DM. Dyslipidemia (especially elevated LDL level) is an important risk factor for atherosclerosis of large vessels, whereas its influence on developing LA is less well known. In some studies, lower HDL values and hypertriglyceridemia were associated with higher risk for developing LA, in others obviously not. Smoking tobacco has been associated with LA in some studies only.

The association between LA and atherosclerosis of large vessels is controversial. Some studies have failed to demonstrate any significant association, whereas in others the association between the two existed [15, 16]. The possible common denominator might be VRF, meaning that atherosclerosis and LA occur independently but contemporarily. On the other hand, it is known that narrowing of lumina of large vessels leads to higher risk for chronic ischaemia and LA [1]. The association between ischaemic heart disease (IHD) and LA could not be regarded as causative but merely as the consequence of the fact that the two share the same VRF. Some studies have succeeded in showing the association between LA and IHD, whereas others have not [17, 18]. The association between lower values of vitamin B_{12} and especially periventricular LA has been shown in some studies. It is known that lower values of vitamin B_{12} and hyper-homocysteinaemia, which can be the consequence of vitamin B_{12} depletion, could be associated with LA [19]. However, there are no relevant data, which suggest that supplementing vitamin B_{12} and/or lowering homocysteine levels would improve LA or decelerate its progression.

Cerebral autosomal dominant arteriopathy with subcortical infarctions and leukoencephal-opathy (CADASIL) manifests with LA as well, although it is a very infrequent cause of LA in population [20]. Small arteries in brain, skin and peripheral nerves show granular osmiophilic deposits in tunica media, with arterial lumen being narrowed due to high electronic density deposits [21]. Normal autoregulatory mechanisms are disturbed due to structural changes in smooth muscle cells leading to WM malfunction. Genetic factors may play an important role in LA according to studies where the association between LA and polymorphisms of numerous genes, for instance for angiotensin convertase and apolipoprotein(a) have been found [22]. Such factors are not necessarily directly associated with the presence of LA but could determine subject's proneness to the development of risk factors for LA or his/her susceptibility to develop end organ damage as the consequence of that risk factor. The susceptibility to develop AH and LA as the consequence of AH is partially genetically determined. Far less commonly, LA could be brought about by many different pathological mechanisms such as neurodegenerative diseases (Alzheimer's, inherited amyloid angiopathies), infections (HIV), inflammations (multiple sclerosis, neurolupus), traumatic head injuries, brain irradiation, cerebrospinal fluid disturbances, chemotherapeutics and metabolic disease, including mitochondriopathies, leukodistrophies and others (e.g., Fabry's disease).

4. Pathophysiology

4.1. Cerebral blood flow and autoregulation

Brain is a highly metabolic organ with autonomous autoregulation, which enables constant cerebral blood flow (CBF) despite fluctuations in mean arterial pressure (MAP). Cerebral autoregulation is in the domain of small cerebral arteries and arterioles. Cerebral autoregulation is divided into mechanoregulation and chemoregulation. Mechanoregulation depends on transmural pressure and endothelial vasodilatation, whereas chemoregulation depends on serum CO_2 level [23]. Endothelial vasodilatation in cerebral vascular bed is of much greater amplitude compared to other regions [24]. Mechanoregulation seems to be the main regulatory mechanism of CBF. On the other hand, chemoregulation has an important influence on CBF during metabolic disturbances and is, unlikely to mechanoregulation, independent of fluctuations in MAP [23]. Both autoregulatory mechanisms function independent of each other. Although their cellular mechanisms are not completely understood, NO seems to play the crucial role, since it is needed for maintaining chemoregulation of CBF [25]. A significant mechanism of regulation of majority of vascular beds is preserved endothelial function. Disturbed function of cerebral endothelium results in diminished release of endothelial NO, culminating in attenuated relaxation of vascular smooth muscle cells of small arteries. Animal and human studies have revealed that mechanoregulation is not diminished despite ageing and other diseases affecting endothelium [26]. Contrary to this, many studies have shown that chemoregulation of CBF depends on the integrity of endothelium. Attenuated chemoregulation has been found in patients with cerebral endothelial dysfunction [27].

4.2. Arterial blood pressure deregulation

It is known that all symptomatic patients with LA do not have AH. Arterial blood pressure deregulation is very complicated, putatively adding to the pathogenesis of LA [12]. Patients with LA had higher levels of ABP and distinct circadian rhythm of ABP with large daily fluctuations or absence of nocturnal physiological fall of ABP [28]. Frequent periods of hypotension in symptomatic patients with LA speak in favour of disturbed cerebral autoregulation in patients with AH and higher burden of periventricular LA. Cerebral autoregulatory mechanisms maintain constant CBF in the MAP interval between 60 and 150 mmHg despite swaying of systemic ABP. Unlike other bodily regions, great intracranial arteries as well as extracranial parts of carotid arteries play an important role in regulation of vascular resistance of cerebral circulation. We should not overlook physiological responses of small cerebral vessels, which are crucial for autoregulation. Their response to ABP depends on their diameter. In cats, fluctuations in MAP between 110 and 160 mmHg provoke only pial arteries wider than 200 μm to respond. Arterioles narrower than 100 μm only dilate at MAP less than 90 mmHg [29]. In MAP less than 70 mmHg, the rate of their widening is larger than in wider vessels.

We presume similar mechanisms are at play in humans. In patients with AH and arteriolosclerotic arteries, fall of ABP brought about by cardiac arrhythmia or disturbed autoregulation can lead to fall of CBF due to the inability of sclerotic vessels to dilate [30]. In patients with AH, autoregulatory boundaries are shifted upwards [31]. Quick fall of ABP in physiological boundaries can significantly lower CBF in WM of patients with chronic AH [32]. In this way, WM of AH patient develops ischaemia at ABP levels which could still be regarded as normal in normotensives [32]. Furthermore, autoregulatory responses of vessels in WM of experimental animals are less efficient as in GM vessels, so at lower values of ABP, falls of CBF are more pronounced in WM compared to GM [33].

4.3. Pathological hallmarks of leukoaraiosis

Oedema, ischaemia and degenerative changes of subcortical WM are principal pathologic characteristics reflecting LA on CT or MRI. Ischaemia probably involved in LA formation includes transitory events characterised by falls of regional CBF culminating in incomplete infarction, a scenario which can be tested in experimental models. Histopathologic studies on rat brain show that oligodendrocytes and myelinated axons are very prone to ischaemic damage. Chronic cerebral hypoperfusion leads to progressive rarefaction and glial activation of WM. Occlusion of rat middle cerebral artery lasting more than 24 hours leads to swelling of oligodendrocytes in subcortical WM after 30 minutes [34]. After 3-hour duration of the occlusion, oligodendrocytes already show irreversible signs of injury like pyknosis and rupture of plasmalemma. Vacuolisation of WM is the consequence of spaces which emerge by the separation of internal myelin sheath from axolemma and also from an increase of extracellular space and swelling of astrocytic processes. All changes described appear prior to irreversible neuronal injury with eosinophilia which implies that early damage of WM is independent of injury to the neuronal perikaryon. In rat models with bilateral occlusion of internal carotid arteries, two consistent types of WM changes have been noted, namely reactive astrogliosis and unspecific rarefaction of WM [35]. It is very important that increased accumulation of extracellular fluid and astrogliosis are also two main pathohistological changes in those areas where CT and MRI reveal LA in humans.

4.4. Leukoaraiosis in different regions of cerebral white matter

Progression of LA follows a uniformed pattern. In the beginning, periventricular lesions on top of horns of lateral ventricles develop (capping) progressing around the ventricles. The LA changes in deep WM initially appear in frontal lobes, then parietooccipital lobes, far less frequently in brainstem and basal ganglia. They very seldom affect temporal lobes, which are typically affected in CADASIL. At first the changes are punctiform, single, but in time they merge and become confluent affecting the whole area. The mechanisms of LA development depend on local blood circulation of a particular subcortical WM region.

4.4.1. Blood supply of different parts of cerebral white matter

The majority of cerebral hemispheric WM is supplied by long penetrant arteries stemming perpendicularly from subarachnoid arteries of pial network on the brain surface. They travel through cortical layers perpendicularly relative to brain surface and enter WM together with myelinated fibres [12]. Penetrant arteries are 20–50 mm long and 100–200 μm wide [12]. They give rise to tiny branches supplying a cylindrical section of WM, known as metabolic unit [12]. Juxtaventricular WM is supplied by ventriculofugal branches of subependymal arteries, which are 15 mm in length, stemming from choroid arteries or end branches of striatal arteries.

4.4.2. Juxtaventricular leukoaraiosis

This form of LA is up to 3 mm away from lateral ventricles and starts ventricularly where there is redundant blood supply, so it is not primarily caused by ischaemia, but demyelination with resultant subependymal gliosis and disruption of ependyma, less frequently granular ependymitis or venous congestion due to collagenosis of veins. Studies support the hypothesis of "leaking" of ventricular walls. Comparable type of LA around horns of lateral ventricles develops in patients with hydrocephalus.

4.4.3. Periventricular leukoaraiosis

Ventriculofugal branches supplying parts of basal ganglia, internal capsule and thalamus stem from arteries of circle of Willis [36]. Ventriculofugal branches travel towards penetrant centripetal arteries of the pial system but seldom, if ever, form anastomoses with them [37]. Leukoaraiosis more than 3 mm away from lateral ventricles is normally ischaemic in origin and emerges as the consequence of microcystic infarctions and local myelin rarefactions [38]. Periventricular WM 3–13 mm away from lateral ventricles represents the border zone between ventricular and cortical blood supply, which is prone to ischaemic impairment due to local or systemic lowering of CBF [39]. Arteriolosclerosis, tortuosity and arterial elongation in elderly people with AH are a probable cause for decrease of CBF in WM [40]. Periventricular WM is prone to ischaemia already at moderate falls of CBF due to the scarcity of anastomoses between the branches of long medullary penetrant arteries [37]. Such periventricular LA is often associated with large vessel disease, atherosclerosis of the aorta or internal carotid artery, smoking, hypercholesterolemia, myocardial infarction or peripheral artery disease [41].

4.4.4. Leukoaraiosis in deep white matter and juxtacortical leukoaraiosis

Deep WM more than 13 mm away from lateral ventricles is supplied by medullary arteries stemming without collaterals from cortical branches of middle cerebral arteries and are substrate of CSWD pathologically associated with fibrohyalinosis and arteriolosclerosis due to hyperhomocysteinaemia and AH [42]. Lacunar infarctions are more frequent in this part of WM than elsewhere. White matter directly beneath cerebral cortex and up to 3 to 4 mm away (U fibres) is supplied by medullary as well as corticomedullary arterioles and arteries showing juxtacortical LA [43]. Mechanisms of its development are far more diverse (demyelination) and not always of ischaemic origin. In ischaemic LA, the U fibres are typically spared [12].

4.5. Ischaemic hypothesis

A strong epidemiologic association between LA and many cerebrovascular diseases speaks in favour of ischaemia playing a significant role in LA emergence and progression [12]. Ageing, chronic AH and DM share a common substrate for the type of changes these conditions trigger in small penetrant WM arteries and arterioles. These changes include substitution of smooth muscle cells with fibrohyalinous material together with thickening of vessel wall and narrowing of vessel lumen (arteriolosclerosis) [44]. Arteriolosclerosis found almost universally in LA areas is probably one of the reasons for altered blood flow in WM leading to localised ischaemic regions of necrosis and cavitations—lacunar infarctions—or diffuse rarefaction of WM-LA. In LA, diminished CBF in WM has been found. Some authors describe changes of CBF in the whole brain or only in the GM of patients with LA [12]. There are, however, only few studies comparing regional CBF in areas with and without LA. One of these found lowered CBF in regions of LA compared to normal WM [45]. Similarly, diminished regional CBF has been found applying SPECT and xenon CT imaging [46]. Decreased regional CBF in LA regions needs to be proven at first. This leaves an open question whether fall of CBF is the cause of LA or just reflects lower metabolic needs of WM, which has atrophied due to other reasons. Therefore, it is difficult to claim whether lower CBF is the cause or just a consequence of tissue damage. Decreased CBF in non-demented patients with LA has been found in frontal and parietal WM but not in occipital lobes [47]. This may reflect the fact that LA pathogenesis probably depends on its topographic localisation in the brain. In patients with less extensive, localised LA, the changes of CBF have not been shown; probably due to the fact that pathogenesis of initial LA stages differs from that of extensive diffuse lesions. It is interesting that CBF in WM measured by MRI perfusion was decreased even in the regions where there are no changes in T2-sequences [3]. Hence, the whole picture is much more complex than one might think at the first glance. Applying new imaging techniques, significant alterations of WM integrity have been discovered in regions appearing normal on T2-weighted sequences [48]. Structurally normal WM does not necessarily imply it functions properly, so it is possible that CBF is decreased secondarily.

4.6. Hypothesis of a leaky blood-brain barrier

The second hypothesis states that malfunctioning BBB leads to injury of WM due to the toxic effects of serum proteins [4]. The diseased endothelium enables serum proteins to enter into the vessel wall causing its swelling leading to hyaline degeneration and fibrosis. This further leads to thickening of vessel wall, narrowing of vessel lumen, decreased blood flow and chronic ischaemia of WM. On the other hand, endothelial dysfunction leads to decomposition of BBB [49]. The plasma constituents to which BBB is normally impermeable can now pass through BBB and enter cerebral interstitium and brain parenchyma, harming neurones and glial cells. These regions manifest as LA on CT/MRI and in pathologic specimens. In regions of LA, WM was full of extravasated serum proteins like IgG, complement and fibrinogen [50]. This may show that the diseased WM can be the place where BBB is leaking. Magnetic resonance imaging with contrast medium showed diminished integrity of BBB which is associated with the stage of LA expression [51]. What is more, BBB permeability is enhanced even in those regions not showing frank LA on imaging [50]. In longitudinal studies, new LA areas have been found in the regions with abnormal blood perfusion or altered BBB permeability [52].

4.7. Endothelial hypothesis

4.7.1. Endothelium

Vasomotor role of endothelium has already been proven. Mediators of cerebral endothelium have been determined functioning through endothelial G-protein coupled receptors (acetylcholine, bradykinin, ATP), intermediary mediators, like NO, some prostanoids and endothelially derived hyperpolarising factor (EDHF). Endothelium releases not only vasodilator but also vasoconstrictive substances, such as endothelin-1. It is not surprising that in light of the complexity of endothelial vasomotor activity, one can conclude that any endothelial injury may lead to its aberrant function. The preserved endothelial function is crucial for undisturbed function of cerebrovascular circulation. Endothelial dysfunction is best researched in patients with VRF such as AH and DM. Both conditions have detrimental impact on endothelially derived NO [53]. It is clear that defective endothelial release of NO is the main indicator of endothelial dysfunction. The same holds true for the influence of ageing on endothelial dysfunction, which could represent an important part of LA pathogenesis. Recently, focus has turned to immune response playing a significant role in LA (neuroinflammation) [52]. It has been shown that cerebral tissue in the vicinity of LA regions includes many foamy macrophages, activated astrocytes and microglia, which speaks in favour of vivid communication between astroglia, pericytes and endothelium [54]. Increased expression of inflammatory indicators in these areas like apolipoprotein E, alfa2-microglobuline and IgG possibly adds to pathophysiological processes leading to LA [55].

4.7.2. Endothelial dysfunction

Recently, the role of endothelial dysfunction in different vascular diseases has been highly debated. It is known that endothelial dysfunction can be brought about by different VRF, metabolic diseases, systemic and local inflammation [7]. Even in LA, there are more and more data showing that endothelium is implicated in its beginning and progression. Hypotheses of decreased blood flow in WM and diseased BBB are mutually exclusionary but could be coupled through endothelial dysfunction. Endothelial dysfunction might play an important role and can be one of the first steps in developing ischaemia due to CSWD [56]. Probably endothelial dysfunction is not specific to LA and occurs in other cerebrovascular diseases as well [57]. Endothelial dysfunction leads to BBB malfunction, diseased autoregulation of CBF and prothrombotic changes. During endothelial activation, some molecules are released to the blood in higher quantities. These can be determined laboratorially, such as intercellular adhesion molecule 1, thrombomodulin and tissue factor and tissue factor pathway inhibitor [58]. Indicators of endothelial dysfunction are lipoprotein-associated phospholipase A2, myeloperoxidase and high-sensitivity C-reactive protein, as well as tumour necrosis factor alpha and interleukin-6 [59]. Inflammation in vessel wall obviously plays an important role in formation and progression of LA [60]. Asymmetric dimethylarginine is a circulating endogenous inhibitor of NO and as such implicated in endothelial dysfunction, especially together with hyperhomocysteinaemia [61]. Homocysteine concentrations correlate with the degree of LA. Hyperhomocysteinaemia is an independent risk factor for LA, since homocysteine is toxic to endothelium [19]. Some studies mention the role of endothelial germ cells implicated in repairing endothelium. A special type of haptoglobin (phenotype 1-1) was associated with decreased ability of endothelium to repair its damage [62].

In a preliminary study conducted by the author of this review and his co-workers, it was found that cerebrovascular reactivity to L-arginine (CVR), an estimate of cerebral endothelial function, and flow-mediated dilatation (FMD) of the right brachial artery, an estimate of systemic endothelial function, were significantly diminished in patients with LA compared to control subjects with identical VRF without LA [7]. Moreover, CVR and FMD correlated positively in LA patients and the degree of cerebrovascular as well as systemic endothelial dysfunctions correlated with the degree of LA [7]. Overall, these results suggest that in patients with LA, both cerebral and systemic endothelial functions are impaired to the degrees that are much higher than could be expected based on present VRF. These results seem to reveal a so far unreported, more than expected additional impairment of cerebral endothelial function alongside systemic endothelial function, which is probably involved in LA pathophysiology.

4.7.3. L-arginine

Up until now, some studies have been performed about the effects of L-arginine on cerebral vasculature, in majority of cases on animal models [63]. L-arginine serves as a donor of NO through NO synthetase (NOS). L-arginine is also known as the most potent vasodilator and is the primary determinant of vascular tone, especially in cerebral vasculature [63]. Among the three isoforms of NOS, the endothelial (eNOS) seems to be of utmost importance in NO-mediated dilatation of cerebral arteries and arterioles [63]. NO forms endogenously as well as exogenously *in vivo*. L-arginine is the main source of endogenous NO. Contrary to endogenous L-arginine, exogenously derived L-arginine not only releases NO in this way but also through releasing other vasoactive substances [64]. The main exogenous sources of NO are NO donors releasing NO through NOS-independent mechanisms. Examples are organic nitrates and sodium nitroprusside. Endothelially derived NO is released constantly in basic quantities (tonically), whereas diverse stimuli dynamically increase its formation. After forming, NO merges with the nearby vascular smooth muscle and other cells. NO effect is short-lived due to quick inactivation. In target cells, NO activates guanylate cyclase with resultant rise of intracellular concentration of cyclic guanosine monophosphate (cGMP). Higher concentration of cGMP leads to lower intracellular calcium concentration in vascular smooth muscle cells and resultant vasodilatation.

L-arginine influences vascular endothelial cells and consequentially blood flow. L-arginine infusion causes vasodilatation and enhanced blood flow in many vascular beds [49]. Animal and clinical studies have shown that L-arginine not only leads to vasodilatation through endothelially derived NO but also decelerates thrombotic activity, cell proliferation, inflammation and other processes, which culminate in cardiovascular diseases. L-arginine prevents and diminishes the consequences of already present atherosclerosis, decelerating adhesion of monocytes on endothelium, lowers ABP in some patients with AH and returns normal endothelial function in hypercholesterolemia [65]. Its application seems to be safe [66].

4.8. Alternative hypotheses of leukoaraiosis pathophysiology

Patients with normotensive hydrocephalus (NTH) have a high prevalence of WM changes. Experimental hydrocephalus in dogs leads to reversible WM changes after shunting has been performed [12]. This was the base for hypothesising that disturbances in cerebrospinal fluid (CSF) circulation may play an important role in pathogenesis of LA, especially of extensive periventricular changes [67]. The increased accumulation of CSF in ventricles leads to higher interstitial pressure in periventricular parenchyma and resultant ischaemia of WM. This is supported by observations that in NTH, blood flow in WM returns to normal values after CSF shunting with resultant diminishing of intraventricular pressure. Leaking of CSF into adjacent brain parenchyma may be the consequence of structural changes of ependymal cells.

White matter changes similar to those in LA (myelin pallor sparing U fibres with reactive astrogliosis and thickened small vessels) have been described in circumstances where brain oedema represents a precursor of LA [12]. In this way, transitory cerebral oedema might be additional cause of WM changes. Higher content of interstitial fluid in WM of patients with LA giving the appearance of hypodensity on CT images can be the consequence of AH and resultant changes of BBB becoming more permeable. In AH patients, capillary permeability to proteins may also be increased. Simultaneously, apart from long-term effects of AH, even short-lived hypertensive outbursts may provoke transudation of fluid and transfer of proteins into brain interstitium [12].

It is known that a substantial proportion of patients with Alzheimer's disease (AD) has radiological and pathohistological changes of WM resembling LA, albeit to a lesser degree compared to patients with cerebrovascular diseases [68]. It is highly unlikely that LA in AD only reflects Wallerian degeneration due to cortical neuronal loss. It is known that histological markers of Wallerian degeneration such as lipid-laden macrophages are missing in the majority of LA lesions. The mismatch between the degree of changes in adjacent cortical GM and WM speaks against this hypothesis. In AD patients, LA can be the consequence of ischaemia due to structural changes in small cerebral vessels in the scope of amyloid angiopathy present in 90% of AD patients [69]. The hypothesis of amyloid angiopathy in AD being causally associated with LA is further supported by the fact that LA has been found in patients with cerebral amyloid angiopathy without changes typical of AD.

5. Intervention studies: a possibility to influence the natural path of leukoaraiosis

In the light of undoubted clinical consequences, understanding LA pathophysiology is important from the viewpoint of its prevention and decelerating its progression [70]. Patients with risk factors for LA could be treated with medications to prevent its occurrence. It is presently thought that LA changes already present seem to be irreversible. It is believed that in order to prevent LA occurrence and decelerate its progression, optimal control of all VRF in a given person is crucial [71]. There is at present relatively scarce evidence that any type of intervention would decelerate or halt the progression of LA. These data come mostly from observational studies and far less frequently from controlled randomised studies. Antihypertensives turned out to postpone the occurrence of LA and decelerate its progression regarding the results of the EVA MRI study [72]. In the PROGRESS study, treatment with diuretic and ACE inhibitor was efficient in halting or decelerating the rate of LA progression in patients with baseline extensive LA [73]. For the time being, there is no compelling evidence that lowering ABP triggers ischaemia in WM alongside disturbed autoregulation.

Regarding the association between stroke and LA, it seems reasonable to lower the risk for stroke by standard medications in its secondary prevention, namely antiaggregation agents and statins. Statins have long been known for their enhancement of endothelial function and cerebral vasomotor reactivity, but there is little clinical evidence for their efficacy in LA. Statins turned out to be associated with deceleration of LA progression at already progressed LA but not in cases with mild initial stages of LA [74]. On the other hand, in the PROSPER study, beneficial effects of pravastatin on LA progression in elderly patients with high risk for vascular complications were not found [75]. Some recent studies report beneficial effects of low doses of fluvastatin and valsartan on the compliance of large arteries or arterial aging [76–78]. In these studies, the research focused on large arteries, whereas in LA small cerebral vessels are affected. Despite this, there is a growing body of evidence that large vessel disease characterised by decreased compliance of vessel wall reflects in pathological changes of cerebral small vessels. This is summed up in the concept of pulse-wave encephalopathy [79]. One could hypothesise that enhancing the compliance of a large artery may lead to halting effects on LA progression. This may offer sound basis for future intervention studies in LA.

The use of acetylsalicylic acid (ASA) inhibiting cyclooxygenase has potential benefits in LA. Cyclooxygenase catalyses biochemical reactions in which superoxide free radicals form inside endothelial cells. In this way, ASA may decrease endothelial impairment and simultaneously inhibit matrix metalloproteinases which are probably involved in progression of LA changes [21]. Dipyridamole, an antiaggregation agent together with its vasodilator effect, may be involved in decelerating LA progression since it lowers ABP [80]. However, at present, relevant data showing undoubted efficiency of antiaggregation agents on LA progression or improved clinical outcomes in LA patients are missing. Substituting L-arginine has been safe and efficient in many other vascular diseases. On the basis of L-arginine's known effects, it is an interesting presumption that long-term oral administration of high doses of L-arginine could result in decelerating LA progression as well as having a positive influence on clinical consequences [81–83].

6. Conclusion

Leukoaraiosis represents the most common phenotype of CSWD of undoubted clinical significance. It has been associated with increasing age and conventional VRF. Despite huge efforts, the LA pathogenesis is still incompletely understood. The hypotheses of ischaemia and malfunctioning BBB seem to oppose each other. Endothelial dysfunction seems to be at the core of LA pathogenesis, leading to chronic ischaemia in WM and BBB dysfunction. The genetic susceptibility to harmful effects of VRF on endothelial function seems to play an important role. Interventional approaches should aim at decelerating or even halting the progression of the disease.

Author details

Matija Zupan

Address all correspondence to: matija.zupan@kclj.si

Department of Neurology, University Medical Centre Ljubljana, Ljubljana, Slovenia

References

[1] Grueter BE, Schulz UG. Age-related cerebral white matter disease (leukoaraiosis): a review. *Postgrad Med J* 2012, 1036:79–87. doi: 10.1136/postgradmedj-2011-130307.

[2] The LADIS study group. Deterioration of gait and balance over time: the effects of age-related white matter change – the LADIS study. *Cerebrovasc Dis* 2013, 35:544–53.

[3] O'Sullivan M, Lythgoe DJ, Pereira AC et al. Patterns of cerebral blood flow reduction in patients with ischaemic leukoaraiosis. *Neurology* 2002, 59:321–6.

[4] Wardlaw JM, Sandercock PA, Dennis MS et al. Is breakdown of the blood-brain barrier responsible for lacunar stroke, leukoaraiosis, and dementia? *Stroke* 2003, 34:806–12.

[5] Birns J, Jarosz J, Markus HS et al. Cerebrovascular reactivity and dynamic autoregulation in ischaemic subcortical white matter disease. *J Neurol Neurosurg Psychiatry* 2009, 80:1093–8.

[6] Markus HS. Genes, endothelial function and cerebral small vessel disease in man. *Exp Physiol* 2008, 93:121–7.

[7] Zupan M, Šabović M, Zaletel M et al. The presence of cerebral and/or systemic endothelial dysfunction in patients with leukoaraiosis – a case control pilot study. *BMC Neurol* 2015, 15:158. doi: 10.1186/s12883-015-0416-z.

[8] Fazekas F, Chawluk JB, Alavi A et al. MR signal abnormalities at 1.5 T in Alzheimer's dementia and normal aging. *AJR Am J Roentgenol* 1987, 149:351–6.

[9] Hachinski VC, Potter P, Merskey H. Leuko-araiosis. *Arch Neurol* 1987, 44:21–3.

[10] Binswanger O. The definition of general progressive paralysis. Berl Klin Wochenschr 1894, 31:1180–6.

[11] van Swieten JC, Hijdra A, Koudstaal PJ et al. Grading white matter lesions on CT and MRI: a simple scale. *J Neurol Neurosurg Psychiatry* 1990, 53:1080–3.

[12] Pantoni L, Garcia JH. Pathogenesis of leukoaraiosis: a review. *Stroke* 1997, 28(3):652–9.

[13] Goldstein IB, Bartzokis G, Hance DB et al. Relationship between blood pressure and subcortical lesions in healthy elderly people. *Stroke* 1998, 29(4):765–72.

[14] Levine D, Galecki A, Langa K et al. Systolic and diastolic blood pressure and cognitive decline over six years. Abstract from "9th International Congress on Vascular Dementia 2015", Oct 16–18 2015, Ljubljana, Slovenia.

[15] Khan U, Porteous L, Hassan A et al. Risk factor profile of cerebral small vessel disease and its subtypes. *J Neurol Neurosurg Psychiatry* 2007, 78:702–6.

[16] Ohmine T, Miwa Y, Yao H et al. Association between arterial stiffness and cerebral white matter lesions in community-dwelling elderly subjects. *Hypertens Res* 2008, 31:75–81.

[17] Ikram MA, van Oijen M, de Jong FJ et al. Unrecognized myocardial infarction in relation to risk of dementia and cerebral small vessel disease. *Stroke* 2008, 39:1421–6.

[18] Streifler JY, Eliasziw M, Benavente OR et al. Lack of relationship between leukoaraiosis and carotid artery disease. The North American Symptomatic Carotid Endarterectomy Trial. *Arch Neurol* 1995, 52:21–4.

[19] Hassan A, Hunt BJ, O'Sullivan M et al. Homocysteine is a risk factor for cerebral small vessel disease, acting via endothelial dysfunction. *Brain* 2004, 127:212–19.

[20] van Den Boom R, Lesnik Oberstein SA, van Duinen SG et al. Subcortical lacunar lesions: an MR imaging finding in patients with cerebral autosomal dominant arteriopathy with subcortical infarcts and leukoencephalopathy. *Radiology* 2002, 224:791–6.

[21] Baudrimont M, Dubas F, Joutel A et al. Autosomal dominant leukoencephalopathy and subcortical ischemic stroke: a clinicopathological study. *Stroke* 1993, 24:122–5.

[22] Turner ST, Jack CR, Fornage M et al. Heritability of leukoaraiosis in hypertensive sibships. *Hypertension* 2004, 43:483–7.

[23] Strandgaard S, Paulson OB. Regulation of cerebral blood flow in health and disease. *J Cardiovasc Pharmacol* 1992, 19(suppl 6):S89–93.

[24] Traystman RJ. Regulation of cerebral blood flow by carbon dioxide. In: Welch KMA, Caplan RL, Reis JD et al, ed. *Primer on Cerebrovascular Diseases*. New York, NY: Academic Press; 1997:55–8.

[25] Lavi S, Egbarya R, Lavi R et al. Role of nitric oxide in the regulation of cerebral blood flow in humans: chemoregulation versus mechanoregulation. *Circulation* 2003, 107:1901–5.

[26] Serrador JM, Sorond FA, Vyas M et al. Cerebral pressure-flow relations in hypertensive elderly humans: transfer gain in different frequency domains. *J Appl Physiol* 2005, 98:151–9.

[27] Lavi S, Gaitini D, Jacob VMG. Impaired cerebral CO_2 vasoreactivity: association with endothelial dysfunction. *Am J Physiol Heart Circ Physiol* 2006, 291:1856–61.

[28] McQuinn BA, O'Leary DH. White matter lucencies on computed tomography, subacute arteriosclerotic encephalopathy (Binswanger's disease), and blood pressure. *Stroke* 1987, 18:900–5.

[29] Kontos HA, Wei EP, Navari RM et al. Responses of cerebral arteries and arterioles to acute hypotension and hypertension. *Am J Physiol* 1978, 234:H371–83.

[30] Heistad DD, Mayhan WG, Coyle P et al. Impaired dilatation of cerebral arterioles in chronic hypertension. *Blood Vessels* 1990, 27:258–62.

[31] Strandgaard S. Autoregulation of cerebral blood flow in hypertensive patients: the modifying influence of prolonged antihypertensive treatment on the tolerance to acute, drug-induced hypotension. *Circulation* 1976, 53:720–7.

[32] Miller JD, Bell BA. Cerebral blood flow variations with perfusion pressure and metabolism. In: Wood JH, ed. *Cerebral Blood Flow: Physiologic and Clinical Aspects*. New York, NY: McGraw-Hill Book Co; 1987:119–29.

[33] Young RSK, Hernandez MJ, Yagel SK. Selective reduction of blood flow to white matter during hypotension in newborn dogs: a possible mechanism of periventricular leukomalacia. *Ann Neurol* 1982, 12:445–8.

[34] Pantoni L, Garcia JH, Gutierrez JA. Cerebral white matter is highly vulnerable to ischemia. *Stroke* 1996, 27:1641–7.

[35] Ni JW, Matsumoto K, Li HB et al. Neuronal damage and decrease of central acetylcholine level following permanent occlusion of bilateral common carotid arteries in rat. *Brain Res* 1995, 673:290–6.

[36] van den Bergh R. Centrifugal elements in the vascular pattern of the deep intracerebral blood supply. *Angiologica* 1969, 20:88–98.

[37] Ravens JR. Anastomoses in the vascular bed of the human cerebrum. In: Cervós-Navarro J, ed. *Pathology of Cerebral Microcirculation*. Berlin, Germany: Walter de Gruyter; 1974:26–38.

[38] van Swieten JC, van den Hout JH, van Ketel BA et al. Periventricular lesions in the white matter on magnetic resonance imaging in the elderly. A morphometric correlation with arteriolosclerosis and dilated perivascular spaces. *Brain* 1991, 114 (Pt 2):761–74.

[39] de Reuck J. The human periventricular arterial blood supply and the anatomy of cerebral infarctions. *Eur Neurol* 1971, 5:321–34.

[40] Spangler KM, Challa VR, Moody DM et al. Arteriolar tortuosity of the white matter in aging and hypertension: a microradiographic study. *J Neuropathol Exp Neurol* 1994, 53:22–6.

[41] Saba L, Sanfilippo R, Pascalis L et al. Carotid artery abnormalities and leukoaraiosis in elderly patients: evaluation with MDCT. *AJR Am J Roentgenol* 2009, 192(2):W63–70. doi: 10.2214/AJR.07.3566.

[42] Fassbender K, Mielke O, Bertsch T et al. Homocysteine in cerebral macroangiography and microangiopathy. *Lancet* 1999, 353(9164):1586–7.

[43] Rowbotham GF, Little E. A new concept of the circulation and the circulations of the brain. The discovery of surface arteriovenous shunts. *Br J Surg* 1965, 52:539–42.

[44] Ostrow PT, Miller LL. Pathology of small artery disease. *Adv Neurol* 1993, 62:93–123.

[45] Meguro K, Hatazawa J, Yamaguchi T et al. Cerebral circulation and oxygen metabolism associated with subclinical periventricular hyperintensity as shown by magnetic resonance imaging. *Ann Neurol* 1990, 28:378–83.

[46] De Cristofaro MT, Mascalchi M, Pupi A et al. Subcortical arteriosclerotic encephalopathy: single photon emission computed tomography-magnetic resonance imaging correlation. *Am J Physiol Imaging* 1990, 5:68–70.

[47] de Reuck J, Decoo D, Strijckmans K et al. Does the severity of leukoaraiosis contribute to senile dementia? A comparative computerized and positron emission tomographic study. *Eur Neurol* 1992, 32:199–205.

[48] O'Sullivan M, Summers PE, Jones DK et al. Normal-appearing white matter in ischemic leukoaraiosis: a diffusion tensor MRI study. *Neurology* 2001, 57:2307–10.

[49] Morikawa E, Rosenblatt S, Moskowitz MA. L-arginine dilates rat pial arterioles by nitric oxide-dependent mechanism and increases blood flow during focal cerebral ischemia. *Br J Pharmacol* 1992, 107:905–7.

[50] Topakian R, Barrick TR, Howe FA et al. Blood-brain barrier permeability is increased in normal-appearing white matter in patients with lacunar stroke and leucoaraiosis. *J Neurol Neurosurg Psychiatry* 2010, 81:192–7.

[51] Starr JM, Wardlaw J, Ferguson K et al. Increased blood-brain barrier permeability in type II diabetes demonstrated by gadolinium magnetic resonance imaging. *J Neurol Neurosurg Psychiatry* 2003, 74:70–6.

[52] Lin Q, Huang WQ, Tzeng CM. Genetic associations of leukoaraiosis indicate pathophysiological mechanisms in white matter lesions aetiology. *Rev Neurosci* 2015, 26(3): 343–58. doi: 10.1515/revneuro-2014-0082.

[53] Dandona P, Chaudhuri A, Aljada A. Endothelial dysfunction and hypertension in diabetes mellitus. *Med Clin North Am* 2004, 88:911–31, x–xi.

[54] Fazekas F, Kleinert R, Offenbacher H et al. Pathologic correlates of incidental MRI white matter signal hyperintensities. *Neurology* 1993, 43:1683–9. Doi: 10.1212/WNL.43.9.1683.

[55] Nag S. Blood–brain barrier permeability using tracers and immunohistochemistry. *Methods Mol Med* 2003, 89:133–44.

[56] Knottnerus ILH, Ten Cate H, Lodder J et al. Endothelial dysfunction in lacunar stroke: a systematic review. *Cerebrovasc Dis* 2009, 27:519–26.

[57] Stevenson SF, Doubal FN, Shuler K et al. A systematic review of dynamic cerebral and peripheral endothelial function in lacunar stroke versus controls. *Stroke* 2010, 41:434–42.

[58] Hassan A, Hunt BJ, O'Sullivan M et al. Markers of endothelial dysfunction in lacunar infarction and ischaemic leukoaraiosis. *Brain* 2003, 126:424–32.

[59] Wright CB, Moon Y, Paik MC et al. Inflammatory biomarkers of vascular risk as correlates of leucoaraiosis. *Stroke* 2009, 40(11):3466–71.

[60] Di Napoli M, Papa F. Present insights in the cerebral small vessel disease physiopathology: the role of C-reactive protein. *Recenti Prog Med* 2006, (5):246–56.

[61] Khan U, Hassan A, Vallance P et al. Asymmetric dimethylarginine in cerebral small vessel disease. *Stroke* 2007, 38(2):411–3.

[62] Rouhl RP, van Oostenbrugge RJ, Damoiseaux JG et al. Haptoglobin phenotype may alter endothelial progenitor cell cluster formation in cerebral small vessel disease. *Curr Neurovasc Res* 2009, 6(1):32–41.

[63] Andresen J, Shafi NI, Bryan RM Jr et al. Endothelial influences on cerebrovascular tone. *J Appl Physiol* 2006, 100:318–27.

[64] Kaposzta Z, Baskerville PA, Madge D et al. L-arginine and S-nitrosoglutathione reduce embolization in humans. Circulation 2001, 103(19):2371–5.

[65] Maxwell AJ, Anderson B, Zapien MP et al. Endothelial dysfunction in hypercholesterolemia is reversed by: nutritional product designed to enhance nitric oxide activity. *Cardiovasc Drugs Ther* 2000, 14(3):309–16.

[66] Fideleff HL, Frigeri AE, Sobrado PG in sod. Reproducibility and safety of the arginine test in normal adults. *Medicina (B Aires)* 1999, 59(3):249–53.

[67] Murata T, Handa H, Mori K et al. The significance of periventricular lucency on computed tomography: experimental study with canine hydrocephalus. *Neuroradiology* 1981, 20:221–7.

[68] Brun A, Englund E. A white matter disorder in dementia of the Alzheimer type: a pathoanatomical study. *Ann Neurol* 1986, 19(3):253–62.

[69] Bornebroek M, Haan J, van Buchem MA et al. White matter lesions and cognitive deterioration in presymptomatic carriers of amyloid precursor protein gene codon 693 mutation. *Arch Neurol* 1996, 53:43–8.

[70] Ovbiagele B, Saver JL. Cerebral white matter hyperintensities on MRI: current concepts and therapeutic implications. *Cerebrovasc Dis* 2006, 22:83–90.

[71] Schwartz GL, Fornage M, Mosley T et al. Treatment of leukoaraiosis. *Curr Treat Options Cardiovasc Med* 2005, 7(3):173–7.

[72] Dufouil C, de Kersaint-Gilly A, Besancon V et al. Longitudinal study of blood pressure and white matter hyperintensities: the EVA MRI Cohort. *Neurology* 2001, 56:921–6.

[73] Dufouil C, Chalmers J, Coskun O et al. Effects of blood pressure lowering on cerebral white matter hyperintensities in patients with stroke: the PROGRESS (perindopril protection against recurrent stroke study) magnetic resonance imaging substudy. *Circulation* 2005, 13:1644–50.

[74] Mok VC, Lam WW, Fan YH et al. Effects of statins on the progression of cerebral white matter lesion: post hoc analysis of the ROCAS (regression of cerebral artery stenosis) study. *J Neurol* 2009, 256:750–7.

[75] ten Dam VH, van den Heuvel DM, van Buchem MA et al. Effect of pravastatin on cerebral infarcts and white matter lesions. *Neurology* 2005, 64:1807–9.

[76] Janić M, Lunder M, Šabovič M. A low-dose combination of fluvastatin and valsartan: a new "drug" and a new approach for decreasing the arterial age. *Biomed Res Int* 2015, 2015:235709. doi: 10.1155/2015/235709.

[77] Hanžel J, Piletič Ž, Turk M et al. A combination of low doses of fluvastatin and valsartan decreases arterial stiffness in patients after myocardial infarction: a pilot study. *Curr Ther Res Clin Exp* 2015, 77:63–5. doi: 10.1016/j.curtheres.2015.06.001.

[78] Janic M, Lunder M, Cerkovnik P et al. Low-dose fluvastatin and valsartan rejuvenate the arterial wall through telomerase activity increase in the middle-aged men. Rejuvenation Res 2016; 19(2):115–9. doi: 10.1089/rej.2015.1722. Epub 2016 Jan 22.

[79] O'Rourke MF, Safar ME. Pulse wave encephalopathy. *J Hypertens* 2012, 30(2):429. doi: 10.1097/HJH.0b013e32834c7bd9.

[80] Aktas B, Utz A, Hoenig-Liedl P et al. Dipyridamole enhances NO/cGMP-mediated vasodilator-stimulated phosphoprotein phosphorylation and signaling in human platelets: in vitro and in vivo/ex vivo studies. *Stroke* 2003, 34:764–9.

[81] Calabrò RS, Gervasi G, Bramanti P. L-Arginine and vascular diseases: lights and pitfalls! *Acta Biomed* 2014, 85(3):222–8.

[82] Calabrò RS, Gervasi G, Bramanti P. Does L-arginine supplementation play a role in cerebral small vessels disease? Implication in the treatment of leukoaraiosis. *Med Hypotheses* 2011, 77(4):671–3. doi: 10.1016/j.mehy.2011.07.012.

[83] Calabro RS, Gervasi G, Baglieri A et al. Is high oral dose L-arginine intake effective in leukoaraiosis? Preliminary data, study protocol and expert's opinion. *Curr Aging Sci* 2013, 6(2):170–7.

Chapter 8

Noninvasive Evaluation of Microcirculation under Normal and Pathological Conditions Using Contrast-Enhanced Ultrasonography (CEUS)

Attila Tamas-Szora, Mihai A. Socaciu,
Alexandru Florin Badea, Iulian Opincariu and
Radu I. Badea

Additional information is available at the end of the chapter

http://dx.doi.org/10.5772/64622

Abstract

The present chapter highlights the most important information about microcirculation and its evaluation using contrast-enhanced ultrasonography (CEUS). In the beginning it outlines some general considerations about microcirculation, together with its morphological and physiological particularities under normal and pathological circumstances. The ultrasonographic (US) evaluation of vascularity is based on the Doppler technique and the harmonic technique using contrast agents. Then it presents briefly the Doppler ultrasound (DUS) and discusses its most important current and emerging indications. CEUS is presented extensively, covering the fundamentals of sonographic contrast agents, harmonic imaging and quantification techniques. A special focus is placed not only on the current and emerging indications of CEUS but also on the advantages and limitations of the method. This chapter also incorporates information about experimental CEUS applications and future perspectives. CEUS is the recommended US method for the characterization of microcirculation. The results of the examination are displayed in real-time, under the eyes of the examiner, while the quantitative assessment of the contrast agent kinetics parameters is easy to perform. This method allows a precise definition of the healthy or pathologic state of an organ and the follow-up of treatment response.

Keywords: microcirculation, contrast agent, ultrasonography, Doppler ultrasonography, microvascular kinetics

1. Introduction

1.1. Microcirculation: general considerations: morphological and physiological particularities under normal circumstances

Microcirculation (MC) represents the segment of the circulatory system that includes vascular structures with a diameter <150 μm; it is present in all tissues and organs (except for cornea and intervertebral disks). This dimensional threshold corresponds to small arteries, arterioles, capillaries and venules. The consensus on this definition is still under debate, therefore in the case of the small arteries (anatomically defined as small, but with a caliber >150 μm) it is unclear whether they should be regarded as part of the MC [1]. The capillaries are organized as a circulatory network (bed) which provides an enormous access area for the blood to the parenchyma (**Figure 1**). There is an ordered distribution pattern of the capillaries, which is also organ-specific. The ordered spatial distribution of the capillaries, correlated with the degree of specialization of the structured cells into the parenchyma, represents the premise for the complex functions specific to each organ: liver, spleen, kidney, thyroid, etc. The main function of MC is to allow and modulate the transfer of nutrients and oxygen to the tissues according to their needs. An adequate operation of this process is a prerequisite for the structural and functional integrity of various tissues and organs. Another function of MC is to prevent the variations of hydrostatic pressure at the level of the capillaries, variations which interfere with normal tissue exchanges. Under normal circumstances, there are significant variations of the vessel caliber and blood volume. These are determined by a number of physiological parameters, such as temperature, arterial pressure, physical and mental activity, age. Other factors that influence MC are feeding, stress, medication, smoking and finally pathological changes. MC alterations include various pathological processes since they may represent both the determining factors and their consequences.

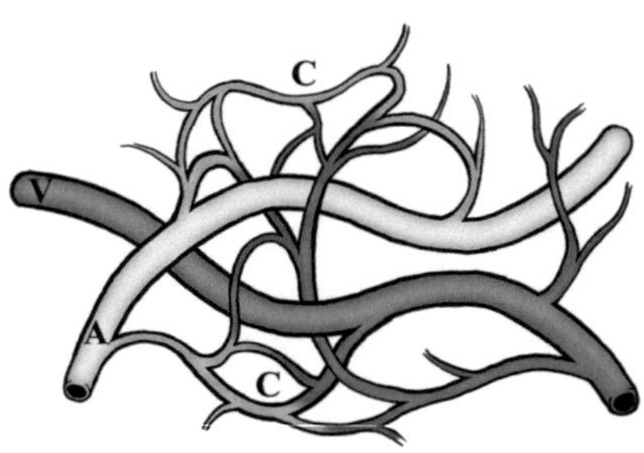

Figure 1. Microcirculation outline. A – arteriole; V – venule; C – capillaries.

1.2. Morphological and physiological particularities under pathological circumstances

Microcirculation, as described above, is an important element of the ensemble that makes up the different tissues and organs. Pathological states have a significant influence on MC.

Inflammation represents the first line of defense against traumatic, pathogenic or toxic injuries and is based on a complex local process that involves microvascular structures, cellular and immunological events. The consequences of these local changes may have an impact at a systemic level. During acute inflammation the alterations of the vascular caliber and blood flow occur immediately after the injury. The transient vasoconstriction of the arterioles represents the initial change and is followed by vasodilation and thus increased blood flow. Increased vascular permeability causes afterwards the slowing of the blood flow, stasis and interstitial edema. The extension of the inflammatory process in time (weeks, months) is characteristic for chronic inflammation. Within this process the active inflammatory alterations, tissue damage and tissue repair happen simultaneously (**Figure 2**).

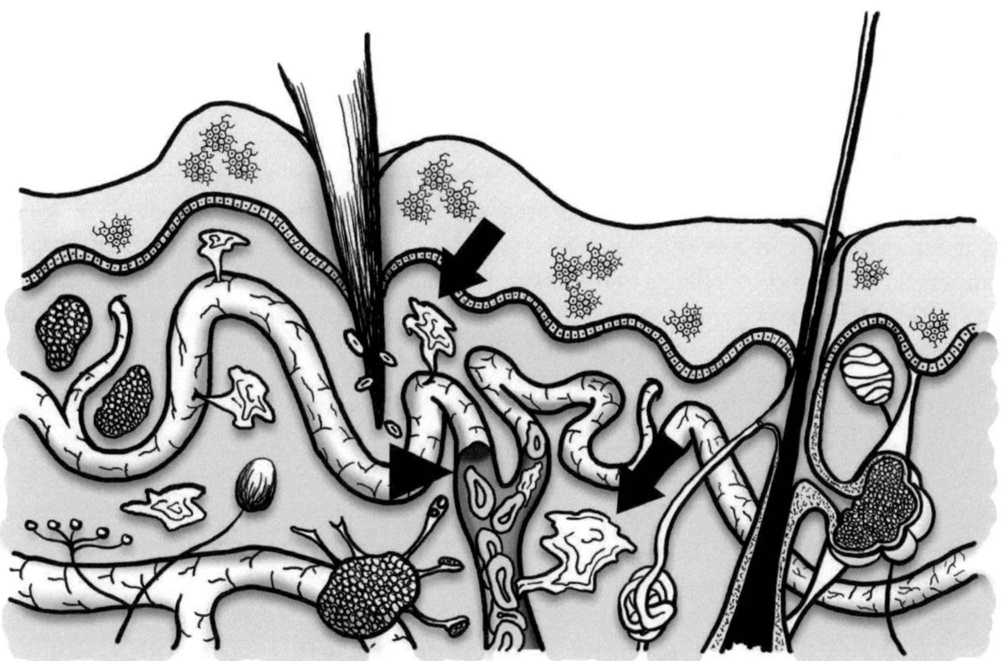

Figure 2. Inflammation of the skin. Dilation (arrowhead) and increased permeability of the vessels are shown (arrows).

Angiogenesis (formation of new vessels) is a central phenomenon in chronic inflammation and represents the development of new vessels from the pre-existing vascular structures. The event is complex and involves various types of cells, growth factors, cytokines, adhesion molecules and signal transformation processes [2]. These factors thus contribute to blood vessels development, maintenance and remodeling.

In physiological processes such as wound healing or during menstrual cycle, angiogenesis is temporarily activated. On the other hand, it also plays an important role in the onset, development and spread of malignancies [3, 4]. Tumors under 1–2 mm receive oxygen and nutrients by diffusion, but their further growth requires the development of new feeding vessels.

Without angiogenesis tumors cannot grow beyond this size and cannot metastasize. The development of benign tumor masses also requires a transient activation of angiogenesis. In their case the resulting vessels have a relatively linear pattern and ordered ramifications. Conversely, the progression of malignant tumors involves a permanent activation of angiogenesis in order to sustain tumor growth. As a result, new vessels are quickly multiplying and developing chaotically, forming a wide, tree-like spatial structure. This structure penetrates into the tumor and ensures a large diffusion area, in contact with the neoplastic cells. Even though the tumor vasculature originates from the normal vessels of the host tissue, the architecture is significantly different. Tumors present an anarchic, inhomogeneous, vascular network, often with dilated, saccular, tortuous structures and irregular ramifications (**Figure 3**). Tumor cells may be found in the endothelium and the blood flow is chaotic, bidirectional and unsteady [5–7]. From a functional point of view, the vessels present an abnormal permeability for large macromolecules, while tissue oxygenation and metabolic residue removal are inefficient. The perfusion rate in many of these tumors is slower than in normal tissues and the average flow rate of erythrocytes may be one level of magnitude lower than in physiologic conditions [8]. Unlike in normal vessels, in neoplastic vessels the characteristic relationship between vessel size and the erythrocyte flow rate is missing. Blood flow through the tumor bed is restrained by the increased downstream resistance and focal leakage. The heterogeneous features of tumor vascularity generate obstacles for the penetration of therapeutic agents and contribute to the development of the abnormal tumor environment. In this way the efficiency of various therapies is reduced while the most aggressive and potentially metastatic cancerous cells are being selected [8].

The main promoter of angiogenesis is the vascular endothelial growth factor (VEGF). In normal circumstances it is suppressed by the Von Hippel-Lindau (VHL) protein, while in the case of tumors it is overexpressed [9]. With the use of immunohistochemistry methods, the CD34 endothelial antigen is marked with specific antibodies and a parameter called microvascular density (MVD) is calculated by means of automatic measurement methods. This is an indicator of the degree of angiogenesis, and some studies indicate a correlation between MVD and cancer patients' survival [10]. The emerging use of MVD is represented by the evaluation of the tumor's response to systemic treatment. Studies performed to this date revealed the utility of MVD for the measurement of the effect of tumor angiogenesis disrupting therapies [11]. These therapies, called antiangiogenic therapies, are designed to reverse vascular and tumoral environment abnormalities and to determine the "normalization" of the tumor vessels' function [12]. As a consequence, there is an improvement in the cytotoxic agents' penetration and the radiation therapy outcome.

Ischemia represents the partial reduction (chronic ischemia) or complete suppression (acute ischemia) of the arterial flow in an organ or anatomical region. The causes are manifold: circulatory alterations such as embolism and thrombosis; degenerative and inflammatory arterial conditions—atherosclerosis and arteriosclerosis; arterial spasm; arterial hypotension. In acute ischemia there is a sudden and complete suppression of the circulation and the evolution toward infarction is variable, depending on the existence of collateral circulation. Chronic ischemia begins with the reduction of the capillaries caliber and blood flow in a more or less well-defined area, depending on the feeding arterial network which may or may not be terminal. There are also associated phenomena to collateral feeding vessels formation. Within the necrotic, infarction area, there is no circulatory bed, only a more or less liquefied tissue, completely or partially replaced by fibrotic structures.

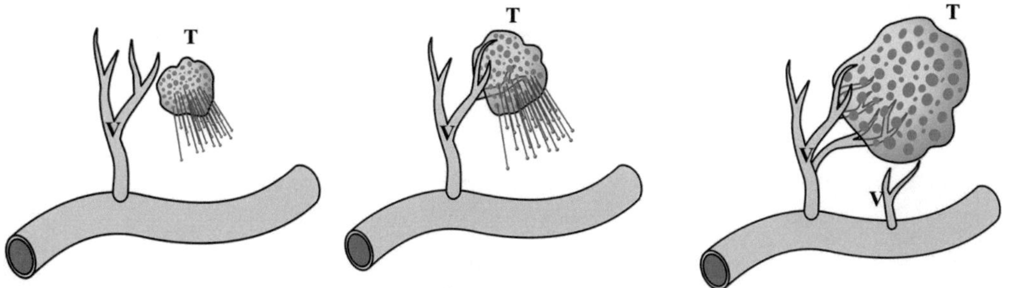

Figure 3. Angiogenesis outline. A small tumor (T) receives nutrients and oxygen by diffusion (a). As the tumor grows normal adjacent vessels (V) multiply quickly and penetrate into the tumor (b, c).

2. Current ultrasonographic techniques used for the evaluation of microcirculation: Doppler ultrasonography

2.1. General principles

This technique detects blood flow down to velocities of 2 cm/s, allows the color coding of the flow ("color flow map" technique – CFM; "power Doppler"- PD), velocity and flow measurements (spectral Doppler). Only vascular structures with a diameter over 100 μm can be analyzed [13, 14]. The physical principle that governs this method is the Doppler effect. For all types of waves (including sound waves) it entails the change of the received signal frequency, when the source of the wave and/or the receiver is moving toward or away from one another

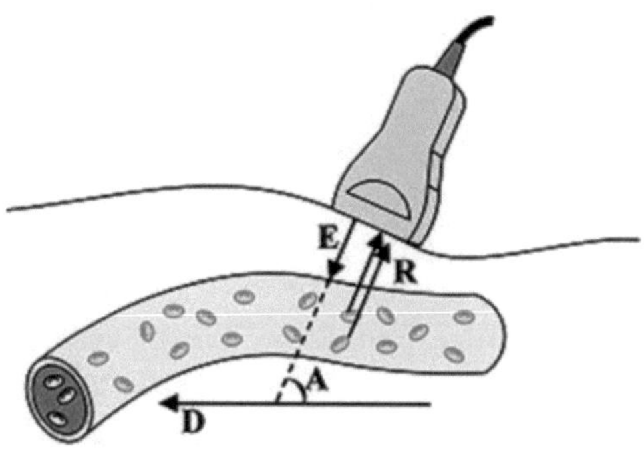

Figure 4. Doppler effect outline. E – emitted sound wave fascicle; R – reflected fascicle; D – direction of movement of blood cells; A – angle between sound wave fascicle and blood cells direction of movement.

(**Figure 4**). The receiver's movement toward a stationary source leads to the detection of higher frequencies. If the receiver moves away from the source it encounters less cycles per second and it will register a wave with a lower frequency than that emitted by the source. In ultrasonographic (US) equipment both the source and the receiver are positioned close to one another inside the transducer. The emitted sound wave fascicle is reflected from the interfaces existing between/in various tissues and afterwards these waves are received and represent the basis for the formation of the US image (**Figure 5**). The movement of the blood cells toward the transducer determines an increase of the reflected wave's frequency, while the opposite movement determines a frequency decrease.

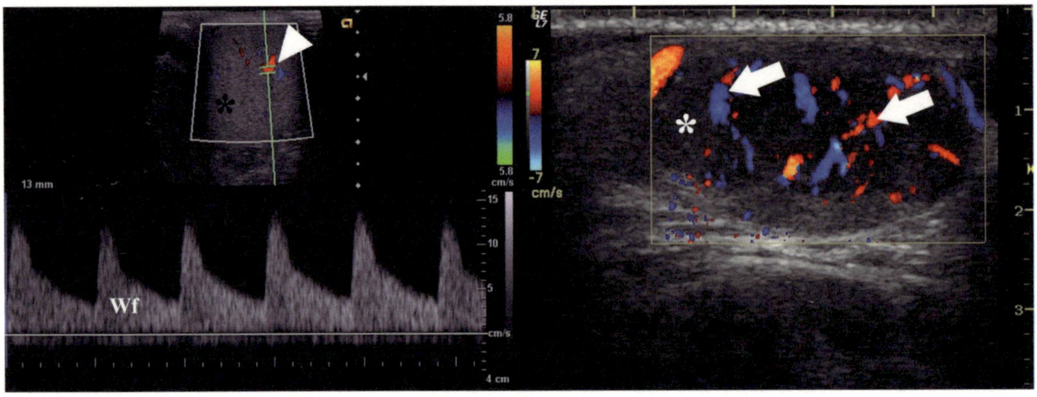

Figure 5. Examples of spectral and color Doppler. On the left: the left testicle (black asterisk) is investigated by spectral Doppler. The measurement sample (arrowhead) is placed inside an artery. The bottom portion of the image displays the spectral Doppler waveform (Wf), in which blood flow velocity (in cm/s) within the Doppler sample is plotted versus time. On the right: a superficial tumoral mass (white asterisk) is investigated with CFM. Flow toward the transducer is represented with shades of red and yellow, whereas flow in the opposite direction is indicated with shades of blue (arrows).

The difference between the received and the emitted sound wave, called differential frequency, is dependent on the emission frequency, propagation velocity of the waves into the tissues, the velocity of the detector and the angle between the detector's direction of movement and the sound wave fascicle. Placing a "measurement sample" inside a vessel will include groups of cells moving at different velocities, each group determining a signal with a particular differential frequency. Therefore, a complex US signal is generated from inside the blood column, which can be analyzed using a specter of frequencies with the help of Fourier techniques. The frequencies which compose the specter are then transformed into velocities using the Doppler equation.

2.2. The applicability of Doppler ultrasonography for the evaluation of normal and pathological circumstances

Within the limits of the spatial and temporal resolution offered by the latest equipment, DUS allows the characterization of the circulatory bed. The normal circulatory bed consists of fine vessels with a radial orientation, from the organ's hilum toward the capsule. This pattern is more obvious in the case of large organs such as the liver or the spleen. Other organs such as the kidney, the thyroid and the testicle have a different appearance, also characteristic, of the normal vascularity, easy to identify and describe.

The features of the circulatory bed during inflammation have been investigated in various studies aimed to detect and measure vascular changes. Rheumatology is one of the beneficiary fields of these US techniques. The common indications include the evaluation of the inflammation, the appreciation of the therapeutic response and the differentiation between inflammatory and degenerative pathology. DUS may identify the augmentation of the blood flow in the inflammation of the synovial and periarticular structures, tendon insertion and sheath. The increase of the blood flow is associated with the histologic identification of the intra-articular pannus [15]. For the time being the detection of the Doppler signal represents an integrated part of the definitions of musculoskeletal conditions (**Figure 6**). Thus, synovitis is defined as an abnormal, hypoechoic, intra-articular structure that is only slightly compressible and which may present Doppler signal. A fluid collection is defined as an hypoechoic or anechoic intra-articular structure which can be dislodged and does not present Doppler signal. Detection of the Doppler signal is also included in the definitions of tenosynovitis and enthesopathy [15, 16]. The method provides high accuracy in showing active synovitis and accompanied by contrast agent (CA) administration it correlates very well with other imaging methods such as contrast-enhanced magnetic resonance imaging (CE-MRI) [17].

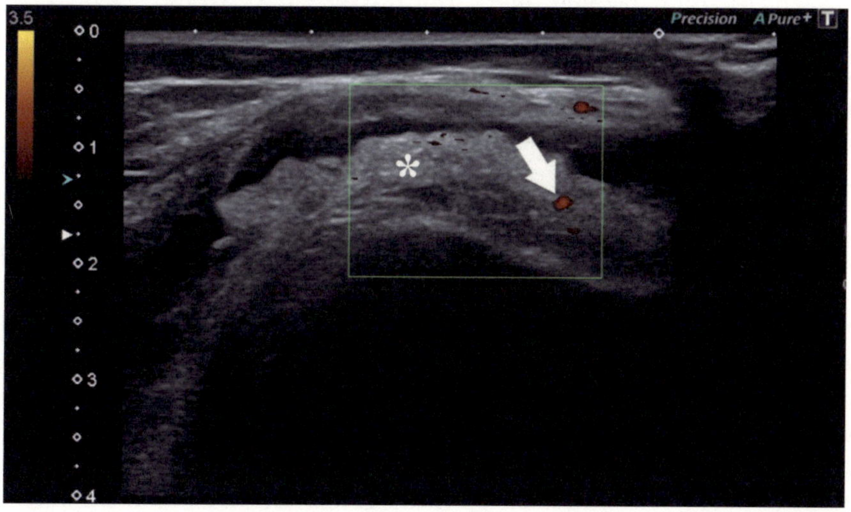

Figure 6. Example of hip synovitis in a child. Synovial thickening is indicated by the asterisk. Power Doppler identifies augmentation of blood flow in the inflamed synovia (arrow).

Another established application of DUS is in the male genital pathology. An increased vascular signal observed upon the CFM or PD examination of an enlarged, hypoechoic epididymis reveals the hyperemia characteristic of acute epididymitis. A similar appearance is identified in the case of acute orchitis. Spectral Doppler shows a high velocity flow and low resistance in these situations (**Figure 7**).

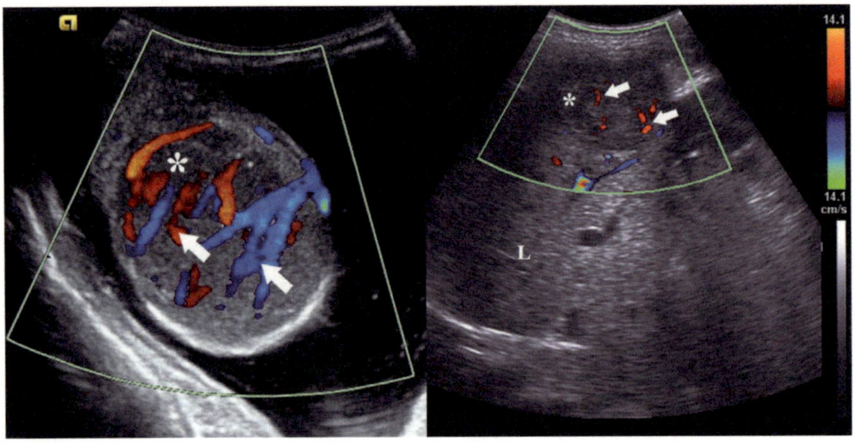

Figure 7. Different alterations of the vasculature identified by CFM. The left image presents a patient with orchitis (acute inflammation). The testicle (asterisk) is examined with CFM and an increased vascular signal is observed (arrows). The right image portrays the evaluation of angiogenesis in a malignant tumor (HCC). The tumor (asterisk) is depicted in a superficial liver (L) segment and CFM identifies the tumor vasculature (arrows).

In tumors, DUS may identify specific circulatory patterns both in benign (e.g., focal nodular hyperplasia [FNH]) and malignant lesions (for instance, the "basket" circulatory pattern is specific to hepatocellular carcinoma (HCC)) (**Figure 7**). The detection of malignancy through DUS depends on the presence of an increased, asymmetric blood flow in a certain region, due to the higher number and size of the vessels. Studies performed on different types of tumors (e.g., skin melanomas) proved that DUS accurately identifies the process of neoangiogenesis and may constitute a prognosis criterion for the recurrence potential of aggressive tumors [18, 19].

As regards the ischemic tissues, the lack of Doppler signal reflects the deficit or absence of blood flow within the vessels of the affected area. This finding must be correlated with the clinical status of the patient and with other investigations, because, for example, in the case of renal infarction, the differentiation from a parenchymal pathology that evolves with hypoperfusion is difficult. This particular situation owes to the DUS limitations in identifying the slow flow at the level of the capillaries when low-frequency US equipment is used (3–5 MHz). Furthermore, the ischemic process is often associated and compensated with the development of a secondary circulatory network which presents reversed flows. Power Doppler mode may overcome this limitation, but it is excessively sensitive and nondiscriminative toward other types of movement such as tissue vibrations and surrounding organs' motility.

Nevertheless, there are situations when DUS may provide indirect information regarding the capillary perfusion status. In a recent study a positive correlation has been established between skin perfusion pressure at the level of the feet and Doppler flow measurements within tibial arteries [20]. This finding has important implications both in the therapeutic approach of leg ulcers and in the evaluation of skin grafts' viability [20]. The situation is identical in the case of organ transplantation.

The quantification of renal vascularity through spectral Doppler is another area that is of interest and up-to-date. There are numerous studies that have succeeded to correlate the alterations of the Doppler parameters with various conditions. The resistivity index (RI, calculated as [peak systolic velocity – end diastolic velocity]/peak systolic velocity) represents the most frequently used parameter to describe the alterations of renal vascularity in relationship with renal impairment. In adults the normal value at the level of the interlobar/arcuate arteries is between 0.6 and 0.7. Renal vasoconstriction encountered in cases of complete pyelocaliceal obstruction is reflected in the elevation of the RI above the normal limits. Although nonspecific, RI > 0.8–0.9 has been demonstrated to be the strongest predictor for renal graft dysfunctionality [21].

Another Doppler application, namely the laser Doppler imaging technique, is still subject to continuous improvement. It is also based on the Doppler principle and uses a light fascicle emitted by a laser source which is reflected by circulating erythrocytes and static tissue structures. There are major advantages to this method in assessing the pathology of superficial structures, such as the skin, since it can measure at 95–100% accuracy the depth of a burn – a value that has not been reached by other methods, thus having implications in the therapeutic conduct [22].

2.3. Limitations and advantages of Doppler ultrasound

Limitations of the Doppler technique consist mainly of the following:

a. the variability from one examination to another, as well as inter- and intraobserver variability;

b. the difficulty in obtaining the Doppler signal from a single target vessel in certain conditions such as a tumor with numerous feeding pedicles and a sinuous spatial trajectory;

c. the dependence of spectral ultrasonography on the insonation angle (it has to be less than 60° in relation to the axis of the vessel);

d. the need to standardize the exploration by using more parameters that must be identical during each examination (wall filter, color gain, scan frequency) in order to ensure the reproducibility of the method [23].

There are ways to quantify the Doppler signal which contribute to the improvement of reproducibility. The main measurable parameters in the case of the spectral method are blood velocity, its relative volume and flow rate. The data obtained by the color-coded technique may be postprocessed by quantifying the number of color pixels within a target area. In situations where an adequate examination protocol is available this information allows the evaluation of tumor response to chemotherapy. The percentage of colored pixels from the total number of pixels present in the target area (called "vascularity index") represents an approach similar to the digital evaluation of MVD used in immunohistochemistry [24]. The new 3D color-coded

Doppler techniques allow the creation of spatial models that illustrate tumoral circulation characteristics [25].

The most important advantages of the Doppler method are:

a. it is noninvasive;

b. it is available on a large scale since most ultrasound machines are equipped with Doppler functions;

c. it offers the possibility to study broad anatomical areas.

3. New ultrasonographic techniques in the evaluation of clinical microcirculation. Intravenous contrast harmonic ultrasound

3.1. Contrast agents used in ultrasonography

Ultrasonographic contrast agents (CAs) are basically echoenhancers that are administered to patients to improve the diagnostic yield.

Joyner mentioned the ultrasonographic contrast effect for the first time in 1960, and during the initial experiments used standard saline solution as a contrast agent for the identification of mitral valve echoes [26]. The saline solution is still used today to evaluate cardiac shunts. Currently the contrast agents consisting of gas microbubbles encapsulated in a lipid, protein or polymer shell are the most widespread and used. These remain strictly intravascular and the encapsulation ensures a longer life of the microbubbles, up to several minutes, unlike the unencapsulated ones which are rapidly dissolved into the blood pool. To ensure the slow diffusion into the blood, gases such as perfluorocarbon, sulfur hexafluoride or nitrogen are found in most of these agents. The size of the microbubbles ranges between 1 and 5 μm and is comparable with that of erythrocytes. The CA is administered intravenously (i.v.), in a bolus dose of 2.4 ml (SonoVue, Bracco, Italy) or by continuous infusion. The newer, more sensitive equipment allows an efficient examination even with lower doses (e.g., 1 ml). For the injection, a special kit is used in which the CA is prepared by mixing with a saline solution and strongly shaking the recipient. The elimination of the CA components is made through the lungs and by hepatic metabolization.

3.2. Harmonics based ultrasound imaging

The high-pressure fluctuations of the sound wave determine a disproportionate change of the microbubbles' radius, thus triggering a nonlinear response. In this situation, the ultrasound waves reflected by the microbubbles are characterized by different frequencies compared to the incident wave, both higher and lower. These are called harmonics, and the second harmonic represents the foundation of "second harmonic imaging" techniques. These detect and convert into image only the second harmonic signal from the scattered ultrasound. To obtain a better contrast-to-tissue ratio, a low mechanical index (MI) is used (**Figure 8**). The MI is always

http://dx.doi.org/10.5772/64622

displayed on the ultrasound machine since it is a critical parameter in contrast-enhanced ultrasonography (CEUS). It represents the amount of negative acoustic pressure within an ultrasonic field. The examiner can modify the MI which in turn will prompt different microbubble responses and modulate the output signature of CAs.

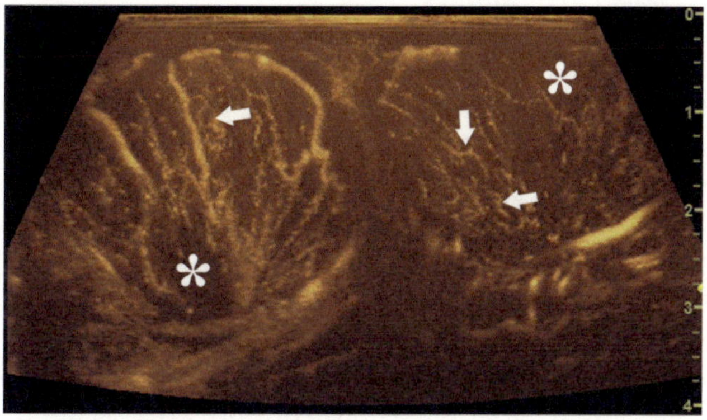

Figure 8. Spectacle view of the testes (asterisks) after administration of CA. Harmonic imaging with low mechanical index (MI = 0.1) sharply identifies testicular microcirculation (arrows).

3.2.1. Techniques with a variable mechanical index

These incorporate two different approaches, based on low and high MI. The low MI technique (MI < 0.2) reduces the microbubble destruction and thus the evaluation of the perfusion can be performed over a relatively long period of time. The high MI (MI > 0.4) approach enables a more accurate characterization of the CA kinetics but could generate adverse biological responses.

Techniques with a low MI include pulse inversion imaging; amplitude/power modulation; power-modulated pulse inversion. The pulse inversion implies the emission down the same transmit line of two consecutive pulses, the second one being identical but 180° inverted with respect to the first pulse. Given the nonlinear response of the CA, the reflected ultrasound waves will be nonidentical and their sum will cause the cancellation of the fundamental part of the signal, the image being formed from the remaining signal. Although the technique has the advantage of sparing the microbubbles, it has the disadvantage of a decreased frame rate which is synonymous to a decreased temporal resolution.

The amplitude/power modulation technique requires the transmission of 2–3 pulses with identical phase and different magnitude. The signals received are combined in such a way that the sum of the pulses with low amplitude is subtracted from the high-amplitude pulse. Since pulses with low amplitude are weak harmonic generators, the difference between the received pulses is due to the nonlinear response of the CA. The technique of power-modulated pulse inversion is a combination of the two techniques described above. The pair of pulses transmitted in the same direction differs both in amplitude and phase, thereby providing a better detection of the nonlinear signals.

High MI-based techniques cause a rapid destruction of most of the microbubbles inside the examination window. The low and high MI techniques are commonly combined ("destruction-replenishment" technique); the examination starts with low MI and after the homogenization of the CA perfusion, the high MI mode is activated.

3.3. The safety of contrast microbubbles

Ultrasonographic contrast agents present a high safety profile and a low incidence of side effects. Compared to other imaging techniques (CT, MRI) they do not lead to renal toxicity and do not alter the thyroid function. The incidence of anaphylactic reactions is very low (<0.002%) [27]. The most important circumstances in which CA administration is forbidden are breast-feeding; recent acute coronary syndrome; right-to-left shunts and unstable ischemic heart disease. The *in vitro* studies have identified a number of possible biological effects resulting from the interaction of the ultrasound wave with microbubbles and cells; as such sonoporation (the appearance of small cracks in the cell membrane), hemolysis and cell death may be encountered. Studies in animal models have shown that the use of high MI (≈0.4) may cause glomerular hemorrhage, but in the current clinical practice MI is set around a value of 0.1 [28]. Mortality associated with CA administration is low (1: 500,000) and studies that included large groups of patients concluded that there is no higher risk of death for patients who underwent CA administration compared to controls [29, 30].

4. The evaluation of microcirculation using i.v. contrast-enhanced harmonic ultrasound: experimental and animal models: clinical applications

4.1. General considerations

CEUS allows the assessment of microcirculation down to the level of very small diameter vessels – such as 40 μm [31]. Although in the capillary bed the blood flow velocity is very low and sometimes interrupted, CEUS allows the visualization of the CA even in these situations.

Before CA administration, the system is set as follows: MI between 0.09 and 0.11; the 'Time Gain Compensation' buttons aligned in the middle position; the overall gain is reduced to the value at which tissue echoes begin to disappear; a single focus set under the region of interest (ROI) is used. The intravenous administration (e.g., through the cubital vein) of the extemporaneously prepared CA is followed by the administration of 10 mL of saline solution bolus. The assessment of the ultrasound images is continuous, beginning from the time of injection until the appearance of the first echoes – called "arterial phase" (10–20 s later), and afterwards until the echoes disappear completely (called "late" venous, tissue or combined phase). The use of the dual image, B mode and contrast mode, is recommended since it helps maintain the area of interest within the insonation plane. To correctly assess the lesions, the examination must be centered on a single structure which will be continuously evaluated for several minutes. To obtain additional information on synchronous lesions, a new CA injection must be administered (CA does not present toxic/lethal doses).

4.2. The analysis of the CA progression

It consists of continuous and real time observation, of the CA transition pattern through the ROI for at least 60–90 s, allowing the characterization of the CA kinetics, from the moment it enters into the circulatory bed (wash-in) and ending with its complete exit (wash-out). The separation between the two is given by the moment when the signal reaches maximum intensity. The digital recording of the examination as video clips facilitates the CA kinetics analysis through ROI, which can be quantified based on qualitative and quantitative parameters. Thus, the CA transition through the region of interest is divided into different temporal phases. The first is the arterial phase (from 10–20 to 30–45 s), which is marked by an abrupt increase of the signal intensity caused by the appearance of the microbubbles. The examination continues with the venous phase, which begins 30–45 s after the injection, and during which the signal intensity reaches a plateau and then gradually drops until it completely disappears. With the exception of the liver and lungs, most organs have a single blood supply (arterial). In the case of the liver the blood supply is ensured through the hepatic artery and the portal vein. This means that after the arterial phase there is an additional vascular intake phase – the portal venous phase (60–120 s) [32]. The liver and spleen display a particular behavior because they have the tendency to retain more microbubbles than other organs. This is due to the accumulation of CA at the level of the sinusoids (in the case of the liver) as well as its capture by the reticulohistiocytic system (in the case of liver and spleen). Consequently, the CA washing phase ('wash-out') is longer compared to other organs, and is called the late phase (up to 4–6 min).

4.2.1. The semiqualitative analysis of the CA progression

Throughout a particular region it is performed by evaluating the following [33]:

a. the moment of arterial phase occurrence (depends on the cardiac activity as well as on the distance between the vein wherein CA is administered and the organ subject to examination);

b. the celerity and length of the arterial phase (conditioned by the capillary bed compliance);

c. the direction of the CA penetration from the organ's hilum toward the capsule;

d. the penetration and spatial distribution characteristics of the CA in the ROI (in relation with the size and number of the feeding vessels and their spatial distribution);

e. the enhancement pattern (homogeneous or nonhomogeneous in relation to the permeability of the capillary bed);

f. the time and speed of the contrast wash-out (in relationship with the arteriovenous shunts that may indicate the malignant nature of the region of interest);

g. the wash-out direction;

h. the wash-out pattern.

4.2.2. The quantitative analysis of the CA progression

It is based on the graphic representation of the variation in time of the CA signal intensity within the blood column (**Figure 9**). This can be done using the ultrasound system or third-party software (e.g., ImageArena, TomTec). The representation is achieved by applying an equation adapted to the blood flow, which results in a time-intensity curve (TIC). The TIC is traced with utmost accuracy when the ROI is stationary. Because in daily practice, with the exception of superficial organ lesions (e.g., lymph nodes), most lesions are mobile during the examination due to the respiratory movements, postprocessing applications were designed to compensate these movements [34]. The TIC analysis is suitable both for techniques with a low MI (CA administered in bolus) and high MI (CA administered in a continuous infusion coupled with the "destruction-replenishment" technique), as it allows the examiner to set the time when the various parameters of the curve are calculated. The microbubble destruction technique, in the context of continuous infusion, leads to a more accurate characterization of the CA kinetics and allows repeated measurements for the same ROI as well as for other regions. The relative limitations of this technique are the lengthy examination time, the possible biological effects of high MI and the need to use special perfusion pumps [35]. The detailed analysis of the TIC curve is performed automatically by the software and is programmed to calculate mathematical parameters derived from the perfusion equation which are then integrated into the context by the examiner. They provide useful information for determining [36]:

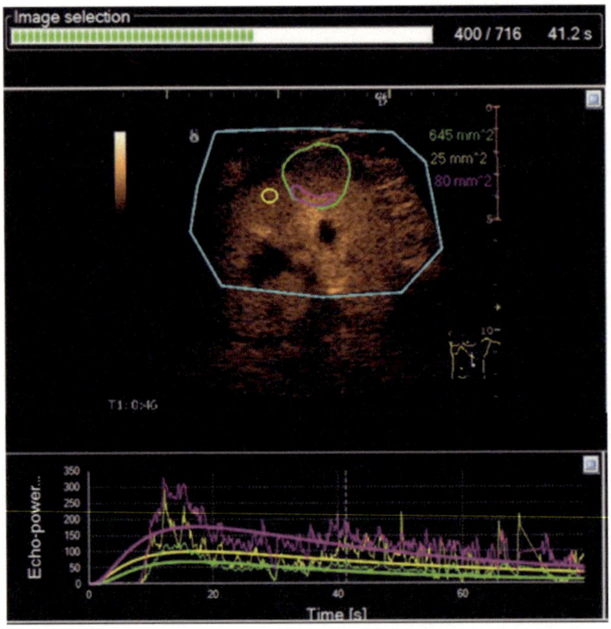

Figure 9. CEUS of a renal tumor. The tumor is depicted in the renal cortex and entirely outlined in green; a smaller region of the tumor parenchyma is outlined in purple; the normal renal cortex is outlined in yellow. In the lower part of the image the TICs were plotted for each of the abovementioned ROIs based on the timing and intensity of the echoes.

http://dx.doi.org/10.5772/64622

a. the circulatory bed volume – the maximum intensity of the signal referred to as "peak intensity" (PI) and respectively the "area under the curve" (AUC);

b. the flow rate – the time elapsed from moment '0' until the point of maximum intensity – "time to peak" (TTP);

c. the enhancement phase of the circulatory bed – "wash in time" (WIT – the time elapsed from the time of 5% enhancement until 95% enhancement);

d. the wash-out phase of the circulatory bed – "wash out time" (WOT – representing the time from the systolic ascension until the full exit of CA from ROI);

e. the rise time –"rise time" (RT);

f. the average transit time through the region of interest – "'mean transit time" (MTT).

4.3. Advantages and limitations of CEUS

Specific CEUS advantages consist of the following:

a. lack of ionizing radiation;

b. repeatability;

c. the possibility to perform a bed-side examination;

d. relatively low costs (as compared to other sectional imaging techniques);

e. time needed for examination is short;

f. the possibility to perform it on patients at risk or with contraindications to iodine agents or gadolinium administration;

g. higher spatial and temporal resolution than CT or MRI;

h. the ability to detect vessels even at very low velocities has been shown in some cases to be superior to contrast-enhanced CT (CECT) [37].

Moreover, CEUS is successful in providing hemodynamic information in areas where the slow flow and insonation angle represent an impediment to Doppler mode.

The limitations of CEUS are:

a. the high costs of the systems able to operate in contrast mode (as compared to basic ultrasound systems);

b. relatively steep and long learning curve;

c. specific artifacts;

d. the dependence on the patient's habitus (especially for deep lesions).

4.4. Experimental animal models

The development of the emerging CEUS applications often involves building a model that is reproducible and based on easily controllable parameters. The animal models play an important role in the development of new therapies, as well as in the validation of the imaging techniques' capability to evaluate the response to treatment. Implementing such a model is a crucial step in the laborious process aimed for the final implementation of new diagnosis and therapeutic strategies in clinical practice. Murine models are the most commonly used. This is due to their relatively low cost, the possibility to obtain a wide range of transgenic animals and the ease of CEUS application to this species. The CEUS examination of the rats follows the same principles as in the case of human subjects. CA administration can be performed through the lateral tail vein [38]. This approach may be sometimes inefficient due to the increased skin rigidity and reduced vein caliber. Other authors have proposed alternative sites of administration, such as intracardiac [39]. Real-time US monitoring of the catheter's progression allows a precise placement of the needle tip and contributes to the success of the technique. This administration route is not without drawbacks, since the rat's accelerated heart rate can lead to catheter displacement outside the heart. Contrast agents developed for humans can be used effectively in animal models (e.g., SonoVue, Bracco Italy). There are also CAs specifically developed for animal studies, such as Micromarker (Bracco, Geneva). They offer the possibility to be combined with various components (e.g., Streptavidin), resulting in a molecular imaging method that addresses specific structures expressed on the endothelium (e.g., VEGFR-2) [40]. One of the basic murine models, which can be easily obtained and has wide applicability, uses the rat carcinosarcoma, known as the Walker 256 tumor. This can be grafted with high success rates in both superficial and intracavitary sites (e.g., intraperitoneal). The application of CEUS in these situations has implications for monitoring and quantifying the natural development of tumor MC and for assessing the success of tumoricidal therapies (**Figure 10**) [39].

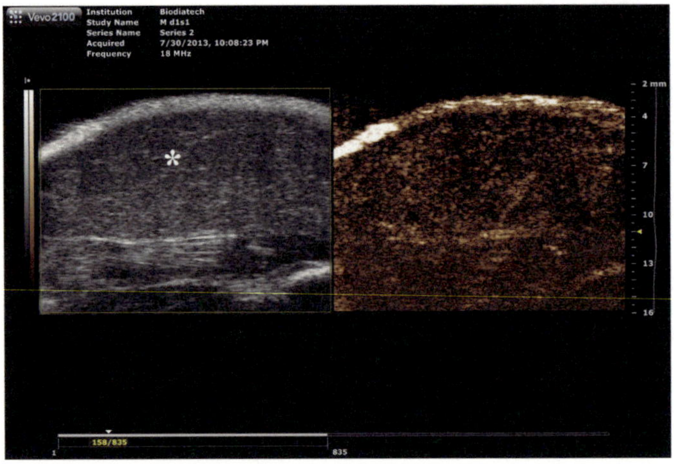

Figure 10. Appearance of an experimentally induced tumor by subcutaneous implantation in a Wistar animal model. On the left the tumor (asterisk) is depicted in B-mode US. On the right the CEUS examination is displayed.

http://dx.doi.org/10.5772/64622

4.5. Modern clinical applications

From 2004 onwards the European Federation of the Societies of Ultrasonography in Medicine and Biology (EFSUMB) together with other entities such as The World Federation of Ultrasonography in Medicine and Biology (WFUMB) has made continuous efforts to publish guidelines and recommendations regarding the application of CEUS in hepatic and nonhepatic pathologies [27, 32].

Its applications in rheumatology, in the form of contrast-enhanced Doppler ultrasonography (Doppler CEUS) have been enhanced especially by the discovery of new treatments for active rheumatoid arthritis that target the microvascularity [41]. Compared to the classic Doppler technique, this application has significantly improved the detection of vascularity and the therapeutic decision in inflammatory pathologies of the small and large joints [42, 43]. However, low MI CEUS is superior to Doppler CEUS in detecting intra-articular microvascularity [44]. Also, the method provides valuable quantitative data through TIC, as revealed by some studies that observed positive correlations between the peak signal intensity and microvascular density (CD105+) in the case of psoriatic arthritis [45].

In the case of orchiepididymitis, the diagnosis is easily established by the clinical and DUS examination of the patient. Additionally, CEUS may point out much earlier an abscess formation, which appears as a nonenhancing structure, and consequently it improves the therapeutic approach [46].

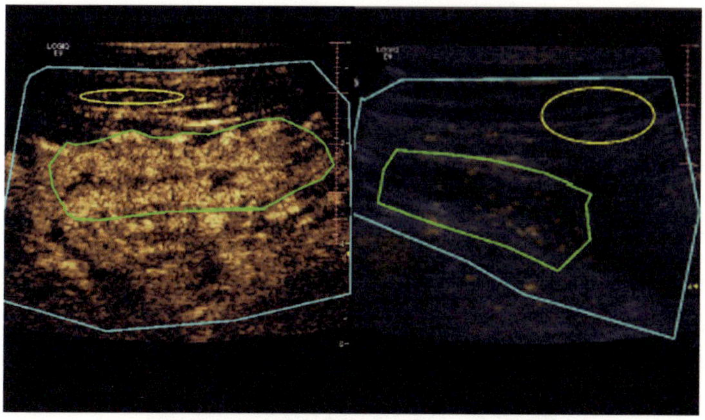

Figure 11. CEUS exploration of the intestinal wall in Crohn's disease, before (left image) and after treatment (right image). The intestinal wall is outlined in green and before treatment it is strongly enhancing, as opposed to the posttreatment findings where the enhancement pattern returned to a normal aspect. The adjacent fat (outlined in yellow) presented similar patterns.

The applications in the pathology of the digestive tract and its glands are numerous and diverse. One of these is the quantification of the intestinal wall vascularity in patients with Crohn's disease [47, 48]. In this particular situation, where angiogenesis is the key element of active disease, CEUS allows the assessment of the intestinal wall as well as of the adjacent fat, the results being strongly correlated with those of the MR [49]. The CA enhancement pattern within the different bowel wall layers is correlated with the clinical parameters that characterize the disease activity. The evaluation of CA behavior through TIC curves allows the quantification of TTP, a parameter that is correlated with the values of the C reactive protein (CRP), which is a surrogate inflammation marker – a short TTP reflects the increased values of CRP encountered during the active stages of the disease [50]. Also, the elevation of TTP is an indicator of the inflammatory changes resolution [50]. The development of strictures is one of the possible complications of Crohn's disease in which CEUS can differentiate between the inflammatory substrate (strong enhancement) and the fibrotic one (weak enhancement) (**Figure 11**) [47, 51].

CEUS holds a distinct role in the appreciation of focal liver lesions since it is frequently successful in establishing an accurate diagnosis or facilitates the decision of further investigations. Benign lesions present a specific and constant enhancement pattern during the arterial and portal phases and no wash-out during the delayed phase [32]. Hemangiomas can be accurately diagnosed in over 95% of the cases since they have a typical CEUS pattern – nodular, peripheral enhancement during the arterial phase which progresses in a centripetal manner, the uptake being partial or complete (**Figure 12**). During the portal venous phase there is constant enhancement. A strong enhancement during the arterial phase is also found in focal nodular hyperplasia (FNH), but the progression is centrifugal and during the delayed phase the lesion may be hyper or isoenhancing compared to the adjacent parenchyma. During the late phases the typical central scar may be identified as a hypoenhancing area (**Figure 12**) [52].

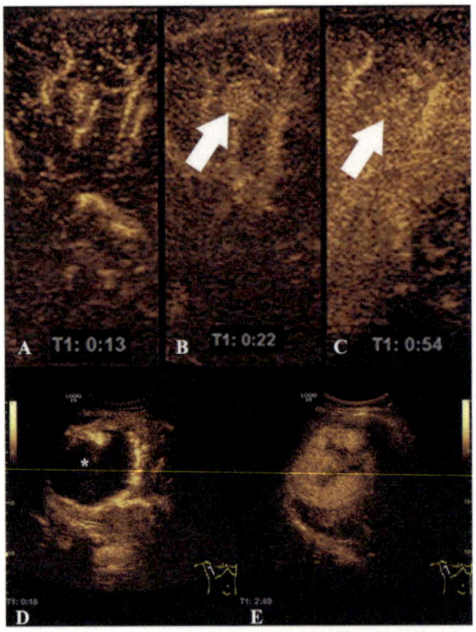

Figure 12. CEUS of liver FNH and hemangioma. The FNH (arrows) presents hyperenhancement during the arterial (A, B) and venous phases (C) that progresses centrifugally. The hemangioma (asterisk) shows intense peripheral enhancement during the arterial phase (D) which progresses centripetally; the tumor is hyperenhanced in the late phase (E).

In malignant liver tumors there is an early and abrupt uptake of the CA within the circulatory bed followed by the CA wash-out from the region of interest in the end of the arterial phase or the beginning of the venous phase. This phenomenon is explained by the existence of arteriovenous communications. In over 97% of the cases HCC is hyperenhancing during the arterial phase and becomes hypoenhancing during the late phase [32]. Highly differentiated tumors may present delayed or absent wash-out, just like in the case of the well-differentiated HCC which can be isoenhancing in these phases. Cholangiocarcinoma displays a different behavior during the arterial phase, but during the subsequent phases a characteristic wash-out is identified. CEUS has implications not only in the diagnosis, but also in the treatment of tumors since it allows the guiding of local ablation techniques (ethanol injection or radio-frequency ablation) by easily identifying the tumor and confirming the efficiency of coagulation necrosis.

Renal tumors also benefit from this method. CEUS allows the differentiation between pseudotumors and tumors and allows the diagnosis of benign and malignant cystic masses [53]. The sensitivity of the method in identifying enhancement at the level of the fine septa is superior to that of CT, even though CT remains the standard method for the staging of malignant cystic tumors. CEUS is also useful in the noninvasive diagnosis of bladder tumors since it can differentiate between a blood clot and a mural tumor which is vascularized and therefore enhances after CA administration.

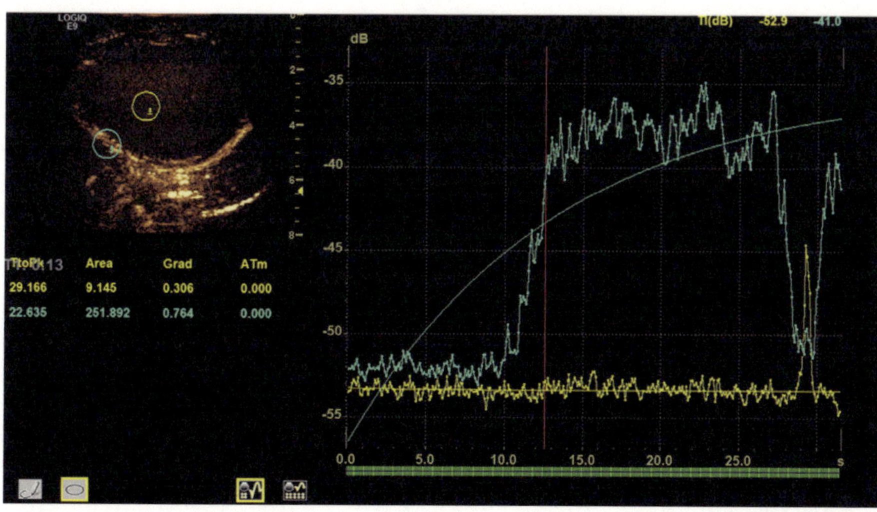

Figure 13. CEUS aspect of testicular infarction. In the upper left image, a yellow ROI is placed inside the testicular parenchyma and a blue ROI is placed upon the scrotal wall. The TICs for each ROI are plotted in the right half of the image. The testicular parenchyma (yellow) shows no enhancement in contrast with the normally enhancing scrotal wall (blue).

Regarding ischemic lesions, CEUS overcomes the limitations of DUS since it can differentiate between a slow circulatory bed and an ischemic area. The accuracy of the method is similar to that of contrast-enhanced CT and superior to DUS in the diagnosis of renal ischemia. Renal infarction appears as a triangular shaped area, with the base toward the renal capsule and which does not enhance with CA, on the background of an enhancing renal parenchyma [54]. Infarction occurring in other organs provides similar CEUS findings (**Figure 13**).

5. Perspectives of the ultrasonographic evaluation of microcirculation

The discovery and use of new biological therapeutic agents not only for cancer treatment but also for other conditions have created the need to evaluate the treatment response in a noninvasive manner. In most cases, the effects of these therapies, especially in the early treatment phases, elude the analysis capacity of the morphological imaging techniques. Identifying the presence or absence of the therapeutic response in the initial phases of the treatment influences decisively the therapeutic itinerary of the patient – functional imaging is capable to assess these early changes. In the case of CEUS, the potential capability derives from the quantitative analysis of TIC. The parameters obtained through TIC before and after the initiation of a treatment with effects on microvascularity have the capacity to become surrogate markers of the therapeutic answer. A series of clinical trials have focused on their analysis and revealed relevant results [55]. For the low MI CEUS technique, the parameters that proved to be useful are WIT; WOT; MTT and AUC [36, 55, 56]. The disadvantage of this method is the lack of control on the CA concentration distributed at the level of the ROI, since it is manually injected. High MI techniques (destruction replenishment) manage to overcome this limitation by the automatic administration of the CA and by obtaining a stable plasmatic CA concentration. Other recent research directions have come to complete the ones already mentioned since they demonstrated the potential of the TIC parameters to become surrogate markers of tumor aggressiveness. The possibility to identify tumor aggressiveness in a noninvasive manner is extremely important due to the potential impact on the efficient individualization of the therapeutic strategy [56].

Recent technological discoveries allowed the development of 4D systems capable to follow the CA kinetics in real-time. These present the advantage of an integrated assessment of the CA kinetics within the whole tumoral mass or region of interest [57].

At the same time, the qualitative and quantitative data obtained through CEUS may be subjected to automatic complex analyses, such as CART (Classification and Regression Trees) that are based on artificial intelligence. They allow an integrated analysis of the CEUS parameters together with those provided by DUS, B mode US, CT/MRI and the creation of a complex, high accuracy, decision protocols [58].

The microbubbles used nowadays may be combined with various antibodies and therefore the technique may target specific structures. The binding may be performed with multiple antibodies at the same time. A recent study succeeded the triple marking of the CA against $\alpha V\beta$-integrin, P-selectin and endothelial growth factor of the human breast cancer endothelium and murinic angiosarcoma [59]. Binding the CA with biomarkers improves the visualization of tumor angiogenesis and in the future these state-of-the-art methods will increase the sensitivity of CEUS in detecting and staging cancers and in evaluating the microcirculation.

6. Conclusions

The ultrasonographic evaluation of vascularity is based on the Doppler technique and the harmonic technique using CAs. CEUS is the recommended US method for the characterization of microcirculation for which it provides a multivariate appreciation. The results of the examination are displayed in real-time under the eyes of the examiner, while the quantitative assessment of the CA kinetics parameters is easy to perform. These features allow a precise definition of the healthy or pathologic state of an organ and the follow-up of treatment response. The method is versatile and in the future it will open new perspectives for individualized, patient-centered therapy, with special benefits for oncologic patients.

Author details

Attila Tamas-Szora[1,2,3*], Mihai A. Socaciu[2,3], Alexandru Florin Badea[1], Iulian Opincariu[1] and Radu I. Badea[2,3]

*Address all correspondence to: tamas-szora.attila@umfcluj.ro

1 Anatomy and Embryology Department, School of Medicine, University of Medicine & Pharmacy "Iuliu Hatieganu", Cluj Napoca, Romania

2 Imaging Department, School of Medicine, University of Medicine & Pharmacy "Iuliu Hatieganu", Cluj Napoca, Romania

3 Ultrasound Research and Education Department, Institute of Gastroenterology and Hepatology "Octavian Fodor", Cluj Napoca, Romania

References

[1] Levy BI, Ambrosio G, Pries AR, Struijker-Boudier HA. Microcirculation in hypertension: a new target for treatment? Circulation. 2001;104(6):735–740. Doi: 10.1161/hc3101.091158.

[2] Alkim C, Alkim H, Koksal AR, Boga S, Sen I. Angiogenesis in inflammatory bowel disease. International Journal of Inflammation 2015;2015:1–10. Doi: 10.1155/2015/970890.

[3] Folkman J. Tumor angiogenesis: therapeutic implications. The New England Journal of Medicine. 1971;285(21):1182–11826. Doi: 10.1056/nejm197111182852108.

[4] Folkman J. Fundamental concepts of the angiogenic process. Current Molecular Medicine. 2003;3(7):643–651. Doi: 10.2174/1566524033479465.

[5] Jain RK. Delivery of novel therapeutic agents in tumors: physiological barriers and strategies. Journal of the National Cancer Institute. 1989;81(8):570–576. Doi: 10.1093/jnci/81.8.570.

[6] Allard WJ, Matera J, Miller MC, Repollet M, Connelly MC, Rao C, et al. Tumor cells circulate in the peripheral blood of all major carcinomas but not in healthy subjects or patients with nonmalignant diseases. Clinical Cancer Research: An Official Journal of the American Association for Cancer Research. 2004;10(20):6897–6904. Doi: 10.1158/1078-0432.ccr-04-0378.

[7] Chaplin DJ, Olive PL, Durand RE. Intermittent blood flow in a murine tumor: radiobiological effects. Cancer Research. 1987;47(2):597–601.

[8] Fukumura D, Duda DG, Munn LL, Jain RK. Tumor microvasculature and microenvironment: novel insights through intravital imaging in pre-clinical models. Microcirculation. 2010;17(3):206–225. doi: 10.1111/j.1549-8719.2010.00029.x.

[9] Vira MA, Novakovic KR, Pinto PA, Linehan WM. Genetic basis of kidney cancer: a model for developing molecular-targeted therapies. BJU International. 2007;99(5):1223–1229. Doi: 10.1111/j.1464-410x.2007.06814.x.

[10] Des Guetz G, Uzzan B, Nicolas P, Cucherat M, Morere JF, Benamouzig R, et al. Microvessel density and VEGF expression are prognostic factors in colorectal cancer. Meta-analysis of the literature. British Journal of Cancer. 2006;94(12):1823–1832. Doi: 10.1038/sj.bjc.6603176.

[11] Medinger M, Esser N, Zirrgiebel U, Ryan A, Jurgensmeier JM, Drevs J. Antitumor and antiangiogenic activity of cediranib in a preclinical model of renal cell carcinoma. Anticancer Research. 2009;29(12):5065–5076.

[12] Jain RK. Normalization of tumor vasculature: an emerging concept in antiangiogenic therapy. Science. 2005;307(5706):58–62. Doi: 10.1126/science.1104819.

[13] Lassau N, Paturel-Asselin C, Guinebretiere JM, Leclere J, Koscielny S, Roche A, et al. New hemodynamic approach to angiogenesis: color and pulsed Doppler ultrasonography. Investigative Radiology. 1999;34(3):194–198. Doi: 10.1097/00004424-199903000-00007.

[14] Yang WT, Tse GM, Lam PK, Metreweli C, Chang J. Correlation between color power Doppler sonographic measurement of breast tumor vasculature and immunohistochemical analysis of microvessel density for the quantitation of angiogenesis. Journal of Ultrasound in Medicine. 2002;21(11):1227–1235.

[15] Schmidt WA. Technology Insight: the role of color and power Doppler ultrasonography in rheumatology. Nature Clinical Practice Rheumatology. 2007;3(1):35–42. Doi: 10.1038/ncprheum0377.

[16] Wakefield RJ, Balint PV, Szkudlarek M, Filippucci E, Backhaus M, D'Agostino MA, et al. Musculoskeletal ultrasound including definitions for ultrasonographic pathology. The Journal of Rheumatology. 2005;32(12):2485–2487.

[17] Szkudlarek M, Court-Payen M, Strandberg C, Klarlund M, Klausen T, Ostergaard M. Power Doppler ultrasonography for assessment of synovitis in the metacarpophalangeal joints of patients with rheumatoid arthritis: a comparison with dynamic magnetic resonance imaging. Arthritis and Rheumatism. 2001;44(9):2018–2023. Doi: 10.1002/1529-0131(200109)44:9<2018::AID-ART350>3.0.CO;2-C.

[18] Botar Jid C, Bolboaca SD, Cosgarea R, Senila S, Rogojan L, Lenghel M, et al. Doppler ultrasound and strain elastography in the assessment of cutaneous melanoma: preliminary results. Medical Ultrasonography. 2015;17(4):509–514. Doi: 10.11152/mu.2013.2066.174.dus/.

[19] Lassau N, Lamuraglia M, Koscielny S, Spatz A, Roche A, Leclere J, et al. Prognostic value of angiogenesis evaluated with high-frequency and colour Doppler sonography for preoperative assessment of primary cutaneous melanomas: correlation with recurrence after a 5 year follow-up period. Cancer Imaging. 2006;6:24–299. Doi: 10.1102/1470-7330.2006.0009.

[20] Sekiya N, Ichioka S. Efficacy of ultrasonography at the ankle level for estimation of pedal microcirculation. Annals of Vascular Diseases. 2015;8(3):198–202. Doi: 10.3400/avd.oa.15-00078.

[21] Gunnar H. Heine, Markus K. Gerhart, Christof Ulrich, Hans Kaler, Matthias Girndt. Renal Doppler resistance indices are associated with systemic atherosclerosis in kidney transplant recipients. Kidney International. 2005;68(2):878–885. Doi: 10.1111/j.1523-1755.2005.00470.x.

[22] Hop MJ, Hiddingh J, Stekelenburg C, Kuipers HC, Middelkoop E, Nieuwenhuis MK, et al. Cost-effectiveness of laser Doppler imaging in burn care in the Netherlands. BMC Surgery. 2013;13(1):1. Doi: 10.1186/1471-2482-13-2.

[23] Ricci S, Matera R, Tortoli P. An improved Doppler model for obtaining accurate maximum blood velocities. Ultrasonics. 2014;54(7):2006–2014. Doi: 10.1016/j.ultras.2014.05.012.

[24] Hsu C, Chen CN, Chen LT, Wu CY, Hsieh FJ, Cheng AL. Effect of thalidomide in hepatocellular carcinoma: assessment with power Doppler US and analysis of circulating angiogenic factors. Radiology. 2005;235(2):509–516. Doi: 10.1148/radiol.235204027.

[25] Kupeli A, Kul S, Eyuboglu I, Oguz S, Mungan S. Role of 3D power Doppler ultrasound in the further characterization of suspicious breast masses. European Journal of Radiology. 2016;85(1):1–6. Doi: 10.1016/j.ejrad.2015.10.019.

[26] Gramiak R, Shah PM. Echocardiography of the aortic root. Investigative Radiology. 1968;3(5):356–366. Doi: 10.1097/00004424-196809000-00011.

[27] Piscaglia F, Nolsoe C, Dietrich CF, Cosgrove DO, Gilja OH, Bachmann Nielsen M, et al. The EFSUMB Guidelines and Recommendations on the Clinical Practice of Contrast Enhanced Ultrasound (CEUS): update 2011 on non-hepatic applications. Ultraschall in der Medizin. 2012;33(1):33–59. Doi: 10.1055/s-0031-1281676.

[28] ter Haar G. Safety and bio-effects of ultrasound contrast agents. Medical & Biological Engineering & Computing. 2009;47(8):893–900. Doi: 10.1007/s11517-009-0507-3.

[29] Piscaglia F, Bolondi L. The safety of Sonovue in abdominal applications: retrospective analysis of 23188 investigations. Ultrasound in Medicine & Biology. 2006;32(9):1369–1375. Doi: 10.1016/j.ultrasmedbio.2006.05.031.

[30] Kusnetzky LL, Khalid A, Khumri TM, Moe TG, Jones PG, Main ML. Acute mortality in hospitalized patients undergoing echocardiography with and without an ultrasound contrast agent: results in 18,671 consecutive studies. Journal of the American College of Cardiology. 2008;51(17):1704–1706. Doi: 10.1016/j.jacc.2008.03.006.

[31] Leen E, Averkiou M, Arditi M, Burns P, Bokor D, Gauthier T, et al. Dynamic contrast enhanced ultrasound assessment of the vascular effects of novel therapeutics in early stage trials. European Radiology. 2012;22(7):1442–1450. Doi: 10.1007/s00330-011-2373-2.

[32] Claudon M, Dietrich CF, Choi BI, Cosgrove DO, Kudo M, Nolsoe CP, et al. Guidelines and good clinical practice recommendations for Contrast Enhanced Ultrasound (CEUS) in the liver – update 2012. Ultrasound in Medicine & Biology. 2013;34(1):11–29. Doi: 10.1016/j.ultrasmedbio.2012.09.002.

[33] Badea R, Ciobanu L. Contrast enhanced and Doppler ultrasonography in the characterization of the microcirculation. Expectancies and Performances. Medical Ultrasonography. 2012;14(4):307–317.

[34] Palmowski M, Lederle W, Gaetjens J, Socher M, Hauff P, Bzyl J, et al. Comparison of conventional time-intensity curves vs. maximum intensity over time for post-processing of dynamic contrast-enhanced ultrasound. European Journal of Radiology. 2010;75(1):149–153. Doi: 10.1016/j.ejrad.2009.10.030.

[35] Wei K, Jayaweera AR, Firoozan S, Linka A, Skyba DM, Kaul S. Quantification of myocardial blood flow with ultrasound-induced destruction of microbubbles administered as a constant venous infusion. Circulation. 1998;97(5):473–483. Doi: 10.1161/01.cir.97.5.473.

[36] Dietrich CF, Averkiou MA, Correas JM, Lassau N, Leen E, Piscaglia F. An EFSUMB introduction into Dynamic Contrast-Enhanced Ultrasound (DCE-US) for quantifica-

tion of tumour perfusion. Ultraschall in der Medizin. 2012;33(4):344–351. Doi: 10.1055/s-0032-1313026.

[37] Tamai H, Takiguchi Y, Oka M, Shingaki N, Enomoto S, Shiraki T, et al. Contrast-enhanced ultrasonography in the diagnosis of solid renal tumors. Journal of Ultrasound in Medicine. 2005;24(12):1635–1640.

[38] Huang YC, Shindel AW, Ning H, Lin G, Harraz AM, Wang G, et al. Adipose derived stem cells ameliorate hyperlipidemia associated detrusor overactivity in a rat model. The Journal of Urology. 2010;183(3):1232–1240. Doi: 10.1016/j.juro.2009.11.012.

[39] Badea AF, Tamas-Szora A, Clichici S, Socaciu M, Tabaran AF, Baciut G, et al. Contrast enhanced ultrasonography (CEUS) in the characterization of tumor microcirculation. Validation of the procedure in the animal experimental model. Medical Ultrasonography. 2013;15(2):85–94. Doi: 10.11152/mu.2013.2066.152.afb1ats2.

[40] Saini R, Sorace AG, Warram JM, Mahoney MJ, Zinn KR, Hoyt K. An animal model allowing controlled receptor expression for molecular ultrasound imaging. Ultrasound in Medicine and Biology. 2013;39(1):172–180. Doi: 10.1016/j.ultrasmedbio.2012.08.016.

[41] Taylor PC. The value of sensitive imaging modalities in rheumatoid arthritis. Arthritis Research & Therapy. 2003;5(5):210–213.

[42] De Zordo T, Mlekusch SP, Feuchtner GM, Mur E, Schirmer M, Klauser AS. Value of contrast-enhanced ultrasound in rheumatoid arthritis. European Journal of Radiology. 2007;64(2):222–230. Doi: 10.1016/j.ejrad.2007.07.011.

[43] Hermann KG, Backhaus M, Schneider U, Labs K, Loreck D, Zuhlsdorf S, et al. Rheumatoid arthritis of the shoulder joint: comparison of conventional radiography, ultrasound, and dynamic contrast-enhanced magnetic resonance imaging. Arthritis and Rheumatism. 2003;48(12):3338–3349. Doi: 10.1002/art.11349.

[44] Klauser A, Frauscher F, Schirmer M, Halpern E, Pallwein L, Herold M, et al. The value of contrast-enhanced color Doppler ultrasound in the detection of vascularization of finger joints in patients with rheumatoid arthritis. Arthritis and Rheumatism. 2002;46(3):647–653. Doi: 10.1002/art.10136.

[45] Fiocco U, Stramare R, Coran A, Grisan E, Scagliori E, Caso F, et al. Vascular perfusion kinetics by contrast-enhanced ultrasound are related to synovial microvascularity in the joints of psoriatic arthritis. Clinical Rheumatology. 2015;34(11):1903–1912. Doi: 10.1007/s10067-015-2894-1.

[46] Moschouris H, Stamatiou K, Lampropoulou E, Kalikis D, Matsaidonis D. Imaging of the acute scrotum: is there a place for contrast-enhanced ultrasonography? International Brazilian Journal of Urology. 2009;35(6):692–702. Doi: 10.1590/s1677-55382009000600008.

[47] Socaciu M, Ciobanu L, Diaconu B, et al. Non-invasive assessment of inflammation and treatment response in patients with Crohn's disease and ulcerative colitis using

contrast-enhanced ultrasonography quantification. J Gastrointestin Liver Dis. 2015;24(4):457–465. Doi: 10.15403/jgld.2014.1121.244.chr.

[48] Neciu C, Badea R, Chiorean L, Badea AF, Opincariu I. Oral and I.V. contrast enhanced ultrasonography of the digestive tract—a useful completion of the B-mode examination: a literature review and an exhaustive illustration through images. Medical Ultrasonography. 2015 Mar;17(1):62–73. Doi: 10.11152/mu.2013.2066.171.cnrb.

[49] Schreyer AG, Finkenzeller T, Gossmann H, Daneschnejad M, Muller-Wille R, Schacherer D, et al. Microcirculation and perfusion with contrast enhanced ultrasound (CEUS) in Crohn's disease: first results with linear contrast harmonic imaging (CHI). Clinical Hemorheology and Microcirculation. 2008;40(2):143–155.

[50] Girlich C, Schacherer D, Jung EM, Schreyer A, Büttner R. Comparison between a clinical activity index (Harvey–Bradshaw-Index), laboratory inflammation markers and quantitative assessment of bowel wall vascularization by contrast-enhanced ultrasound in Crohn's disease. European Journal of Radiology. 2012;81(6):1105–1109. Doi: 10.1016/j.ejrad.2011.02.054.

[51] Wilson SR, Burns PN. Microbubble-enhanced US in body imaging: what role? Radiology. 2010;257(1):24–39. Doi: 10.1148/radiol.10091210.

[52] Piscaglia F, Gianstefani A, Ravaioli M, Golfieri R, Cappelli A, Giampalma E, et al. Criteria for diagnosing benign portal vein thrombosis in the assessment of patients with cirrhosis and hepatocellular carcinoma for liver transplantation. Liver Transplantation. 2010;16(5):658–667. Doi: 10.1002/lt.22044.

[53] Tamas-Szora A, Opincariu I, Manea C, Dobrotă F, Coman I, Buruian M, Badea R. Radiological and imaging features of renal small cell carcinoma: a case report and literature review. Romanian Journal of Functional & Clinical, Macro-& Microscopical Anatomy & of Anthropology. 2015;14(2):275–280.

[54] Bertolotto M, Martegani A, Aiani L, Zappetti R, Cernic S, Cova MA. Value of contrast-enhanced ultrasonography for detecting renal infarcts proven by contrast enhanced CT. A feasibility study. European Radiology. 2008;18(2):376–383. Doi: 10.1007/s00330-007-0747-2.

[55] Hudson JM, Williams R, Tremblay-Darveau C, Sheeran PS, Milot L, Bjarnason GA, et al. Dynamic contrast enhanced ultrasound for therapy monitoring. European Journal of Radiology. 2015;84(9):1650–1657. Doi: 10.1016/j.ejrad.2015.05.013.

[56] Tamas-Szora A, Socaciu M, Crisan N, Dobrota F, Prundus P, Bungardean C, et al. Investigation of renal cell carcinoma by contrast-enhanced ultrasound- predictive value of time intensity curve analysis in establishing local tumor invasion and stage: a pilot study. Urology Journal. 2015;12(3):2173–2181.

[57] Maruyama H, Yoshikawa M, Yokosuka O. Current role of ultrasound for the management of hepatocellular carcinoma. World Journal of Gastroenterology. 2008;14(11): 1710–1719. Doi: 10.3748/wjg.14.1710.

[58] Badea AF, Bran S, Tamas-Szora A, Floareş A, Badea R, Baciut G. Solid parotid tumors: an individual and integrative analysis of various ultrasonographic criteria. A prospective and observational study. Medical Ultrasonography. 2013;15(4):289–298. Doi: 10.11152/mu.2013.2066.154.afb2.

[59] Warram JM, Sorace AG, Saini R, Umphrey HR, Zinn KR, Hoyt K. A triple-targeted ultrasound contrast agent provides improved localization to tumor vasculature. Journal of Ultrasound in Medicine. 2011;30(7):921–931.

Chapter 9

Laser Doppler Flowmetry Evaluation of the Microcirculation in Dentistry

Carmen Todea, Silvana Canjau, Mariana Miron,
Bogdan Vitez and Gheorghe Noditi

Additional information is available at the end of the chapter

http://dx.doi.org/10.5772/64926

Abstract

This chapter presents the most important features of laser Doppler (LD) techniques: LD flowmetry (LDF) and LD imaging (LDI), together with examples of their clinical applications in dentistry. LDF gives a constant estimation of blood flow at a specified point, whereas LDI gives a 'snapshot' of perfusion at a given point. These methods are non-invasive laser-based techniques for monitoring gingival and pulpal blood flow and could be used as a diagnostic tool. In paediatric dentistry and odontology, LDF proved to be an atraumatic real-time method used for determining the tooth vitality by monitoring the pulp microcirculation in traumatized teeth, fractured teeth and teeth undergoing different conservative treatments (e.g. bleaching, dental preparation for prosthetic restorations, etc.). In periodontology, recent studies showed the ability of LDF to evaluate the health of gingival tissue in different types of periodontal diseases. By using LDF, it is also possible to evaluate the outcome after different periodontal treatments. The laser Doppler line scanning can be used for recording the gingival healing process after a surgical procedure in the anterior area of the oral cavity.

Keywords: microcirculation, dental pulp, gingiva, laser Doppler flowmetry, laser Doppler imaging

1. Introduction

The microcirculation consists of vessels with the diameter less than 100 μm. The structure and topological organization of the microcirculation located within organs differ from the larger conduit vessels that distribute blood flow to the organs. The rheological properties of blood in the microcirculation differ from those in the large vessels due to the Fahraeus-Lindqvist effect, which lead to diameter-dependent reduction in hematocrit and effective blood viscosity in microcirculatory vessels [1]. The main function of the microcirculation is to deliver nutrients to and remove waste products from the various tissues as well as support the exchange of respiratory gasses. It also plays an essential role in fluid exchange between blood and tissue, delivery of hormones from endocrine glands to target organs, and bulk delivery between organs for storage or synthesis and provides a line of defence against pathogens [2]. An ideal technique for measurement of tissue oxygenation should provide quantitative, accurate and reproducible real-time information about oxygen supply and utilization in specific tissue beds. For clinical applications, such a device should be safe, non-invasive and easy to use.

Laser Doppler flowmetry (LDF) and laser Doppler imaging (LDI) have been widely used to assess tissue micro-vascular function. These techniques have functioned as clinical surrogate markers. However, the lack of standardization in data expression limits the use of these tests in routine practice. Nowadays, LDF is commonly used to assess tissue blood flow; yet, data exhibit great spatial variability. Another way of getting around spatial variability could be to evaluate tissue blood flow over wider areas by using LDI. Successful wound healing following periodontal surgery is strongly influenced by revascularization rate as well as by preservation and reconstruction of the micro-vascularity of the gingival tissues [3, 4]. Regular post-operative assessment of flap perfusion by members of the microsurgery team trained in the use of laser Doppler line scanning might, therefore, represent a practical alternative to more complex and invasive monitoring techniques.

There are numerous applications where LDF was used to non-invasively monitor changes in blood flow in living tissues. LDF has been used to assess blood flow for intact microvascular systems such as the skin, the retina, gut mesentery, renal cortex and mucous membranes [5, 6]. Dental applications include LDF readings (LDFRs) of periodontal ligament [7], pulpal blood vessels [8–12], gingival or sulcular blood flow in health and disease [13–18], evaluation of the degree in healing and revascularization of surgical wounds [19], the effect of orthodontic treatment [20] or the injection of vasoconstrictive anaesthetics on blood flow [21]. Single-point LDF, the technique mentioned above, shows good temporal resolution, poor spatial resolution and poor reproducibility in low capillary density tissue areas [22, 23]. This latter issue can be overcome by using either integrated probes with several transmitting and/or receiving fibres or full field techniques such as LDI. This technique shows excellent spatial resolution but poor temporal resolution for most devices (especially when scanning large areas) [24], but it provides a more valid measure of tissue blood flow [25].

2. Methods and results

The pulpal and gingival blood flows (GBFs) in the clinical situations described in this chapter were monitored using a MoorLab Laser Doppler (LD) equipment (Moor Instruments Ltd., Axminster, UK) with a straight optical probe, MP3b, 10 mm. A double silicone impression fixed perpendicularly on the buccal cervical surface of the tooth was used for stabilizing the probe. The Moor Instruments MoorLab LD monitor uses laser radiation generated by a semiconductor laser diode operating at a wavelength of 780 + 10 nm and a maximum accessible power of 1.6 mW. The programmed bandwidth of the recorded LD signal was 20 Hz–20 kHz while sampling frequency was 40 Hz. Calibration was performed according to the manufacturer instructions. LDF was recorded and analysed using MoorSoft MoorLab V2.01 software. The physical parameters assessed were flux, expressed in perfusion units (PU) and perfusion measurement (DC). The term used to estimate blood flow is flux—a quantity proportional to the average speed of the blood cells and their concentration. This is expressed in arbitrary perfusion units (AU) that are linearly related to flux. DC gives an indication of the backscattered laser light intensity. The DC signal indicates a correct positioning of the optical probe, showing the reflected laser radiation level from the level of concerned area. The DC signal is the one that indicates the mechanic stability of the optical probe placed at the level of acquisition area. The data were processed using statistical analysis software SPSS v16.0.1.

2.1. Microcirculation of the dental pulp

The tooth vitality preservation is one of the most important aims in conservative dentistry. This is why the reliable vitality assessment of the dental pulp has always been problematic and therefore, many methods have been suggested to test pulp vitality [26]. Pulp vitality tests should attempt to examine the presence of pulp blood flow, offering a precise, objective and quantitative assessment as opposed to the conventional tests that rely on the patient's subjective sensitivity [27, 28].

It is reported in the literature that the LDF technique is reliable for measuring human pulpal blood flow (PBF) to determine pulp vitality [29, 30]. The technique can measure perfusion quantitatively in real time [31]. However, it has also been claimed that signals from human teeth do not necessarily indicate pulpal blood flow and could be confused with a signal obtained from nearby gingival tissues, suggesting that periodontium and other neighbouring tissues can contribute to the signal [32–34]. Polat et al. [34] examined the scattering and penetration properties of the laser used in LDF by using a camera with slow speed shutters. They demonstrated that the laser can densely penetrate up to 4 mm in depth and less densely for up to 13 mm. This also suggests that even with proper isolation of the tooth, some signal contamination from the periodontium is inevitable. They also demonstrated that without isolation, the laser light could scatter from the source tooth to the whole oral cavity, which can also potentially contribute to signal contamination. Karayilmaz and Kirzioglu [35] indicated that LDF could reliably discriminate the vitality of the teeth with a sensitivity and specificity of 1.0 for studied sample. LDF was found to be a more reliable and effective method than pulse oximetry (PO) and electric pulp tester (EPT) in assessing the pulpal status of human teeth.

The isolation method before LDF measurements is crucial for obtaining an accurate signal. Therefore, many authors have used different isolation techniques, thus the different results. This is why many studies suggest that 45–82% of the blood flow recorded with LDF from human teeth may not be from the pulp [36–39]. Soo-Ampon et al. [33] found that up to 80% of the LDF output signal in human incisors may be non-pulp in origin if attempts at tooth isolation are not made. Polat et al. [34] compared teeth that had undergone a pulpectomy with contralateral healthy pulps as controls. They also found that approximately 70% of the LDF readings from teeth with the pulps removed were non-pulp in origin. The results obtained by our group [40] show that about 69% of the acquired LD signal is of non-pulp origin, consistent with the existing literature [38, 39, 41, 42].

For this reason, in our studies investigating dental pulp blood flow, a silicone impression combined with light cure periodontal liquid dam was used in order to reduce the signal contamination. This method offered an excellent isolation certified by the DC values obtained during the measurements. It has been shown that the light from a LDF probe placed at 2 mm above the buccal cement-enamel junction is transmitted apically towards the radicular pulp [41]. There are several studies that have reported the placement of the LDF probe at 1–1.5 [43], 2 [44], 2–3 [45, 46], ~3 [47] and 4–5 mm [48] coronal to the gingival margin. In our studies, the probe was placed on the cervical third of the tooth, at 3 mm away from the gingival margin (**Figure 1**).

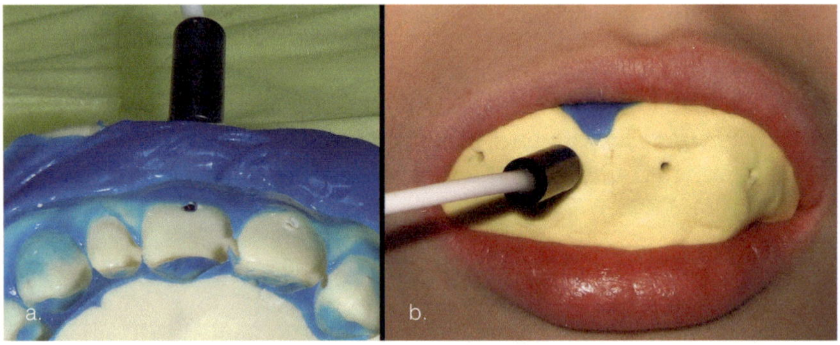

Figure 1. The acquisition technique of laser Doppler signals. (a) Silicone holder with the optical fibre inserted in the canal previously created and (b) intra-oral positioning of the silicone holder together with the stabilized optical fibre.

2.1.1. Bleaching and pulp microcirculation

The treatment of teeth whitening can be performed in the dental office, by the dentist, or at patient's home, and uses whitening agents, such as hydrogen peroxide gel (3–38%), carbamide peroxide (10–30%) or a mixture of hydrogen peroxide and sodium carbonate. Tooth bleaching, as one of the most required dental cosmetic procedures, must imply a consequent tooth vitality assessment. Sensitivity is strongly related to concentration, time and rate of usage of the bleaching gel [39, 42, 49–51]. In general, the activation systems have a role in increasing the temperature of the whitening agent, which penetrates rapidly the dental hard tissues, an aspect that favours the obtaining of an optimal result in a short interval of time but with the risk of increasing the inner pulp temperature. Therefore, this procedure can cause a local irritation to the dental pulp, which affects its micro-vascularization. In one of our studies, we chose the 1064 nm laser instrument for activating the bleaching gel and we compared it with the conventional 'in office' bleaching procedure, using LDF measurements.

In the Nd:YAG (1064 nm) laser-assisted bleaching, the pulp had a much better recovery (**Figure 2**), suggesting that LDF is a suitable method for a continuous monitoring of the dental pulp microcirculation [52].

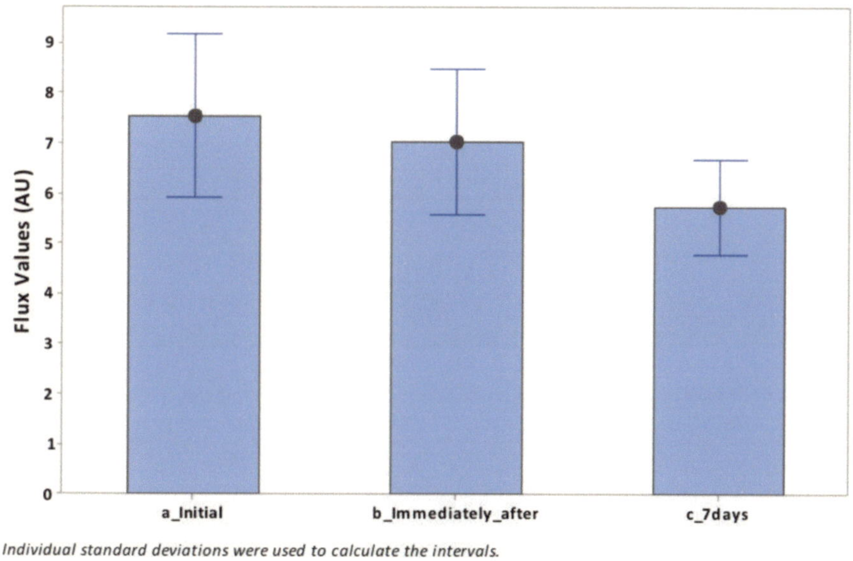

Figure 2. Interval plot of mean recorded before, immediately after and 1 week after treatment, indicating the evolution of the pulp blood flow over time for laser-assisted bleaching procedure.

2.1.2. *Prepared teeth and pulp microcirculation*

Determination of pulpal health represents an objective of endodontic diagnosis. It is important to assess pulp vitality prior to undertaking extensive tooth preparation in order to improve the prognosis of the restoration. It is also desirable to confirm periodically the pulp vitality in teeth that have undergone pulp preservation procedures or have had extensive restorations [53].

Full crown preparation procedures are probably the greatest restorative injury to which the dental pulp is subjected [54, 55]. The extensive cutting during crown preparation, desiccation, thermal injury and bacterial contamination has been implicated in the injury associated with tooth preparation [56]. Crown preparation without water spray causes about 95% reduction in the pulpal blood flow by 1 h after preparation. In contrast, the use of water spray virtually eradicates any alteration in pulpal blood flow. The reduction in coronal pulp blood flow is the result of an increased blood flow through the apically positioned arteriovenous (AVA) shunts and a redistribution of blood flow from the drilled side to the opposite side of the pulp [28, 57].

However, few reports were found in the literature regarding the use of LDF in assessing the pulpal blood flow in teeth that underwent prosthetic preparations [58, 59]. That is why the aim of our study was to evaluate how teeth preparation for full crown coverage may affect the pulpal blood flow.

The results obtained in our study show a linear increase in pulpal blood flow (PBF) values for all samples after dental prosthetic preparation. The values recorded 7 days after the preparation were higher than those recorded at 24 h after the preparation (**Figure 3**), which suggests that the increase in values does not relate only to optical changes due to the reduction of dental hard tissue but rather to the establishment of proper PBF. As a consequence, it may be assumed that a phenomenon of micro-irritation has appeared in the investigated area.

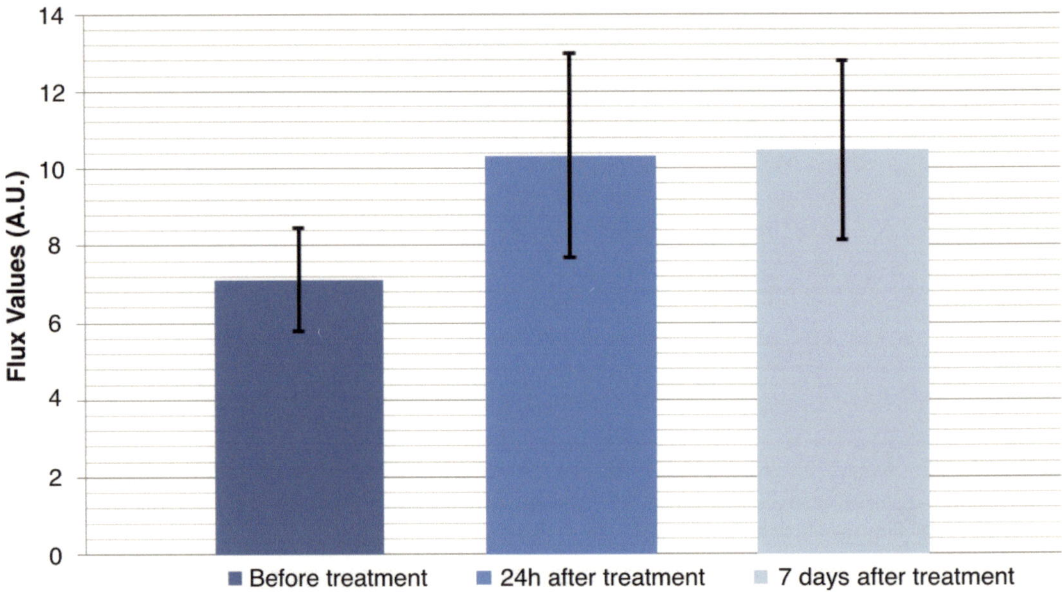

Figure 3. The PBF in time for the prepared teeth.

Only in one sample, the PBF recorded at 24 h was tremendously different from the initial moment and even from the PBF recorded at day 7. The patient did not report clinical symptoms of pulpal inflammation, such as pain and tenderness to percussion.

Yanpiset et al. [43] found LDF measurements to be extremely accurate in differentiating a revascularized (vital) tooth from a necrotic tooth pulp. An exciting finding of their study was that an accurate LDF reading of pulpal revascularization could be established at the fourth week after treatment, which is much earlier than it would be expected from standard sensitivity tests. This finding corresponds to those from the study by Skoglund et al. [60]. The LDF is extremely accurate in non-vital teeth, with almost 100% accuracy, but not as good in vital teeth. The blood vessels, fibroblasts and fibrous connective tissue that occupy the central portion of the pulp chamber can be affected without having a significant inflammatory reaction. While this tissue is vital and would give a radiographic picture of continued root development, the amount of moving blood cells creating a Doppler shift would be minimal. Another reason is that the revascularized teeth containing predominantly osteoid tissue may have a different optical property and the flux value reading from a revascularized tooth may be different from a normal tooth pulp. These teeth might give a false negative result [44]. Clinically, it has to be assumed that one may not rely solely on the LDF, but an estimation of signs of the pulpal or periapical pathology would still be necessary, before initiating endodontic treatment.

2.1.3. Pulp capping and pulp microcirculation

Injuries to permanent anterior teeth account for the most frequent form of orofacial trauma at a young age. According to various epidemiological studies, the permanent central incisors are mostly involved in traumatic events, sustaining nearly 80% of all registered injuries [61, 62].

Crown fractures may be uncomplicated involving enamel and dentin, without pulp exposure, or complicated, with pulp involvement. Therefore, an efficient clinical evaluation of an injured tooth requires symptomatic, visual and radiographic assessment. This is where LDF steps in, allowing a more accurate assessment of vascularization status in injured teeth whenever required, meaning immediately after the traumatic episode, as well as during and after treatment, justified by the method's safeness and non-invasiveness.

In one of our studies, we aimed to investigate the use of LDF, the pulpal healing process in complicated and uncomplicated crown fractures—with and without pulpal exposure when laser-assisted therapy combined with calcium hydroxide was used. After rubber dam placement, indirect pulp capping and preparation for resin composite restoration were performed for the upper right (#1.1) and left (#2.1) central incisors using Er:YAG laser irradiation (wavelength of 2940 nm; energy 240–80 mJ, SSP). Immediately after the treatment, the LDFRs were analysed and the results showed an increase in PBF on both teeth especially for tooth 2.1. After 7 days, the LDFRs evaluation was performed, and it showed a decrease in PBF in both teeth. The decrease was more notable in tooth 2.1 where the indirect pulp capping was performed. The last LDFRs evaluation was performed after 6 weeks, which revealed the recovery of PBF to a normal value, demonstrating that the pulp reached normal healthy status (**Figures 4** and **5**).

After 7 days, the pulp tissue was not restored to a healthy condition, with normal blood flow as shown by LDFRs, but after 6 weeks, the PBF recorded by LDF and the clinical assessment also showed almost a complete restoration of PBF. Vascular changes are essential to the initiation of acute as well as chronic inflammation, and blood flow is essential to its resolution. The inflammation process involves vasodilatation, thus increased circulation and perfusion. Therefore, a successful pulp capping is obtained when the following clinical conditions are met: uninflamed pulp, good antibacterial seal and the use of a capping material tolerated by the pulp tissue; better outcome is mainly registered in young teeth. Consequently, the clinical signs of inflammation correlated with the changes in PBF. LDF may therefore play a key role in clarifying the importance of PBF dynamics in the treatment of young traumatized teeth. Moreover, the recovery of PBF after laser indirect pulp capping was spectacular. This fact has been attributed to laser treatment for preparing the area for a hermetic sealing of the pulp. The practician must pay attention to the cavity preparation as well as to optimal placement of the capping material, which is in the benefit of the formation of tertiary dentine. Laser-assisted pulp capping represents a new treatment opportunity that improves the working conditions and the biological quality of the irradiated surface, thus increasing the effectiveness of the interaction between pulp tissue and capping agent.

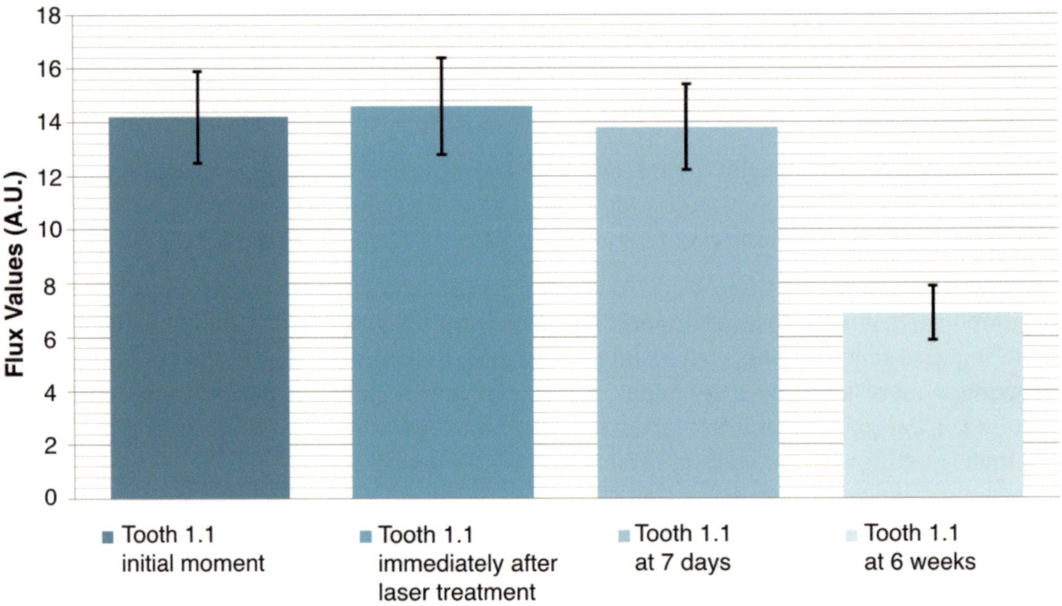

Figure 4. The descriptive graphic for LDFRs in traumatized tooth 1.1.

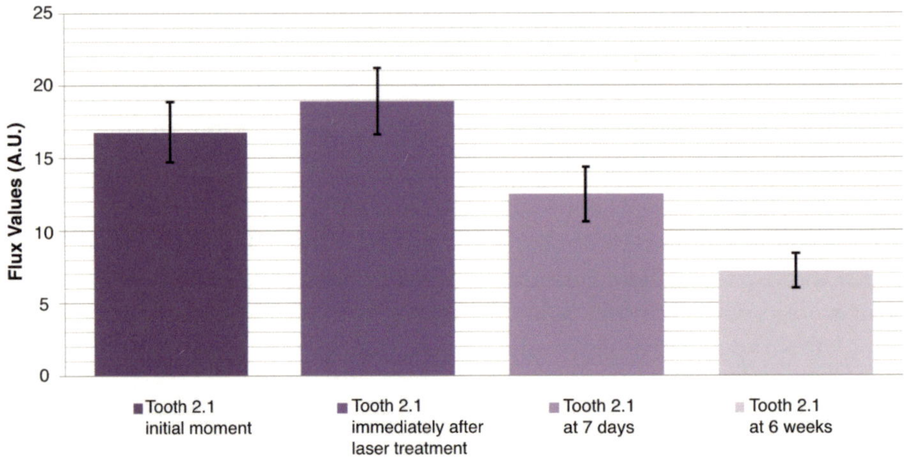

Figure 5. The descriptive graphic for LDFRs in traumatized tooth 2.1.

2.1.4. Traumatology and pulp microcirculation

LDF has been shown to be valuable in monitoring revascularization of teeth following severe dental trauma. During follow-up examinations the traumatized tooth can be unresponsive to traditional vitality testing during the first 6 months; however, LDF indicated that revascularization had occurred much sooner. Until recently, CO_2 ice has been the most effective method for sensitivity testing in trauma cases but LDF is able to give the assurance that we could defer invasive care during critical time period when the root canal therapy might have been initiated for the patient [63]. The information obtained by LDF is of additional importance for the treatment planning. Since the clinical examination of traumatized teeth is sometimes inconclusive, LDF could be regarded as a further diagnostic tool but it cannot replace the radiological or clinical examination [64].

A prospective, cohort study conducted by Emshoff et al. [65] on patients with dental injuries developed prediction rules for the treatment response related to the management of dental injuries. Treatment response (success or failure) was categorized based on findings of clinical and radiographic evaluation after 9 months. The most important variables were sub-luxation, root fracture, baseline PBF level and a change in PBF level at 3-month follow-up. The results show that the outcome following the management of dental injuries may be predicted from variables collected with LDF and physical examination. Predictive modelling may provide clinicians with the opportunity to identify 'at-risk' patients early and initiate specific treatment approaches.

2.2. Microcirculation of the gingiva

There is quite little information in the literature about the vascular dynamics of the gingival circulation in healthy and diseased sites. LDF emerged more than 30 years ago as a non-invasive and real-time method for perfusion measurements [66]. The LD technique made it possible to demonstrate that blood flow wave patterns differ consistently among gingival tissue types [67, 68] and that there are no within-subject differences over time in LDFRs [16].

One of the earliest signs of any inflammatory process is the change in the vascular architecture and microvasculature. This is also true for gingivitis [69]. The healthy gingiva is characterizes by a sub-epithelial vascular plexus consisting of a capillary network with loops arching towards the epithelium [70]. Gingival inflammation presents an increased vascularity with larger vessel size, more capillary loops, [71] slowed blood flow [72] and a restriction of the afferent blood vessels [73]. The capillary units are among the first vessels affected by inflammation in the crestal gingiva [74]. If changes of the vascular morphology in inflammation are related to blood flow changes, they may be the first sign to predict the onset of pathological events in the gingiva [75]. Thus, gingival blood flow (GBF) may serve as a prognostic marker. Gingival microcirculation (GM) has lacked exact evaluation for a long time. This was mainly due to methodological difficulties. Different methods, such as impedance plethysmography or the implantation of microspheres, have been employed to study GBF [76–82]. Unfortunately, most of them were invasive or inapplicable to humans. Other studies on dogs have shown that predictable morphologic changes occur in the blood vessels at the gingival margin with the onset of inflammation. These vascular changes precede recognizable histopathological alterations, starting as early as 2 days after the induction of gingivitis [36, 37, 83].

In our studies, in order to obtain a correct LDF measurement of the gingival blood flow, the probe was positioned 4 mm above the cervical line of the upper incisors and was also distanced using a gingival dam (LC Block-Out Resin, Ultradent Products, Inc.) before creating the silicone holder. This distance was necessary in order to avoid pressure on the gingival tissue when applying and removing the silicone holder during measurements phases. A silicone rubber holder was used in order to secure the gingival LDF probe in position at the studied site. A small hole for the laser probe was placed in the holder at 4 mm away from the gingival margin, using a high-speed handpiece and a 1.5 mm diameter fissure bur. After calibration and disinfection, the laser probe was inserted into a rigid opaque plastic tube with a 1.5 mm diameter and 0.1–0.2 mm longer than the fibre. The plastic tube was used to reduce the movement artefacts of the fibre inside the impression, by increasing adherence and protection of the active optic surface. The plastic tube was forcefully inserted in the canal carved in the impression and positioned afterwards according to study protocol. With the purpose of insuring the reproducibility of LD signal acquisition, a guiding mark was set on the fibre in order to allow its placement in the same position for each testing.

2.2.1. *Healthy and inflamed gingiva*

Previous researchers have shown that an interaction between GBF and gingival health exists [84]. One of our studies [18] aimed at evaluating the microcirculation in subjects with gingivitis compared to healthy gingiva by using LDF. The subjects of the present study were young adults in whom oral hygiene and dietary habits were well established. Ramsay et al. [85] indicated that the reliability of blood flow measurements required accurate repositioning of the measurement probe; that is why the technique used in the study aimed at achieving a correct reproducibility of the LDF measurements.

The results showed that LDF could be a useful non-invasive, sensitive, reproducible and harmless method for measuring GM in humans. LDF may therefore be an important element in clarifying the role of GBF dynamics in clinical gingivitis as well as in understanding the blood flow dynamics in the gingiva. At the seventh day, the gingiva was not restored to a healthy condition, with normal blood flow as shown by LDFRs but after 14 days, the GM recorded by LDF and the clinical assessment also showed almost a complete restoration of the gingivitis group. Consequently, the clinical signs of inflammation correlated with the changes in GBF (**Figure 6**).

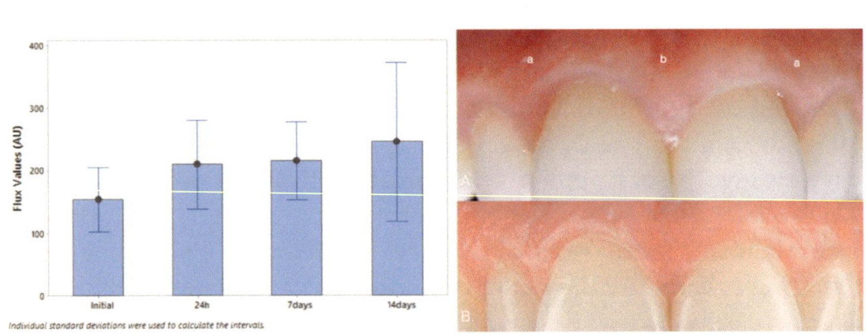

Figure 6. The mean values of the gingival blood flow (GBF) recorded at various moments of time; interval plot of the four moments of time in which the LDF measurements were carried out (*SD* = 74.9411); A. (a) sites with gingivitis; (b) healthy gingival site; B. restored gingival health after 14 days.

The results showed significant statistical differences between the four recordings in time. At 24 h after the initiation of therapy, the GBF was significantly increased compared to the baseline values suggesting local inflammation of the tissues after the initial therapy. No significant differences were noticed between initial moment and 7 days after the treatment and also between initial moment and 14 days after. The GBF values at 14 days were not significantly different compared to the control group (**Figure 7**).

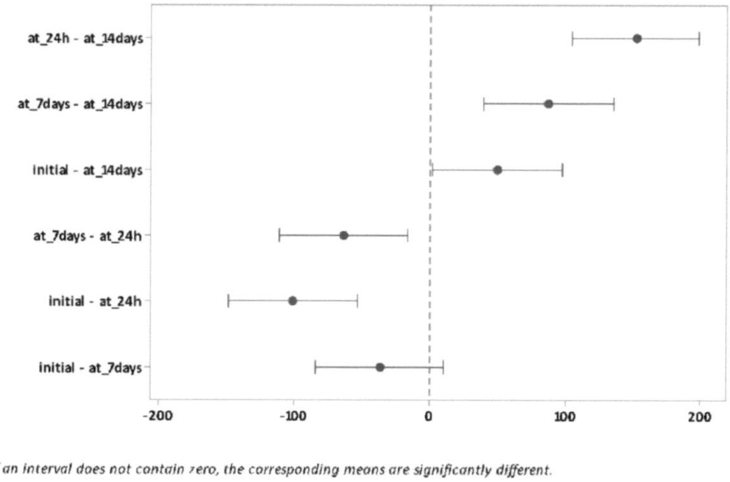

Figure 7. Fisher individual 95% CIs. Comparison of GBF values of the gingivitis group among the four moments of time recorded in the study. Showing that there are no statistical significant differences between the initial and the 7-day groups as well as between the initial and the 14-day groups.

2.2.2. *Laser periodontal surgery and gingival recovery*

When performing gingivoplasty by conventional methods, there are limitations regarding healing by secondary intention, post-operative bleeding, loss of keratinized gingiva and inability to treat the underlying osseous deformities, which leads to the inability to complete the treatment [87]. Performing surgical procedure using laser technology can solve most of these limitations.

LDF found an excellent utility in the evaluation of the gingival recovery after surgery performed with the high-end methods available today.

When using lasers, the depth and amount of soft tissue ablation are more precisely established than with mechanical instruments [88, 89]. In particular, Er:YAG laser is very adequate and useful for aesthetic periodontal soft tissue management because this laser is capable of accurately ablating soft tissues using various handpiece tips, and therefore, the healing process is faster and favourable due to the minimal thermal alteration of the treated surface [90].

Diode lasers act as a useful tool for cutting gingival tissue, producing good haemostasis and reducing bacterial growth in periodontal surgery. There is evidence that this wavelength can reduce gingival inflammation and also the need for local anaesthesia during surgical procedures.

In order to establish the efficiency of one laser in comparison with other, we decided to perform a study where LDF was used to compare GBF after Er:YAG (Fotona Fidelis Plus II) and 980 nm diode laser (Diode Laser Smile Pro 980 Biolitec) gingivectomy.

The evaluation was carried out on 20 anterior teeth that underwent reshaping of gingiva in five female patients (four anterior teeth/patient), aged between 20 and 35, capable of adequate compliance. The Er:YAG laser was used in Long Pulse: 600 μsec (LP) and Very Long Pulse: 1000 μsec (VLP) modes, 140–250 mJ, 10–20 Hz frequency, contact mode and using cylindrical sapphire tips. The parameters were established according to previous research [26] and were found suitable for soft tissue without causing visible major thermal damage to root dentin or bone. The 980 nm diode laser was used in continuous wave mode, 4 W, contact mode and cooling with saline solution using a 360 μm diameter quartz fibre as delivery system (**Figure 8**).

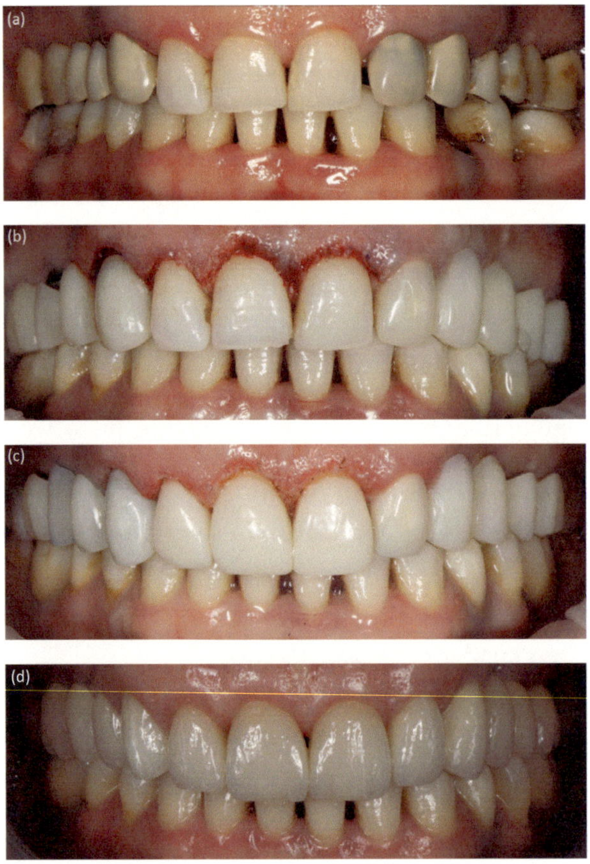

Figure 8. (a). Initial intra-oral status, (b) immediately after laser surgery, (c) 24 h after the laser surgery with indirect provisional restorations, and (d) clinical intra-oral aspect 2 months after treatment with the final ceramic restorations.

At first appointment, the initial measurements were carried out. Post-operative controls and LDF measurements were accomplished after 24 h, 7 and 14 days to evaluate healing and wound evolution on a total of eight points/patient (two points on each tooth) for each patient.

As for the gingival surgery with Er:YAG laser, significant differences in LDF recordings over time were established between different times ($p < 0.001$ with a significant level $\alpha = 0.001$, Friedman test). The results showed that after 24 h the differences are significant compared to the initial moment; 7 days after the treatment, with the Er:YAG, LDF was slightly raised compared to the initial moment ($p = 0.256$), and after 14 days, LDF the values were insignificantly lower compared to pre-treatment ($p = 0.431$) (**Figure 9**).

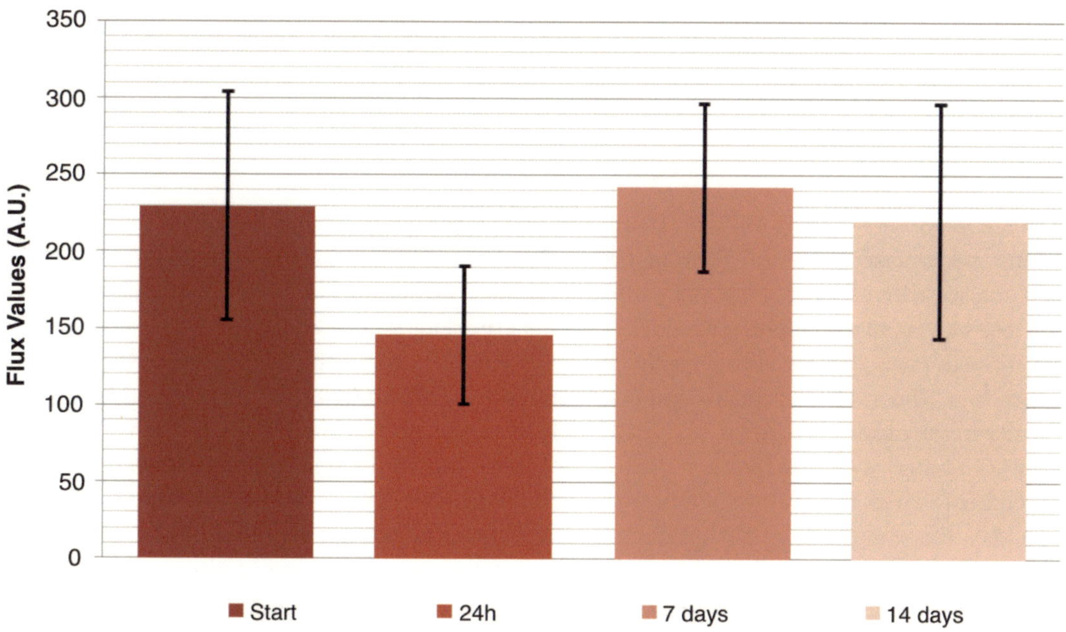

Figure 9. The descriptive graphic for 'Laser 1' method applied at the four moments of time.

Regarding gingival surgery with the diode laser, significant differences between the four tracings over different times were found ($p < 0.001$ with a significant level $\alpha = 0.001$, Friedman test). After 24 h, the differences were significantly lower compared to the initial moment; whereas after 7 and 14 days, the recorded LDF values were significantly raised compared to the initial moment ($p < 0.001$) (**Figure 10**).

The Levene's test for equality of variances was used in order to establish the equal variances assumed at the initial moment as well as after 14 days, and afterwards, the independent sample test was used for comparing the values obtained for the Er:YAG area and for the diode area at the initial moment (insignificant differences $p = 0.897$) and after 14 days (significant difference $p < 0.001$). We established that after 14 days, the recorded fluxes for the diode area were significantly higher compared to the values obtained for the Er:YAG area ($p < 0.001$).

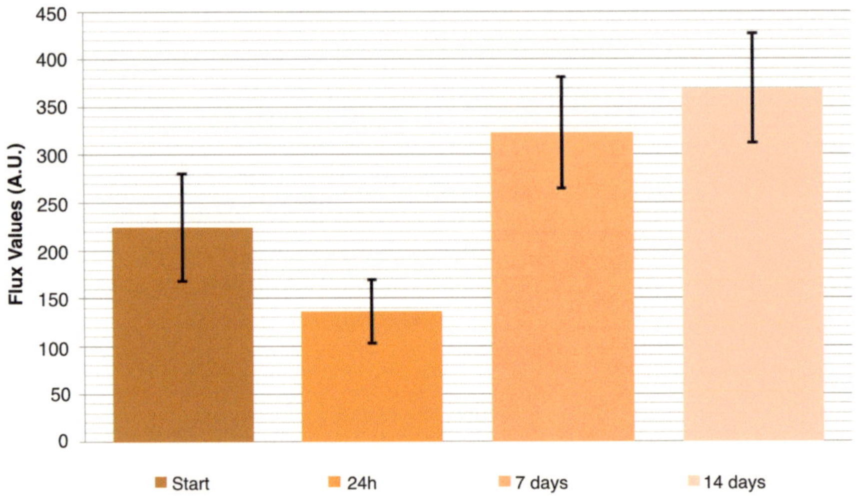

Figure 10. The descriptive graphic for 'Laser 2' method applied at the four moments of time.

The results obtained after the laser treatment on the free gingival area indicate a modification in the micro-vascular blood flow response. Furthermore, our measurements, which are in accordance with other studies [91], indicate that LDF technique can offer information regarding the micro-vascular changes during healing period. These results showed an evident decrease in perfusion for both areas in comparison with the baseline values 24 h after surgical procedure. The micro-vascular blood flow increased significantly after 7 days in both areas but mostly in the diode area. After 14 days, the blood perfusion returned to the initial value in the Er:YAG-treated area. The results in the diode-treated area remained at a higher level, showing that after 14 days, the healing in this area was not complete. The response after laser treatment in both areas was an obviously hyperaemic one. The difference in haemodynamic changes that occurred after 14 days can be explained by the differences in tissue interaction of the different laser procedures applied in our study.

2.2.3. Mucositis and gingival blood flow

In a study [92] conducted by our group, we evaluated the immediate effects of radiotherapy, more precisely, the oral and perioral soft tissue changes that appear after the radiotherapy treatment period. Additionally, we measured the gingival blood flow using LDF, in order to objectively determine any changes of the microvascular system of the gingiva.

Even after the first radiotherapy exposure, the blood flow values increased towards the irradiated area and remained increased throughout the entire treatment. This suggests that the periodontal tissue responds immediately to radiotherapy (as expected), and an inflammatory state is established even after the first exposure and it persists during treatment. What we found interesting was that this increase in vascularity preceded the clinical modifications, which means that with the help of LDF, we can diagnose an inflammation and we can predict the setting of the clinical side effects of radiotherapy. On the other hand, we did not find any numerical correlation between blood flow values and the severity of the clinical manifestation of the radiation-induced side effects.

LD was a useful instrument in establishing the kind of dental procedures we can perform during treatment. Based on our results, we recommend to perform, during this time frame, mostly conservative measures, surgical measures should be performed keeping in mind that the tissues are inflamed and that the bleeding would be greater than normal and wound healing difficult. Prosthetic treatments, if performed, should be done with consideration towards the periodontal tissue that should not be additionally irritated. The clinician should carefully wage the advantages of the treatment against the possible complications that it could bring. The goal of any dental treatment should be increasing the patients' quality of life and decreasing the risks of interrupting radiotherapy, due to the onset of the side effects that it causes.

2.2.4. Smokers and gingival microcirculation

One of our studies [93] aimed at investigating microcirculatory alterations of the gingiva occurring after smoking tobacco compared the periodontal status of both smoker and non-smoker patients and also the registered values between the sexes (**Figure 11**).

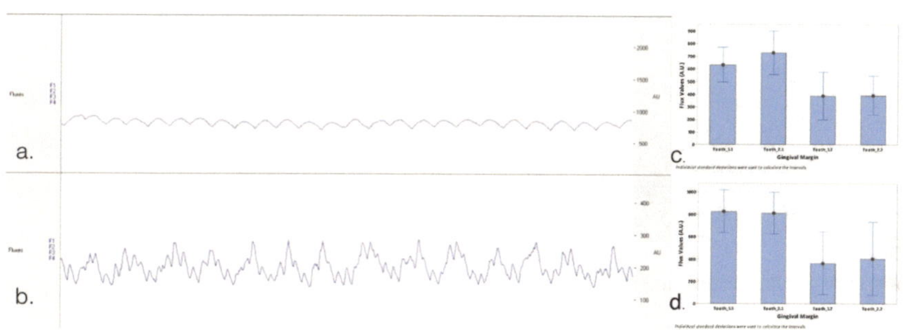

Figure 11. (a) Example of LDF recording from a non-smoker patient; (b) example of LDF recording from a smoker patient; (c) interval plot of flux values (AU) in smoker male group; and (d) interval plot of flux values (A.U.) in smoker female group.

We found no significant differences (*t*-test) between non-smoker male group (I-M) and non-smoker female group (I-F). On the other hand, LDF in the smoker female group (Group II-F) was significantly elevated compared to the smoker male group (Group II-M). The Group II-M LDF values were slightly increased compared to the Group I-M. The LDF values in the Group II-F were significantly higher than the LDF values in Group I-F.

2.2.5. Laser Doppler imaging and gingival microcirculation

Essentially, LDI works by scanning a monochromatic laser across the surface of the tissue. Light, which is backscattered from moving erythrocytes, undergoes a shift in frequency proportional to its velocity, according to the Doppler principle. Most laser Doppler set-ups use a helium-neon laser (RED, 632.8 nm), providing an estimate of perfusion up to a depth of 1–

1.5 mm into the dermis of white skin and thus mainly measure the perfusion in arterioles, venules and capillaries. LDI gives a 'snapshot' of perfusion at a given point.

The objective of one of our studies [19] was to evaluate the applicability of LD line scanning in recording the gingival healing process after a surgical procedure followed by two types of plastic provisional restoration. As a secondary objective, we also aimed at testing two different techniques and materials for performing the plastic temporaries. The results were also validated by clinical examination.

The moorLDI2-IR instrument, infrared diode laser 785 nm nominal, maximum power 2.5 mW with a visible diode laser (target beam for infrared systems) 660 nm nominal, maximum power 0.25 mW, was used in our study. The microcirculation in the investigated areas suffered changes in the analysed period (14 days) and was monitored with the Moor laser Doppler line scanner (**Figure 12**).

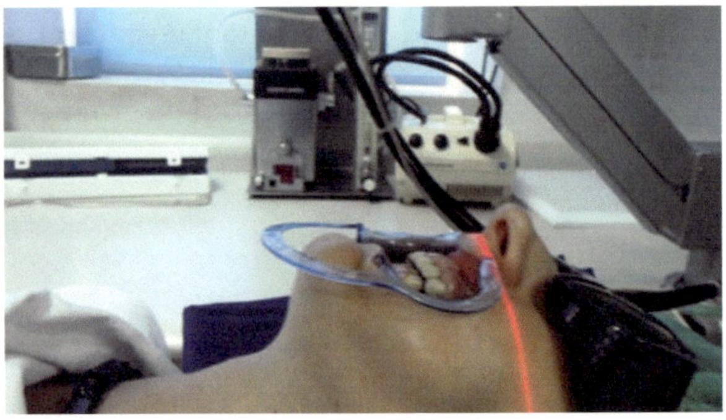

Figure 12. Laser Doppler line scanning procedure.

LDI recordings were performed in the labial regions of the operated areas at the day of the surgery, prior to local anaesthesia, after 24 h, after 7 days and 14 days following the intervention. The scanner used in this study was placed so that it was directed to record the vessels within the selected area. The differences between the four recordings clearly demonstrated adjustments in the micro-vascularity of the region in the healing period. The initial images of the area (**Figure 13(a)**) showed a certain perfusion map that differed completely from the LDI images at 24 h after the surgical procedure and the cementation of the plastic temporaries. The image at 24 h showed increased microcirculation as a reaction to the surgical procedure (**Figure 13(b)**). This situation is represented by an increase in the red colour of the affected areas in the perfusion map. The LDI images, 7 days after the surgical procedure, showed an improvement in the microcirculation healing in the interested area while the LDI images, 14 days after the surgical procedure, confirmed healing by offering a perfusion map similar to the initial one. The clinical examination asserted the changes observed on the perfusion maps in both cases.

With the aid of LDI, it was possible to obtain information regarding the impact of different materials for aesthetic prosthetics temporary restoration after surgical treatment on GM. The two types of plastic materials had no negative influence on the healing process of investigated area.

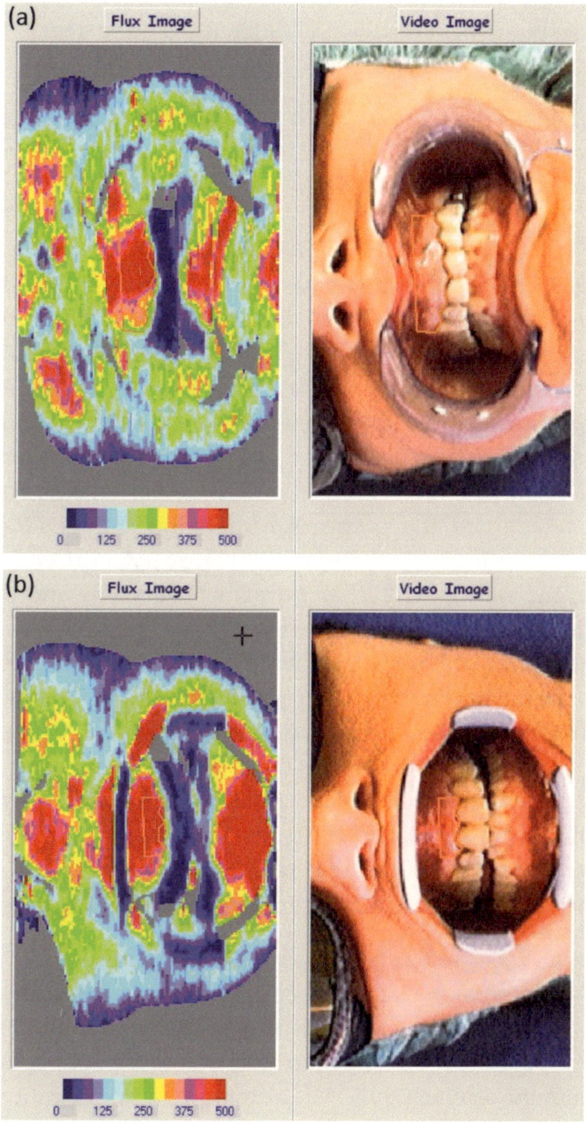

Figure 13. (a) Initial LDI recording and (b) LDI recording at 24 h with an increase in the red colour of the affected areas in the perfusion map.

The major advantages of LDI over LDF are the fact that there is no need for direct contact with the tissue (max. distance 19 cm), the possibility to accomplish multiple measurements allowing to obtaining many images in the area of interest (120 pixel/cm) and most importantly, it allows a global analysis of blood flow in the area of interest.

This technique has been shown to be easy to learn by surgeons. Regular post-operative assessment of flap perfusion by members of the microsurgery team trained in the use of LD line scanning might, therefore, represent a practical alternative to more complex and invasive monitoring techniques. Issues of inter- and intra-examiner reliability have yet to be examined, and in an area where only a low percentage of flaps undergo vascular compromise, this may prove impractical.

One advantage that LDF has over LDI is that it gives a constant measure of blood flow at the specified point, whereas LDI gives a 'snapshot' of perfusion at a given point.

2.3. Limitations

Although LDF has proved valuable for a variety of clinical applications, there are some limitations to its use in oral medicine. A major drawback is that LDF can only detect red blood cell movement in a small volume of tissue (1 mm^3); thus, variables such as the number of vessels with active flow, changes in vessel diameter and flow in individual micro-vessels cannot be analysed. The small measuring area may also influence the reproducibility of the results due to the fact that a minimal displacement of the optical probe would lead to a change in the investigated area [20]. Another source of error in LDF measurements are the artefacts caused by tissue motion in relation to the probe. Additionally, oral LDFRs have demonstrated considerable intra- and inter-individual variability [94, 95]. A part of the limitations is being solved by the fact that the velocity of PBF in humans is very low and that LDF modified for the measurement of slow blood flow is appropriate for PBF measurement in humans [96]. One of the most important limitations of the LDF is that each patient presents variation of blood flow because the measurement is influenced by the thickness of the connective tissue and local distribution of the vessels and also the recording site (free gingivae, inter-dental gingivae, attached gingivae or alveolar mucosae) [35–37, 40]. Other limitation of LDF is that flow readings are not only dependent on the blood flow in the measurement volume but also on the scattering properties of the surrounding tissues. It has been reported that up to 80% of LD blood flow signal recorded from an intact human pulp is of non-pulpal origin [41]. The same could be anticipated for LDF measurements performed on the gingivae.

Originally, iontophoresis was used in conjunction with single-point LDF, as opposed to LDI systems, which measure perfusion over a larger area and produce a detailed perfusion map. Laser Doppler flowmetry typically measures within a small volume ($\sim$1 mm^3) and, as a result, has often suffered from poor reproducibility, mainly due to the spatial heterogeneity of tissue blood flow and movement artefacts [97, 98], although reproducibility has been improved recently by the use of 'integrated probes'. These uses multiple collecting fibres positioned in a ring around a central light delivery fibre, thus increasing the spatial resolution. However, the use of LDI still provides a larger surface area measurement and should be the preferred choice in areas of tissues with high spatial variability, despite the significant difference in costs. This could be detrimental if one is interested in the dynamics of the dilator response. This problem can be partially solved by altering the time taken for a scan. This can be done in two ways: by reducing the area to be scanned and/or increasing the scanning speed of the laser. The latter has the slight disadvantage of producing a slightly less detailed image, but in most cases, it is a compromise worth making. Many studies are not closely concerned with the dynamics of the cutaneous response and are instead focusing more on the maximum response at a given dose, in which case LDI is adequate. The line-of-sight velocity of the moving scatterers is directly proportional to the frequency of the fluctuations. This would suggest that both techniques are linear with respect to velocity. In the case of Doppler, however, it has been accepted for some 30 years that if you take the first moment of the power spectrum of the fluctuations, then it scales linearly with both velocity and concentration (number of moving scatterers) [99]. In the case of blood flow, this is a measure of perfusion. If a Doppler system uses this algorithm (first moment of the power spectrum), then it should be linear with respect to perfusion [100].

3. Conclusions

The major advantage of the laser Doppler techniques in general is their non-invasiveness and their ability to measure the microcirculation flux of the tissue and fast changes of perfusion during provocations. The LDF represents an important instrument to assess gingival and pulpal microcirculation in the oral cavity. In this respect, it enables monitoring of the tooth vitality, establishing the pulp revascularization before these data could be derived from traditional sensitivity tests, which can also add more inflammation to the already irritated pulp. LDF can be used to assess the degree and duration of the pulpal inflammation or ischemic episodes, thereby identifying patients at risk for adverse reactions such as irreversible inflammation, avascular necrosis and tissue loss. Further studies are warranted to assess the validity of pulpal blood flow measurements by comparing them with histological tooth pulp changes, and by determining how well the LDF diagnoses of pulp health may predict the course of pre-prosthetic treatment.

In conclusion, LDF is a suitable technique for determining pulp vitality in most clinical situations and can be used together with other indices to evaluate the marginal gingival health status.

Author details

Carmen Todea[1*], Silvana Canjau[1], Mariana Miron[1], Bogdan Vitez[1] and Gheorghe Noditi[2]

*Address all correspondence to: carmentodea@gmail.com

1 Department of Oral Rehabilitation and Dental Emergencies, Faculty of Dentistry, 'Victor Babes' University of Medicine and Pharmacy, Timisoara, Romania

2 Department of Plastic and Reconstructive Surgery, 'Victor Babeș' University of Medicine and Pharmacy, Timisoara, Romania

References

[1] Pries AR, Neuhaus D, Gaehtgens P. Blood viscosity in tube flow: dependence on diameter and hematocrit. Am J Physiol. 1992;263:H1770–H1778.

[2] Johnson PC. Overview of the microcirculation. In: Tuma RF, Duran VN, Ley K, eds. Handbook of Physiology: Microcirculation. Oxford: Elsevier Science; 2002; pp. xi–xxiv. DOI: 10.1016/B978-0-12-374530-9.00022-X

[3] Patiño-Martin N, Martínez F, Loyola-RodríGuez JP, Tenorio-Govea E, Brito-Orta MD, Rodríguez-Martínez M. A novel procedure for evaluating gingival perfusion status using laser-Doppler flowmetry. J Clin Periodontol. 2005;32:231–237. DOI: 10.1111/j.1600-051X.2005.00655.x

[4] Matsuki M, Xu YB, Nagasawa T. Gingival blood flow measurement with a non-contact laser flowmeter. J Oral Rehabil. 2001;28:630–633. DOI: 10.1046/j.1365-2842.2001.00729.x

[5] Juliusson S, Bende M. Allergic reaction of the human nasal mucosa studied with laser Doppler flowmetry. Clin Allergy. 1987;17:301–305.

[6] Speight EL, Essex TJ, Farr PM. The study of plaques of psoriasis using a scanning laser Doppler velocimeter. Br J Dermatol. 1993;125:519–524. DOI: 10.1111/j.1365-2133.1993.tb00228.x

[7] Sasano T, Kuriwada S, Sanjo D, Izumi H, Tabata T, Karita K. Acute response of periodontal ligament blood flow to external force application. J Periodontal Res. 1992;27:301–304.
DOI: 10.1111/j.1600-0765.1992.tb01682.x

[8] Gazelius B, Olgart L, Edwall B, Edwall L. Non-invasive recording of blood flow in human dental pulp. Endod Dent Traumatol. 1986;2:219–221. DOI: 10.1111/j.1600-9657.1986.tb00148.x

[9] Kim S, Liu M, Markowitz K, Billoto G, Dorscher-Kim J. Comparison of pulpal blood flow in dog canine teeth determined by the laser Doppler and 133Xenon wash- out methods. Arch Oral Biol. 1990;35:411–413. DOI: http://dx.doi.org/10.1016/0003-9969(90)90189-H

[10] Miron MI, Dodenciu D, Sarbescu P, Canjau S, Ardelean L, Rusu L, Todea C. Condensation silicones and light-curing resin used within a laser Doppler pulp vitality testing method. Mater Plast. 2012;49(3):171–175.

[11] Miron MI, Dodenciu D, Calniceanu M, Filip LM, Todea DC. Optimization of the laser Doppler signal acquisition timing for pulp vitality evaluation. Timisoara Med J. 2010;60(1):44–49.

[12] Miron MI, Dodenciu D, Calniceanu M, Lungeanu D, Filip LM, Balabuc CA, Todea C. Evaluation of the effect of ambient light on laser Doppler flowmetry recordings in anterior teeth. Archives Balkan Med Union. 2009;44(4):265–270.

[13] Baab DA, Oberg A, Lundström A. Gingival blood flow and temperature changes in young humans with a history of periodontitis. Arch Oral Biol. 1990;35:95–101.

[14] Baab DA, Oberg PA. Laser Doppler measurement of gingival blood flow in dogs with increasing and decreasing inflammation. Arch Oral Biol. 1987;32:551–555.

[15] Matheny JL, Johnson DT, Roth GI. Aging and micro-circulatory dynamics in human gingiva. J Clin Periodontol. 1993;20:471–475. DOI: 10.1111/j.1600-051X.1993.tb00393.x

[16] Hinrichs JE, LaBelle LL, Aeppli D. An evaluation of laser Doppler readings obtained from human gingival sulci. J Periodontol. 1995;66:171–176. DOI:10.1902/jop.1995.66.3.171

[17] Todea C, Canjau S, Dodenciu D, Miron MI, Tudor A, Bălăbuc C. Laser Doppler flowmetry evaluation of gingival recovery response after laser treatment. Head and Neck Optical Diagnostics, Proc. SPIE 8805, 880508. 2013: DOI: 10.1117/12.2034038.

[18] Canjau S, Miron MI, Todea CD. Laser Doppler flowmetry evaluation of gingival microcirculation recovery in gingivitis. Archives Balkan Med Union. 2015;50(3):354–359.

[19] Noditi G, Todea C. Laser Doppler imaging—as a non-invasive method for assesing regional microcirculation when using plastic materials for guided healing. Mater Plast. 2013;1(50):40–43.

[20] Boutault F, Cadenat H, Hibert PJ. Evaluation of gingival microcirculation by a laser-Doppler flowmeter. J Craniomaxillofac Surg. 1989;17:105–109.

[21] Ketabi M, Hirsch RS. The effects of local anesthetic containing adrenaline on gingival blood flow in smokers and non-smokers. J Clin Periodontol. 1997;24:888–892. DOI: 10.1111/j.1600-051X.1997.tb01207.x

[22] Cracowski JL, et al. Assessment of endothelial and neurovascular function in human skin microcirculation. Trends Pharmacol. Sci. 2006;27:503–508. DOI: 10.1016/j.tips.2013.05.007

[23] Roustit M, et al. A Microvasc Res. 2010;79:102–108.

[24] Roustit M, et al. Excellent reproducibility of laser speckle contrast imaging to assess skin microvascular reactivity. A Microvasc. Res. 2010;80:505–511. DOI: 10.1016/j.mvr.2010.05.012

[25] Kernick DP, Shore AC. Characteristics of laser Doppler perfusion imaging in vitro and in vivo. Physiol Meas. 2000;21:333–340.

[26] Musselwhite JM, Klitzman B, Maixner W, Burkes E. Laser Doppler flowmetry. Oral Surg Oral Med Oral Pathol Oral Radiol Endod. 1997;84:411–419. DOI: http://dx.doi.org/10.1016/S1079-2104(97)90041-X

[27] Chen E, Abbott P. Dental pulp testing: a review. Int J Dent. 2009. DOI: 10.1155/2009/365785

[28] Jafarzadeh H. Laser Doppler flowmetry in endodontics: a review. Int Endod J. 2009;42:476–490. DOI: 10.1111/j.1365-2591.2009.01548.x

[29] Polat S, Er K, Polat N. Penetration depth of laser Doppler flowmetry beam in teeth. Oral Surg Oral Med Oral Pathol Oral Radiol Endod. 2005;100:125–129. DOI: http://dx.doi.org/10.1016/j.tripleo.2004.11.018

[30] Roy E, Alliot-Licht B, Dajean-Trutaud S, Fraysse C, Jean A, Armengol V. Evaluation of the ability of laser Doppler flowmetry for the assessment of pulp vitality in general dental practice. Oral Surg Oral Med Oral Pathol Oral Radiol Endod. 2008;106:615–620. DOI: http://dx.doi.org/10.1016/j.tripleo.2008.05.035

[31] Rajan V, Varghese B. Review of methodological developments in laser Doppler flowmetry. Laser Med Sci. 2007. DOI: 10.1007/s10103-007-0524-0

[32] Ikawa M, Vongsavan N, Horiuchi H. Scattering of laser light directed onto the labial surface of extracted human upper central incisors. J Endod. 1999;25:483–485.

[33] Soo-ampon S, Vongsavan N, Soo-ampon M, Chuckpaiwong S, Matthews B. The sources of laser Doppler blood-flow signals recorded from human teeth. Arch Oral Biol. 2003;48(5):353–360. DOI: http://dx.doi.org/10.1016/S0003-9969(03)00011-6

[34] Polat S, Er K, Akpinar K, Polat N. The sources of laser Doppler blood-flow signals recorded from vital and root canal treated teeth. Arch Oral Biol. 2004;49:53–57. DOI: http://dx.doi.org/10.1016/S0003-9969(03)00197-3

[35] Karayilmaz H, Kirzioglu Z. Comparison of the reliability of laser Doppler flowmetry, pulse oximetry and electric pulp tester in assessing the pulp vitality of human teeth. J Oral Rehab. 2010. DOI: 10.1111/j.1365-2 84of 2.2010.02160.x

[36] Hartmann A, Azérad J, Boucher Y. Environmental effects on laser Doppler pulpal blood-flow measurements in man. Arch Oral Biol. 1996;41(4):333–339. DOI: http://dx.doi.org/10.1016/0003-9969(95)00133-6

[37] Akpinar KE, Er K, Polat S, Polat NT. Effect of gingiva on laser Doppler pulpal blood flow measurements. J Endod. 2004;30(3):138–140. DOI: http://dx.doi.org/10.1097/00004770-200403000-00003

[38] Rajan V, Varghese B, Van Leeuwen T, Steenbergen W. Review of methodological developments in laser Doppler flowmetry. Lasers Med Sci. 2009;24:269–283. DOI: 10.1007/s10103-007-0524-0

[39] Marson FC, Sensi LG. Clinical evaluation of in-office dental bleaching treatments with and without the use of light-activation sources. Operative Dent. 2008;33(1):11–18. DOI: http://dx.doi.org/10.2341/07-57

[40] Miron MI, Dodenciu D, Saarbescu PF, Filip LM, Balabuc CA, Hanigovski E, Todea DC. Optimization of the laser Doppler signal acquisition technique in pulp vitality tests. Archives Balkan Med Union. 2011;46(4):280–284.

[41] Odor T, Watson T, Pitt Ford T, Mcdonald F. Pattern of transmission of laser light in teeth. Int Endod J. 1996;29:228–234. DOI: 10.1111/j.1365-2591.1996.tb01374.x

[42] Wetter NU, Walverde DA, Kato IT, Eduardo C de P. Bleaching efficacy of whitening agents activated by xenon lamp and 960-nm diode radiation. Photomed Laser Surg. 2004;22(6):489–493.

[43] Yanpiset K, Vongsavan N, Sigurdsson A, Trope M. Efficacy of laser Doppler flowmetry for the diagnosis of revascularization of reimplanted immature dog teeth. Dent Traumatol. 2001;17:63–70. DOI: 10.1034/j.1600-9657.2001.017002063.x

[44] Roeykens H, Van Maele G, De Moor R, Martens L. Reliability of laser Doppler flowmetry in a 2-probe assessment of pulpal flow. Oral Surg Med Oral Pathol Oral Radiol Endod. 1999;87:742–748. DOI: http://dx.doi.org/10.1016/S1079-2104(99)70173-3

[45] Ingolfsson A, Tronstad L, Hersh E, Riva C. Effect of probe design on the suitability of laser Doppler flowmetry in vital testing of human teeth. Endod Dent Traumatol. 1993;9:65–70.

[46] Roebuck E, Evans D, Strriups D, Strang R. The effect of wavelength, bandwidth, and probe design and position on assessing the vitality of anterior teeth with laser Doppler flowmetry. Int J Paediatr Dent. 2000;10:213–220. DOI: 10.1046/j.1365-263x.2000.00194.x

[47] Norer B, Kranewitter R, Emshoff R. Pulpal blood-flow characteristics of maxillary tooth morphotypes as assessed with laser Doppler flowmetry. Oral Surg Oral Med Oral Pathol Oral Radiol Endod. 1999;87:88–92. DOI: http://dx.doi.org/10.1016/S1079-2104(99)70301-X

[48] Buckley J, Jones M, Hill M, Sugar A. An evaluation of the changes in maxillary pulpal blood flow associated with orthodontic surgery. Br J Orthod. 1999;26:39–45.

[49] Matis BA, Wang Y, Jiang T, Eckert GJ. Extended at-home bleaching of tetracycline-stained teeth with different concentrations of carbamide peroxide. Quintessence Int. 2002;33(9):645–655.

[50] Deliperi S, Bardwell DN, Papathanasiou A. Clinical evaluation of a combined in-office and take-home bleaching system. J Am Dent Assoc. 2004;135(5):628–634. DOI: http://dx.doi.org/10.14219/jada.archive.2004.0252

[51] Wetter NU, Barroso MC, Pelino JE. Dental bleaching efficacy with diode laser and LED irradiation: an in vitro study. Lasers Surg Med. 2004;35(4):254–258. DOI: 10.1002/lsm.20103

[52] Todea C, Sarpe A, Vitez B, Draganescu G. New method of laser Doppler flowmetry signal processing in pulp vitality evaluation after teeth cosmetic treatment. Proc. SPIE 8925, Fifth International Conference on Lasers in Medicine: Biotechnologies Integrated in Daily Medicine, 892502. 2014. DOI: 10.1117/12.2042778

[53] Ford P, Patel S. Technical equipment for assessment of dental pulp status. Endod Topics. 2004;7:2–13. DOI: 10.1111/j.1601-1546.2004.00063.x

[54] Yuen T, Wilson P. The effect of venting on pulpward pressure transmission and seating on crown cementation: a laboratory study. J Oral Rehabil. 2000;124:38–46. DOI: 10.1111/j.1365-2842.2000.00612.x

[55] Richardson D, Tao L, Pashley DH. Dentin permeability. Effects of crown preparation. Int J Prosthodont. 1991;4:219–225.

[56] Brännström M. Reducing the risk of sensitivity and pulpal complications after the placement of crowns and fixed partial dentures. Quintessence Int. 1996;27:673–678.

[57] Suda H, Ikeda H. The circulation of the pulp. In: Hargreaves KM and Goodis HE, eds. Seltzer and Bender's Dental Pulp. Quintessence Publishing Co. 2002;140–144.

[58] Messer H. Permanent restorations and the dental pulp. In: Hargreaves KM and Goodis HE, eds. Seltzer and Bender's Dental Pulp. Quintessence Publishing Co. 2002;357–359.

[59] Kunt G, Körcü D, Ceylan G, Ylmaz N, Güller A. Pulpal blood flow in abutment teeth of removable partial dentures. Bosn J Basic Med Sci. 2009;9:296–300.

[60] Skoglund A, Tronstad L, Wallenius K. A microangiographic study of vascular changes in replanted and autotransplanted teeth of young dogs. Oral Surg Oral Med Oral Pathol. 1978;45:17–28.

[61] Zerman N, Cavalleri G. Traumatic injuries to permanent incisors. Endod Dent Traumatol. 1993;9:61. DOI: 10.1111/j.1600-9657.1993.tb00661.x

[62] Strobl H, Haas M, Norer B, Gerhard S, Emshoff R. Evaluation of pulpal blood flow after tooth splinting of luxated permanent maxillary incisors. Dent Traumatol 2004;20:36–41. DOI: 10.1046/j.1600-4469.2003.00223.x

[63] Lee J, Yanpiset K, Sigurdsson A, Vann Jr W. Laser Doppler flowmetry for monitoring traumatized teeth. Dent Traumatol. 2001;17:231–235.

[64] Winzap-Kälin C, Chappuis V, von Arx T. Laser Doppler flowmetry for vitality testing of traumatized maxillary incisors. Schweiz Monatsschr Zahnmed. 2005;115(1):12–17.

[65] Emshoff R, Gerhard S, Ennemoser T, Hächel O, Scherl M, Strobl H. The use of likelihood ratio methodology to find predictors of treatment outcome in patients with dental injury diagnoses. J Oral Rehabil. 2010;37(2):107–115. DOI: 10.1111/j.1365-2842.2009.02025.x

[66] Stern MD. In vivo evaluation of microcirculation by coherent light scattering. Nature. 1975;254:56–58. DOI: 10.1038/254056a0

[67] Baab DA, Oberg PA, Holloway GA. Gingival blood flow measured with a laser Doppler flowmeter. J Periodont Res. 1986;21:73–85.

[68] Kerdvongbundit V, Sirirat M, Sirikulsathean A, Kasetsuwan J, Hasegawa A. Blood flow and human periodontal status. Odontol. 2002;90(1):52–56.

[69] Kerdvongbundit V, Vongsavan N, Soo-Ampon S, Hasegawa A. Microcirculation and micromorphology of healthy and inflamed gingivae. Odontol. 2003;91(1):19–25. DOI: 10.1007/s102660200007

[70] Kindlová M. The blood supply of the marginal periodontium in *Macacus rhesus*. Arch Oral Biol. 1965;10:869–874.

[71] Egelberg J. The blood vessels of the dento-gingival junction. J Periodont Res. 1966;1:163–179.

[72] Hansson BO, Lindhe J, Branemark PI. Microvascular topography and function in clinically healthy and chron- ically inflamed dentogingival tissues—a vital microscopic study in dogs. Periodontics. 1968;6:264–271.

[73] Hock J, Nuki K. A vital microscopy study of the morphology of normal and inflamed gingiva. J Periodontal Res. 1971;6:81–88. DOI: 10.1111/j.1600-0765.1971.tb00592.x

[74] Nuki K, Hock J. The organization of the gingival vasculature. J Periodontal Res. 1974;9:305–313. DOI: 10.1111/j.1600-0765.1974.tb00686.x

[75] Vág J, Fazekas A. Influence of restorative manipulations on the blood perfusion of human marginal gingiva as measured by laser Doppler flowmetry. J Oral Rehabil. 2002;29(1):52–57. DOI: 10.1046/j.1365-2842.2002.00818.x

[76] Forsslund G. The structure and function of the capillary system in the gingiva in man. Acta Odontol Scand. 1959;17:S1–144

[77] Vandersall DC, Zander HA. Experimental obstruction of the periodontal blood circulation. Helv Odontol Acta. 1967;11:74–79

[78] Hock J, Nuki K. Erythrocyte velocity in vascular networks of young non-inflamed dog gingiva. J Dent Res. 1976;55:1058–1060. DOI: 10.1177/00220345760550060801

[79] Kinnen E, Goldberg HJ. The application of electrical impedance plethysmography to the study of gingival circulation. J Periodontol. 1978;49:528–533. DOI:10.1902/jop.1978.49.10.528

[80] Hock J, Nuki K, Schlenker R, Hawks A. Clearance rates of Xenon-133 in non-inflamed and inflamed gingiva of dogs. Arch Oral Biol. 1980;25:445–449. DOI: 10.1016/0003-9969(80)90050-3

[81] Clarke NG, Shepherd BC, Hirsch RS. The effects of intra-arterial epinephrine and nicotine on gingival circulation. Oral Surg Oral Med Oral Pathol. 1981;52:577–582. DOI: 10.1016/0030-4220(81)90071-2

[82] Kaplan ML, Jeffcoat MK, Goldhaber P. Blood flow in gingiva and alveolar bone in beagles with periodontal disease. J Periodontal Res. 1982;17:384–389. DOI: 10.1111/j.1600-0765.1982.tb01169.x

[83] Matsuo M, Okudera T, Takahashi SS, Wada-Takahashi S, Maeda S, Iimura A. Microcirculation alterations in experimentally induced gingivitis in dogs. Anat Sci Int. 2016;91:1–6. DOI: 10.1007/s12565-015-0324-8

[84] Develioglu H, Ozcan G, Taner L, Ozgören O. A limited and useful approach to determine proximal periodontal health. West Indian Med J. 2010;59(2):215–218.

[85] Ramsay DS, Artun J, Martinen SS. Reliability of pulpal blood-flow measurements utilizing laser Doppler flowmetry. J Dent Res. 1991;70:1427–1430. DOI: 10.1177/00220345910700110601

[86] Phillips R. Skinner's science of dental materials. Philadelphia: WB Saunders; 1982;149–153.

[87] Cohen ES. Atlas of Cosmetic and Reconstructive Periodontal Surgery, Third Edition. Hamilton: BC Decker Inc. 2007.

[88] Ishikawa I, Aoki A, Takasaki AA. Potential applications of erbium: YAG laser in periodontics. J Periodont Res. 2004;39:275–285. DOI: 10.1111/j.1600-0765.2004.00738.x

[89] Walsh LJ. The current status of laser applications in dentistry. Aust Dent J. 2003;48(3): 146–155. DOI: 10.1111/j.1834-7819.2003.tb00025.x

[90] Kenneth S, Magid R, Strauss A. Laser use for esthetic soft tissue modification. Dent Clin N Am. 2007;51:525–545. DOI: 10.1016/j.cden.2006.12.005

[91] Donos N, D'Aiuto F, Retzepi M, Tonetti M. Evaluation of gingival blood flow by the use of laser Doppler flowmetry following periodontal surgery. A pilot study. J Periodontal Res. 2005;40(2):129–137. DOI: 10.1111/j.1600-0765.2005.00777.x

[92] Petre LC, Miron MI, Ianes E. Laser Doppler flowmetry—an early diagnosis instrument in detecting the soft tissue changes that occur during radiotherapy to the head and neck area. Proc. SPIE 9670, Sixth International Conference on Lasers in Medicine, 96700E. 2016. DOI: 10.1117/12.2191426

[93] Vitez B, Todea C, Velescu A, Șipoș C. Evaluation of gingival vascularisation using laser Doppler flowmetry. Proc. SPIE 9670, Sixth International Conference on Lasers in Medicine, 96700J. 2016. DOI: 10.1117/12.2191859

[94] Hoke JA, Burkes EJ, White JT, Duffy MB, Klitzman B. Blood-flow mapping of oral tissues by laser Doppler flowmetry. Int J Oral Maxillofac Surg. 1994;23:312–315.

[95] Sasano T, Shoji N, Kuriwada S, Sanjo D. Calibration of laser Doppler flowmetry for measurement of gingival blood flow. J Periodontal Res. 1995;30:298–301. DOI: 10.1111/j.1600-0765.1995.tb02138.x

[96] Qu X, Ikawa M, Shimauchi H. Improvement of the detection of human pulpal blood flow using a laser Doppler flowmeter modified for low flow velocity. Arch Oral Biol. 2014;59(2):199–206. DOI: 10.1016/j.archoralbio.2013.11.009

[97] Fagrell B, Nilsson G. Advantages and limitations of one-point laser Doppler perfusion monitoring in clinical practice. Vasc Med Rev. 1995;6:97–101.

[98] Morris SJ, Shore AC. Skin blood flow responses to the iontophoresis of acetylcholine and sodium nitroprusside in man: possible mechanisms. J Physiol. 1996;496:531–542. DOI: 10.1113/jphysiol.1996.sp021704

[99] Bonner R, Nossal R. Model for laser Doppler measurements of blood flow in tissue. Appl Opt. 1981;20:2097–2107. DOI: 10.1364/AO.20.002097

[100] Tew GA, Klonizakis M, Crank H, Briers JD, Hodges GJ. Comparison of laser speckle contrast imaging with laser Doppler for assessing microvascular function. Microvasc Res. 2011;82:326–332. DOI: 10.1016/j.mvr.2011.07.007

Chapter 10

Vascular Regeneration by Endothelial Progenitor Cells in Health and Diseases

Estefanía Nova-Lamperti, Felipe Zúñiga,
Valeska Ormazábal, Carlos Escudero and
Claudio Aguayo

Additional information is available at the end of the chapter

http://dx.doi.org/10.5772/64529

Abstract

Human endothelial progenitor cells (hEPCs) are adult stem cells, located in the bone marrow and peripheral blood. These cells can be differentiated into mature endothelial cells, which are involved in processes of angiogenesis and vessel regeneration. Different phenotypes and subtypes of endothelial progenitor cells (EPCs), such as early and late EPCs, have been described according to their functionality. Thus, it has been shown that early EPCs release cytokines that promote tissue regeneration and neovasculogenesis, whereas late EPC and endothelial colony forming cells (ECFCs) contribute to the formation of blood vessels and stimulate tube formation. It has been demonstrated that the number of circulating hEPC is decreased in individuals with hypercholesterolemia, hypertension, and/or diabetes. In addition, the number and the migratory activity of these cells are inversely correlated with risk factors such as hypertension, hypercholesterolemia, diabetes, and metabolic syndrome. On the other hand, the number of circulating hEPC is increased in hypoxia or acute myocardial infarction (AMI). hEPCs have been used for cell-based therapies due to their capacity to contribute in the re-endothelialization of injured blood vessels and neovascularization in ischemic tissues. This chapter provides an overview of the key role of hEPC in promoting angiogenesis and their potential use for cell therapy.

Keywords: stem cell, endothelial progenitor cells, angiogenesis, vascular regeneration, cell therapy

1. Introduction

Stem cells are characterized by their ability to proliferate and self-renew in response to signals or stimuli generated by the microenvironment. These signals can also induce the differentiation of stem cells into diverse cell types with specialized features and functions [1, 2]. According to their differentiation potential, stem cells can be classified as either embryonic or adult. The characteristics of both cell populations are summarized in **Table 1**. In this chapter, we will focus on adult stem cell. This subtype of stem cells is present in several tissues and is thought to be a part of the natural tissue repair system (**Figure 1**). Adult stem cells can be present not only in tissues with high regeneration potential, such as the skin, intestinal epithelium [3], and vascular tissue [3] but also in tissues with lower cell turnover like the brain [4]. They are responsible for tissue regeneration, and they can be classified as hematopoietic stem cells (HSCs), mesenchymal stem cells (MSCs), and endothelial progenitor cells (EPCs).

Characteristics	Embryonic stem cells	Adult stem cells
Proliferation capacity	+++	+
Potential differentiation	+++	++
Cellular availability	+++	+
Immunogenicity allogenic	++	+++
Teratogenicity	Yes	No
Ethical acceptability	No	Yes
Complexity of isolation	+++	++
Clinical practice	No	Yes

+++: high; ++: medium; +: low.
Adapted with permission from Smart and Riley [127] and Adams et al. [128].

Table 1. Main characteristics of human stem cells.

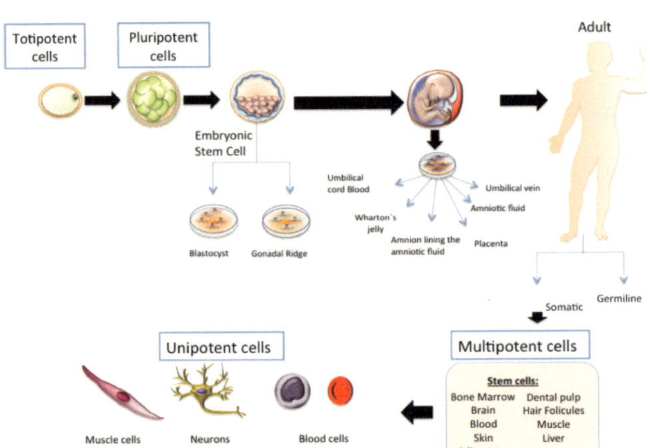

Figure 1. Types of stem cell and their potential differentiation.

http://dx.doi.org/10.5772/64529

2. Hematopoietic stem cells (HSCs)

HSCs are multipotent tissue-specific stem cells that give rise and maintain lifelong hematopoiesis [5]. HSCs only comprise approximately 0.001–0.01% of total bone marrow cells in mice and approximately 0.01–0.2% of total bone marrow mononuclear cells in humans [6]. Moreover, HSCs express cytokines receptors, allowing them to respond to signals from immune cells and to sense pathogens during inflammation or infection. This capacity allows them to adapt their cycling and differentiation behavior according to the requirements of the body [7].

3. Mesenchymal stem cells (MSCs)

MSCs are bone marrow–derived stem cells that have the capacity to form plastic-adherent colony forming unit-fibroblasts (CFU-f) [8]. They exhibit a well-known phenotype ($CD73^{+}CD90^{+}CD105^{+}CD34^{-}CD45^{-}$), and they have the capacity to differentiate into osteoblasts, adipocytes, and chondroblasts [9]. Furthermore, they can be also differentiated into numerous cell types derived from all three embryonic layers, which include muscle, vascular, nervous, hematopoietic, and bone cells, among others. MSCs can be isolated from bone marrow, adipose tissue, synovium, skeletal muscle, dermis, pericytes, amniotic fluid, umbilical cord, and even human peripheral blood [10–13]. These cells are indeed promising candidates for tissue engineering and cell-based therapies not only because of their multipotent differentiation potential but also due to their low immunogenicity [14].

4. Human endothelial progenitor cells (hEPCs)

hEPCs are adult stem cells characterized by the capacity to proliferate [15], self-renew and repair endothelial tissue [16]. They have been successfully isolated from peripheral blood [16], placenta, and bone marrow [17]. Several cell surface markers have been described to identify hEPC, such as CD34 [18], vascular endothelial growth factor (VEGF) receptor-1 or Flt-1 [19, 20], CD133 or prominine-1 (surface glycoprotein), Tie-2 (endothelial receptor tyrosine kinase), Von Willebrand factor, Nanog, and Oct-4 (Octámer-4) [21].

The original description of hEPCs by Asahara et al. was based on (1) the ability of hEPC to adhere to fibronectin-coated surfaces and (2) the surface expression of both immature stem cells (CD34, CD45, VEGFR2, or Flk-1) and mature endothelial cell (EC) markers (CD31, E-selectin, and angiopoietin receptor Tie-2) [20]. In addition, the expression of endothelial nitric oxide synthase (eNOS), the synthesis of nitric oxide (NO), and the ability to incorporate low-density lipoproteins (LDL) have been also associated with differentiation of hEPC toward endothelial cells [22].

4.1. Origin of hEPCs

To date, at least four cell sources of circulating hEPCs have been described: (1) HCSs (hemangioblast and myeloid cell), (2) bone marrow–derived MSCs, (3) hEPC not derived from bone marrow (fat and resident cells in tissues such as heart, liver, intestine, and nervous system), and (4) mature ECs migrating from the vascular wall [16, 23]. The best-characterized and most abundant hEPC are hematopoietic-derived hEPC, which can be isolated from peripheral blood mononuclear cells (PBMCs), umbilical cord, and placenta [16, 24]. Despite the fact that hematopoietic-derived hEPC are identified in different tissues, they have similar features, for example, hEPCs from umbilical cord exhibit the same surface markers (CD34, CD146, vWF, and VEGFR2) as hEPC from peripheral blood [25]. Other similarities between hematopoietic-derived hEPC include the ability to uptake modified LDL and the capacity to form capillary type structures in matrigel [26]. It has been shown that circulating monocytes have also the potential to differentiate into a variety of cell types (transdifferentiation), including EPCs [27]. Schmeisser et al. showed that $CD14^+CD34^-$ cells, isolated from PBMCs and cultured for 2–4 weeks on fibronectin-coated plates with VEGF supplemented medium, were able to express markers of ECs, such as von Willebrand factor (vWF) [20], vascular endothelial (VE)-cadherin, and eNOS [28]. In addition, these $CD14^+$ cells changed their phenotype toward endothelial morphology and were able to form capillary type structures on matrigel [29, 30]. The principal surface markers of hEPC are shown in **Table 2**.

Hemangioblast	Early hEPC	Late hEPC	Endothelial cell
CD 34^+	CD 34^+	CD 34^+	CD 34^+
CD $133^\pm$	CD 133^+	CD 31^+	CD 31^+
$VEGFR2^+$	CD 31^+	$VEGFR2^+$	$VEGFR2^+$
	$VEGFR2^+$	VE-cad^+	VE-cad^+
		E-$selectin^+$	E-$selectin^+$
		e-NOS^+	e-NOS^+
		vWF^+	vWF^+

VEGFR2, vascular endothelial growth factor receptor; vWF, von Willebrand factor, eNOS, endothelial nitric oxide synthase; VE-Cad, vascular endothelial cadherin.
Adapted with permission from: Hur et al. [56].

Table 2. Surface markers of hEPC.

Hematopoietic-derived hEPCs are maintained in a particular niche in the bone marrow, and they can be released into circulation by cytokines such as VEGF or stromal-derived factor 1 (SDF-1), synthesized by ischemic tissues and hormonal stimuli. Once in circulation, hEPCs are recruited to repair damaged endothelium and/or induce blood vessel formation. In target tissues, they can be differentiated into mature ECs to lead re-endothelialization processes and neovascularization [16].

Circulating hEPCs can be isolated and cultured from PBMCs by three different methods:

a. Cell-culture on fibronectin matrix in the presence of VEGF [20]. Under these conditions, hEPCs are selected by their ability to bind fibronectin. After removing PBMCs in suspension, early hEPC can be identified after 3 days of culture, whereas late hEPCs are observed after 2 weeks of culture.

b. Successive cell-cultures on fibronectin matrix [31]. This method takes into consideration a preliminary cell-culture of PBMCs in fibronectin-coated plates with medium without VEGF for 48 h. After that, cells in suspension are cultured for 5 days in a second fibronectin-coated plate to induce the adherence of hEPCs to the matrix and the generation of colony forming units of endothelial cells (CFU-ECs). Recent studies indicate that this technique selects a mixture of hematopoietic cells, including monocytes, lymphocytes, and progenitor cells [29].

c. Cell-culture on collagen matrix. For this method, PBMCs are cultured in basal medium for 24 h in collagen-coated plates to induce the adherence of hEPCs to the collagen. hEPCs are then recovered and cultured again for 14 days to obtain mature ECs with high proliferative capacity called CFU-ECs [31]. These cells were initially considered as "real" hEPCs because they do not express myeloid or hematopoietic markers and have the ability to form capillary-type structures similar to mature ECs. CFU-ECs express high levels of CD34 and KDR and low levels of CD45 on their cell membrane. The origin of the ECFCs has not been described yet, but it has been suggested that these cells could be derived from the vascular wall [30].

4.2. Quantification of circulating EPCs

Since EPCs can be identified from peripheral blood samples, their detection, quantification, and characterization may be considered as potential diagnostic and prognostic biomarkers and as a novel therapeutic option for cardiovascular disorders. The main methods to quantify EPCs in human studies can be divided into two approaches: flow cytometry and CFU assays; these are also the two most widely used methods for EPCs quantification. Flow cytometry offers the advantage of a multiparameter approach that allows the identification of both endothelial and stem cell markers. However, the gating strategies used to interpret the flow cytometric events are still highly variable and dependent on the criteria of each research group; therefore, a well-defined and uniform gating strategy to identify these cells has not been fully established yet.

The quantification of EPCs by flow cytometry requires a combination of antibodies that recognize antigens of both progenitor and endothelial cells. This technique has allowed to identify that *in vitro* cultured $CD34^+/KDR^+$ cells home to sites of neovascularization. Based on a review of studies using EPC phenotypes as biomarker in different diseases, the $CD34^+/KDR^+/CD45^{dim}$ phenotype appears to be the best option to identify these cells in terms of sensitivity, specificity, and reliability to quantify EPC in the clinical settings [32].

In terms of absolute quantification, it has been shown that peripheral blood samples from healthy donors ($n = 10$) have a median value of 1.88 $CD45^{dim}CD34^+VEGFR2^+$ EPCs per microliter. Similar data reported by Van Craenenbroeck et al. showed that the median value of $CD34^+VEGFR\text{-}2^+CD133^+$ EPCs was 1.95 per microliter [33]. Other authors have reported similar values of peripheral blood EPCs [34–36].

The different absolute numbers obtained for circulating EPC quantification could be explained by the use of different gating strategies and phenotypes to identify EPC subpopulation.

4.3. Migration, recruitment, and differentiation toward EPCs

In healthy individuals, hEPC correspond to the 0.0001–0.01% of the total cells in blood circulation [37]. The majority of these cells are located in the bone marrow as stem cells in a quiescent state. In this tissue, hEPCs are surrounded by stromal cells in a microenvironment characterized by low oxygen tension and high levels of chemoattractant molecules [29, 38]. Different factors such as hypoxia, trauma, physical exercise, estrogen, or cytokines can access to the bone marrow from circulation and induce the release of stem cells with the potential to differentiate toward hEPCs. Once released, stem cells migrate via circulatory system to the injury zone. How these cells reach the site of injury is not totally understood; however, it has been described that cells can be guided by the concentration gradient of different chemoattractant molecules [39].

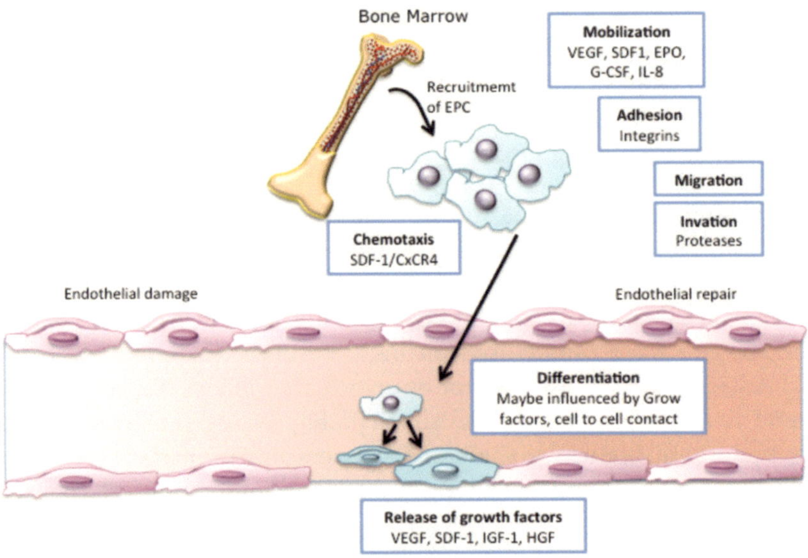

Figure 2. Recruitment and incorporation of hEPCs into ischemic tissue.

It has been shown that hEPC migration and mobilization is related to the secretion of angiogenic growth factors such as VEGF-A, VEGF-B, stromal cell-derived factor 1 (SDF-1), and insulin-like growth factor-I (IGF-1) that attract cells to the site of injury [40]. SDF-1 is a potent chemoattractant molecule released by platelets during endothelial damage [41], and its effects are dependent on the activation of the CXCR4 receptor. VEGF exerts its effect via tyrosine kinase receptors, VEGFR1 or VEGFR2, VEGFR3, which are mainly expressed in ECs from blood and lymph vessels. VEGF is produced by different cell types, such as ECs and smooth muscle cells, and is a potent angiogenic agent that regulates key steps in the process of angiogenesis, including proliferation and migration of ECs [42] and hEPC [43]. Cytokines, such

http://dx.doi.org/10.5772/64529

as tumor necrosis factor alpha (TNF-α), granulocyte-macrophage colony-stimulating factor (GM-CSF), granulocyte colony-stimulating factor (G-CSF), interleukin (IL)-6, and IL-3, trigger the mobilization and recruitment of hEPC. *In vivo* studies by Jin et al. in animal models subjected to ischemia demonstrated that the release of soluble proteins such as thrombopoietin (TPO), sKitL hematopoietic cytokines (soluble ligand kit), erythropoietin (EPO), and GM-CSF induced the release of SDF-1 from platelets, enhancing neovascularization via mobilization of $CXCR4^{+}VEGFR1^{+}$ hemangiocytes [44]. Another study observed that there is an early vascular response involving platelet adhesion to exposed subendothelium, which represents a critical step in the homing of hEPCs to the site of endothelial disruption [45] (**Figure 2**).

As mentioned, hEPCs migrate and home to specific sites following ischemic via growth factor and cytokine gradients. Some growth factors are unstable under acidic conditions of tissue ischemia; therefore, synthetic analogues stable at low pH may provide a more effective therapeutic approach for inducing hEPC mobilization and cerebral neovascularization after an ischemic stroke [46, 47].

Also, the release of hEPC from the stem cell niche in the bone marrow has been associated with the activation of proteinases such as elastase, cathepsin G, and matrix metalloproteinases (MMP) [48]. It has been shown that stromal cells can maintain precursor stem cells or hEPCs in the bone marrow via the interaction of c-Kit ligand (cKitL), expressed on stromal cells and their receptors expressed on precursor hEPCs. The mechanism of this interaction is under investigation; however, it is known that stromal cells induce the synthesis of nitric oxide (NO) and MMP-9 in response to VEGF, SDF-1, and GM-CSF. The production of these two proteins has been associated with the cleavage of cKitL in stromal cells, allowing the release of hEPCs toward circulation [49–51].

4.4. EPCs and angiogenesis *in vivo*

Angiogenesis and re-endothelialization are required for the maintenance of vascular homeostasis. Initially, it was thought that these processes occurred exclusively by the migration and proliferation of mature ECs surrounding the endothelial injury. Nowadays, new vascular repair mechanisms involving precursor cells from bone marrow, such as hEPCs have been proposed [52–54]. *In vitro* studies conducted in matrigel angiogenesis have shown that hEPCs have the ability to form capillary structures, depending on their maturation stage [55, 56]. For example, early hEPCs can migrate into a tubular network already formed and secrete IL-8 and VEGF, but they cannot form new capillary structures [57]. On the other hand, late hEPC lose their secretory capacity, but they can form capillary structures *in vitro* [56]. The ability of hEPC to form capillary structures *in vitro* and *in vivo* allowed the development of new treatments for vascular diseases. It has been demonstrated that cell therapy performed with *in vitro*-cultured EPCs, successfully promote neovascularization in ischemic tissues without the coadministration of angiogenic growth factors [58]. Several studies have shown that hEPCs from peripheral blood can induce endothelial cells turnover, via differentiation into functional mature ECs [59–62]. Kalka et al. performed this therapeutic strategy of neovascularization for the first time in 2000 [63]. They showed improved neovascularization and functional recovery when hEPCs were injected intravenously in immunodeficient mice suffering from ischemia in the lower limbs. In rat models of myocardial ischemia, the treatment with hEPC improved the migration of cells into the neovascularization area, as well as their ability to differentiate into mature ECs, which in turn was associated with the recovery of ventricular function and reduction of the ischemic area size [64, 65]. In another study, Cui et al. injected green fluorescent protein-tagged EPCs (GFP-EPCs) in murine models exhibiting damaged endothelium by ligation of the left carotid artery. In these animals, GFP-EPCs were detected at the site of injury contributing to the process of re-endothelialization [59]. The presence of GFP-EPCs in the injury enhances re-endothelialization associated with decreased neointimal formation, demonstrating that EPCs have an active role in tissue repair [59] (**Figure 3**). Other research groups have also shown that EPCs have been associated with improvements in the re-endothelialization and neointimal formation in animal models [60, 62, 65].

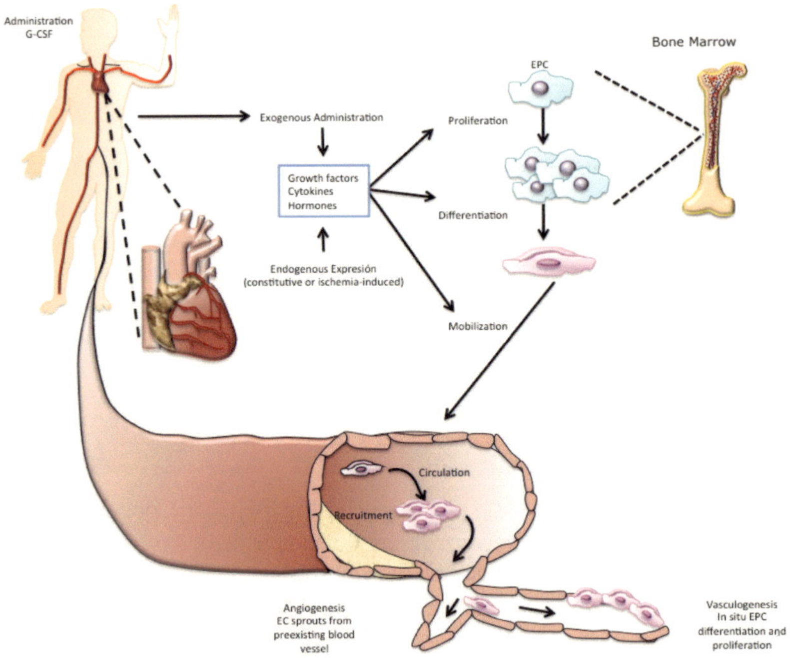

Figure 3. Mobilization of hEPCs from the bone marrow.

All these studies have shown that hEPC are crucial for vascular repair, and it has been observed that the number and migratory activity of these cells in blood are inversely correlated with the presence of risk factors for coronary artery disease [66]. Therefore, an adequate number and a correct functional state of hEPCs are required for the maintenance of the endothelium and vascular remodeling.

4.5. Mobilization mechanisms of EPCs in ischemia

One of the main transcription factors induced during acute and chronic ischemia in response to hypoxia is the hypoxia inducible factor 1 (HIF-1). In general, the activation of the HIF-1 pathway has been associated with protective responses during ischemia. The mechanism of activation of HIF-1 has been extensively described by Agani and Jiang [67]. HIF-1 is a transcription complex formed by two subunits, alpha (Hif-1α) and beta (Hif-1β). While Hif-1β is constitutively expressed, Hif-1α levels are highly regulated by cellular oxygen partial pressure, thus Hif-1α-mediated cellular responses depend on oxygen levels [68]. After Hif-1α induction, in response to low oxygen partial pressure, the ECs undergo prosurvival signals, which include the increased expression of VEGF and angiogenesis. HIF-1α is the main direct regulator of EC function and its upregulation in EPCs promoted differentiation, proliferation, and migration in a model of hindlimb ischemia [69].

HIF-1α-transfected EPCs exhibited higher revascularization potential, as increased capillary density was observed at the site of injury. This study suggests that siRNA-mediated downregulation of the HIF-1 α gene can effectively sensitize EPCs to hypoxic conditions. It can also significantly blunt early EPC growth and differentiation into ECs [70]. The underlying mechanisms of the effect of HIF-1α in EPC have been well described [69–72].

It has been shown that hypoxia-induced HIF-1 is reduced in patients with chronic heart failure (CHF) [73]; however, it has been also observed that exercise transiently increases circulating hEPCs in CHF patients. This transient effect can be sustained for approximately 4 weeks when exercise is combined with statins and/or VEGF treatment [43, 63, 74, 75].

This evidence suggests that EPCs mobilization and recruitment could also be mediated by hypoxic conditions via HIF-1-induced expression of VEGF.

4.6. Cardiovascular risk factors and hEPC function

hEPCs number and functional status are important for their repair capacity; however, these parameters are greatly influenced by clinical condition and risk factors. Indeed, several studies have shown that patients with cardiovascular risk factors such as age, gender, smoking habits, hypertension, diabetes mellitus (DM), and dyslipidemia have reduced number and function of hEPCs in peripheral blood. In contrast, some cytokines, hormones, drugs, and physical activity can increase not only the circulating number of hEPC but also their function [30, 49, 74, 76] (**Figure 4**).

Vasa et al. showed that the number of hEPC inversely correlates with cardiovascular risk factors (age and LDL cholesterol levels). According to these results, patients with higher cardiovascular risk factors have lower number of circulating hEPC compared with the control group [66]. Studies by Hill et al. showed a positive correlation between hEPC colony numbers in culture and endothelium-dependent vasodilatation and a negative correlation between hEPC colony number and the Framingham index [31]. Moreover, a negative correlation between the severity of atherosclerosis and hEPC levels has been described, showing decreased circulating hEPCs levels as an early risk factor of subclinical atherosclerosis [77]. Furthermore, reduced number of circulating hEPCs has been found in patients with hypercholesterolemia, which correlates with the fact that increased plasma cholesterol levels have been linked with endothelial damage. In the same study, the number of hEPCs was negatively correlated with total cholesterol and low-density lipoprotein (LDL) cholesterol level [78]. On the other hand, it has been also observed that the number of circulating hEPCs increases significantly after exercise [79] and in response to statins [80], antidiabetic (Pioglitazone, Sitagliptin) [81], and antihypertensive drugs (Ramipril and Enalapril) [82, 83].

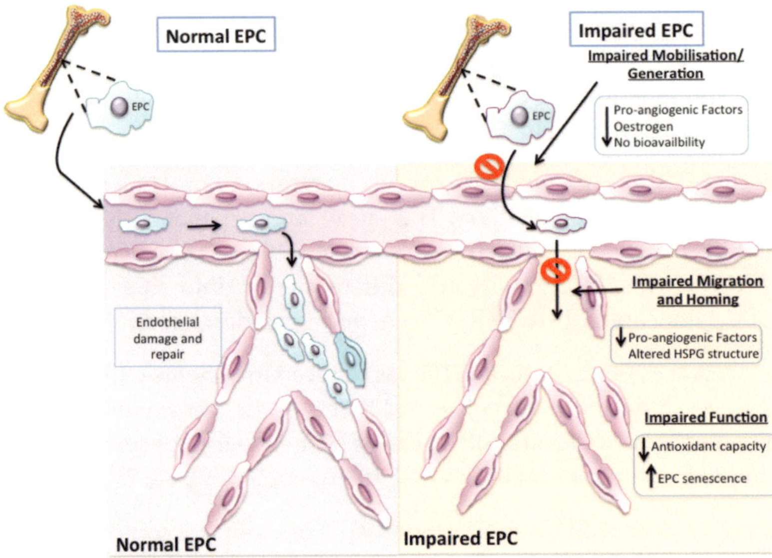

Figure 4. Mechanism of contributes EPC to the repair of injured vessels.

4.7. Correlation of EPC and clinical conditions

In addition, lower numbers of circulating hEPCs have been observed in individuals with stable and unstable angina [84], erectile dysfunction [85], and atherosclerosis [86] compared with healthy volunteers. Patients with type 1 and 2 diabetes also show lower number and functionality of hEPC than healthy individuals [87]. For instance, poor glycemic control, determined by HbA1c levels, appears to be associated with a reduction in the number of circulating EPCs, whereas an adequate control of glycemia seems to increase their numbers [88]. Several mechanisms seem to be involved in that, including advanced glycation end products formation [89], reduced activity of silent information regulator 1 (SIRT1), and increased synthesis of platelet-activating factor (PAF) [90].

Patients with familial hypercholesterolemia and hypertension [91, 92] also showed lower number and function of circulating hEPC. However, this last effect was reversed when angiotensin-converting-enzyme inhibitor (ACE-inhibitor) was used, a phenomenon associated with reduction in the progress of vascular damage [93]. Imanishi et al. have reported that hEPCs senescence is accelerated in both experimental hypertensive rats and in patients with essential hypertension, which may be related to telomerase inactivation [94, 95]. They also found that the hypertension-induced EPC senescence decreases vascular remodeling process [95].

Other conditions affecting the functionality of hEPC are ischemic heart disease and nonalcoholic fatty liver disease (NAFLD) [96]. Also, in patients with stable coronary artery disease (CAD [66, 97]), heart failure deterioration has been correlated with low number of circulating hEPC.

Furthermore, EPCs play an important role in the development and regulation of vascularization in pregnancy. Luppi et al. reported a progressive increase of circulating CD133$^+$/VEGFR-2$^+$ cells from the first trimester onwards, with a significant rise of CD34$^+$/VEGFR$^+$ cells near-term [98]. In preeclampsia for example, a pregnancy condition associated with hypertension, Matsubara et al. reported no difference in the number of circulating EPCs [99]. In contrast, studies from Sugawara et al. and Lin et al. showed lower cell numbers of circulating hEPCs in this condition compared with normal pregnancies [100, 101].

Conditions	Number hEPC	Function hEPC	Reference
Rheumatoid arthritis *in vitro*	Increased CD34$^+$/CD133$^+$/KDR$^+$	Decreased migration	[129, 130]
Atherosclerosis/heart attacks	Increased colony forming units	Increased migration in patients	[131]
Gestational diabetes 3rd trimester	Decrease in CD34$^+$/CD133$^+$	ND	[132]
Diabetes mellitus type II	Increased in CD34$^+$	Decreased vasculogenesis and adhesion capacity	[133, 134]
Erectile dysfunction	Decreased number of CD34$^+$/KDR$^+$	ND	[135]
Exercising	Increased in CD34$^+$ cells in vitro	Increased migration, proliferation	[136]
		Angiogenic capacity	[137, 138]
Erythropoietin	Increased CD34+	Increased migration	[139, 140]
		Angiogenesis	[140]
Statins	Increase proliferation	Increased migration	[66, 74]
Estradiol	Increased CD34+	Increased mobilization	[141]
Hyperhomocysteinemia	Increased CD34+ in vitro	Decreased proliferation, migration, adhesion and vasculogenic capacity	[76, 92, 142]
Acute myocardial infarct	Increased colony forming units	Increased migration and proliferation	[43, 75]
Low-density lipoprotein	CD34$^+$/KDR$^+$	Decreased migration	[31, 66]
Hypertension			[31, 143]
Prostaglandin E	Increased CD34$^+$	Increased migration and improves the function	[144]
C-reactive protein	Decreased CD34$^+$ in vitro	Decreased angiogenic capacity	[145]

Table 3. Physiological and pathological conditions and their effect on hEPC.

Patients with obesity were reported to have reduced numbers of circulating hEPCs, and this was inversely associated with an increased intima-media thickness [102]. Obesity was a more prominent predictor of the number of hEPC than any other cardiovascular risk factors, and weight loss was associated with an increased hEPC count and an improved brachial artery flow-mediated dilation. Similar evidence suggests that overweight is associated with reduced capacity to produce colony-forming units [103].

Altogether these studies support the idea that hEPCs play an important role in the maintenance of vasculature homeostasis. Thus, new therapeutic strategies should aim to increase their number and functionality in circulation. A summary of the main physiological and pathological conditions associated with functionality of hEPC is shown in **Table 3**.

4.8. Clinical translation of EPC therapy

Stem cell therapy holds great promise to restore damaged vessels. Researchers have made significant progress in cell transplantation in preclinical and clinical settings. For example, initial preclinical studies have reported favorable improvements in left ventricular function in a rat model of acute myocardial infarction (AMI) after intravenous injection of *ex vivo* expanded human $CD34^+$ cells [104]. In another study, the intramyocardial injection of EPC in a swine model of AMI reduced the scar formation and prevented the left ventricular dysfunction after AMI, providing encouraging outcomes in favoring the application of EPCs as a potential therapy in clinical trials [105, 106] (**Figure 5**).

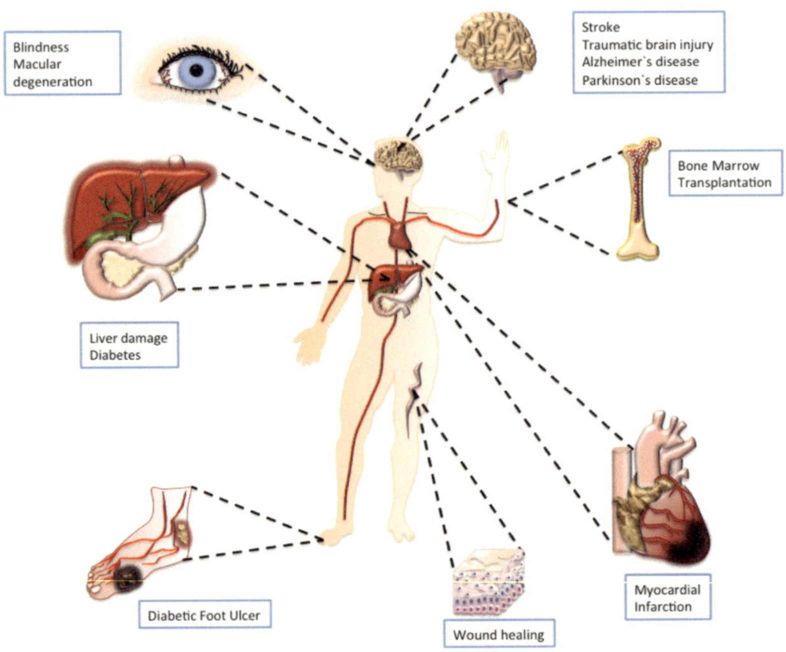

Figure 5. Potential therapeutic features and the sources of their extraction of EPC.

In the human studies performed by Li et al. [108] and Lasala et al. [107] it has been shown that intracoronary infusion of hEPC in patients with AMI were associated with the migration and incorporation of hEPCs in the infarcted tissue, a reduction of infarct size, and secretion of angiogenic growth factors including VEGF, SDF-1, and IGF-1, which produced more capillarity and higher transdifferentiation of cells to cardiac progenitor cardiomyocytes [107, 108]. Moreover, these hEPCs also reduced apoptosis of endothelial cells and increased myocardial viability in the infarcted area [109, 110]. Studies from Dobert et al. described increased myocardial viability in patients receiving intracoronary infusion of peripheral blood bone marrow-derived hEPCs 4 days after myocardial infarction [111]. In addition, other studies [112, 113] suggest that adhesion and differentiation of hEPC into mature ECs in infarcted tissue is partially modulated by fibrin, which in turn promotes angiogenesis. Similar studies have been conducted in patients with chronic critical limb ischemia of the lower extremities. In a Phase II clinical study, patients who received $CD133^+$ cells, obtained from peripheral blood and mobilized with G-CSF, experienced limb salvage, symptomatic relief, appearance of blood flow, and significant functional improvement at the site of injury [114–116]. Similarly, treatment with autologous G-CSF-mobilized peripheral blood $CD34^+$ cells in nonhealing diabetic foot patients have been promising [117].

Bone marrow-derived EPCs may be mobilized to stimulate angiogenesis and may attenuate tissue ischemia CAD and peripheral arterial disease (PAD). For instance, intramyocardial transplantation of autologous $CD34^+$ cells improved survival in patients with cardiovascular diseases [118]. In another study, patients with refractory angina who received autologous $CD34^+$ cells showed a reduction of angina frequency and improvement of exercise tolerance [119].

In addition, hEPCs may contribute to liver repair and regeneration by promoting the secretion of supportive factors to induce host's endogenous repair mechanisms [120]. EPC treatment has been shown to halt the progression of liver fibrosis in rats by suppressing hepatic cell activation by increasing the MMP activity and regulating hepatocyte [121].

Similar evidence has suggested that hEPCs are involved in the recovery after deep vein thrombosis (DVT). DVT is characterized by a fibrotic vein injury with loss of venous compliance and subsequent venous hypertension [122]. In this disease, hEPCs were involved in blood vessel recanalization in organized venous thrombi [123]. Human studies suggest that children with idiopathic pulmonary arterial hypertension (IPAH) had no severe adverse events after hEPCs infusion and improved pulmonary functions [124, 125]. In animal models, Baker et al. (2013) described the use of autologous bone marrow-derived EPCs in a rat model of pulmonary arterial hypertension (PAH) [126]. They found that EPCs reduced the hemodynamics and ventricular weight, at the same time that they increased connexin, eNOS expression and activity, Bcl-2 expression, and the number of alveolar sacs and small lung arterioles.

5. Concluding remarks

Vascular regeneration is a dynamic area of research showing remarkable medical advances, both in basic science and in the clinical application field. The preclinical and clinical studies reviewed here strongly support a therapeutic potential use of EPCs in the treatment of cardiovascular diseases; however, the very low number of these cells limits their use for cell-based therapies. The number of EPCs needed for therapy in human adults is relatively large, that is, about 3×10^8 to 6×10^8 cells, which means that 8.5–120 L of peripheral blood are required to isolate an adequate number of EPCs. Therefore, protocols aimed to expand EPCs will be needed for future therapies. However, EPCs can be used in the present as a biomarker to identify the state of diverse diseases.

The mechanisms by which EPCs mediate vessel growth and repair could potentially be ascribed to a variety of angiogenic factors produced by EPCs. However, optimal quality/quantity of EPCs is essential to set up a successful therapeutic EPC-based approach. In order to get this, it is important to improve the isolation, characterization, and expansion methods to obtain the optimal numbers and functionality of EPCs. In addition, it is also relevant to improve the administration of these cells and the cellular application techniques such as quantification of EPC. Finally, a positive clinical outcome will be the main indicative to demonstrate whether these are able to repair the disease-based dysfunction by the different mechanism already mentioned in this chapter.

Author details

Estefanía Nova-Lamperti[1], Felipe Zúñiga[2], Valeska Ormazábal[3], Carlos Escudero[4,5] and Claudio Aguayo[2,4*]

*Address all correspondence to: caguayo@udec.cl

1 MRC Centre for Transplantation, King's College London, London, UK

2 Department of Clinical Biochemistry and Immunology, Faculty of Pharmacy, University of Concepción, Concepción, Chile

3 Department of Physiopathology, Faculty of Biological Sciences, University of Concepción, Concepción, Chile

4 Group of Research and Innovation in Vascular Health (GRIVAS Health), University of Bío-Bío, Chillán, Chile

5 Vascular Physiology Laboratory, Group of Investigation in Tumor Angiogenesis (GIANT), Department of Basic Sciences, University of Bío-Bío, Chillán, Chile

References

[1] Pomerantz J, Blau HM. Nuclear reprogramming: a key to stem cell function in regenerative medicine. Nature Cell Biology. 2004;6(9):810–6.

[2] McCulloch EA, Till JE. Perspectives on the properties of stem cells. Nature Medicine. 2005;11(10):1026–8.

[3] Chia LA, Kuo CJ. The intestinal stem cell. Progress in Molecular Biology and Translational Science. 2010;96:157–73.

[4] Gage FH. Mammalian neural stem cells. Science. 2000;287(5457):1433–8.

[5] Kondo M, Wagers AJ, Manz MG, Prohaska SS, Scherer DC, Beilhack GF, et al. Biology of hematopoietic stem cells and progenitors: implications for clinical application. Annual Review of Immunology. 2003;21:759–806.

[6] Oguro H, Ding L, Morrison SJ. SLAM family markers resolve functionally distinct subpopulations of hematopoietic stem cells and multipotent progenitors. Cell Stem Cell. 2013;13(1):102–16.

[7] Riether C, Schurch CM, Ochsenbein AF. Regulation of hematopoietic and leukemic stem cells by the immune system. Cell Death and Differentiation. 2015;22(2):187–98.

[8] Friedenstein AJ, Chailakhyan RK, Latsinik NV, Panasyuk AF, Keiliss-Borok IV. Stromal cells responsible for transferring the microenvironment of the hemopoietic tissues. Cloning in vitro and retransplantation in vivo. Transplantation. 1974;17(4): 331–40.

[9] Halfon S, Abramov N, Grinblat B, Ginis I. Markers distinguishing mesenchymal stem cells from fibroblasts are downregulated with passaging. Stem Cells and Development. 2011;20(1):53–66.

[10] Mitrano TI, Grob MS, Carrion F, Nova-Lamperti E, Luz PA, Fierro FS, et al. Culture and characterization of mesenchymal stem cells from human gingival tissue. Journal of Periodontology. 2010;81(6):917–25.

[11] Salvolini E, Lucarini G, Zizzi A, Orciani M, Di Benedetto G, Di Primio R. Human skin-derived mesenchymal stem cells as a source of VEGF and nitric oxide. Archives of Dermatological Research. 2010;302(5):367–74.

[12] Battula VL, Bareiss PM, Treml S, Conrad S, Albert I, Hojak S, et al. Human placenta and bone marrow derived MSC cultured in serum-free, b-FGF-containing medium express cell surface frizzled-9 and SSEA-4 and give rise to multilineage differentiation. Differentiation; Research in Biological Diversity. 2007;75(4):279–91.

[13] Aguilera V, Briceno L, Contreras H, Lamperti L, Sepulveda E, Diaz-Perez F, et al. Endothelium trans differentiated from Wharton's jelly mesenchymal cells promote tissue regeneration: potential role of soluble pro-angiogenic factors. PLoS One. 2014;9(11):e111025.

[14] Pittenger MF, Mackay AM, Beck SC, Jaiswal RK, Douglas R, Mosca JD, et al. Multilineage potential of adult human mesenchymal stem cells. Science. 1999;284(5411):143–7.

[15] Schmidt A, Brixius K, Bloch W. Endothelial precursor cell migration during vasculogenesis. Circulation Research. 2007;101(2):125–36.

[16] Mayr M, Niederseer D, Niebauer J. From bench to bedside: what physicians need to know about endothelial progenitor cells. The American Journal of Medicine. 2011;124(6):489–97.

[17] Levesque JP, Winkler IG, Larsen SR, Rasko JE. Mobilization of bone marrow-derived progenitors. Handbook of Experimental Pharmacology. 2007(180):3–36.

[18] Sipos PI, Crocker IP, Hubel CA, Baker PN. Endothelial progenitor cells: their potential in the placental vasculature and related complications. Placenta. 2010;31(1):1–10.

[19] Timmermans F, Van Hauwermeiren F, De Smedt M, Raedt R, Plasschaert F, De Buyzere ML, et al. Endothelial outgrowth cells are not derived from CD133+ cells or CD45+ hematopoietic precursors. Arteriosclerosis, Thrombosis, and Vascular Biology. 2007;27(7):1572–9.

[20] Asahara T, Murohara T, Sullivan A, Silver M, van der Zee R, Li T, et al. Isolation of putative progenitor endothelial cells for angiogenesis. Science. 1997;275(5302):964–7.

[21] Romagnani P, Annunziato F, Liotta F, Lazzeri E, Mazzinghi B, Frosali F, et al. CD14 + CD34 low cells with stem cell phenotypic and functional features are the major source of circulating endothelial progenitors. Circulation Research. 2005;97(4):314–22.

[22] Diaz-Perez F, Radojkovic C, Aguilera V, Veas C, Gonzalez M, Lamperti L, et al. L-arginine transport and nitric oxide synthesis in human endothelial progenitor cells. Journal of Cardiovascular Pharmacology. 2012;60(5):439–49.

[23] Alexandru N, Popov D, Dragan E, Andrei E, Georgescu A. Circulating endothelial progenitor cell and platelet microparticle impact on platelet activation in hypertension associated with hypercholesterolemia. PLoS One. 2013;8(1):e52058.

[24] Kim J, Jeon YJ, Kim HE, Shin JM, Chung HM, Chae JI. Comparative proteomic analysis of endothelial cells progenitor cells derived from cord blood- and peripheral blood for cell therapy. Biomaterials. 2013;34(6):1669–85.

[25] Sudchada S, Kheolamai P, Y UP, Chayosumrit M, Supokawej A, Manochantr S, et al. CD14-/CD34+ is the founding population of umbilical cord blood-derived endothelial progenitor cells and angiogenin1 is an important factor promoting the colony formation. Annals of Hematology. 2012;91(3):321–9.

[26] Shin JW, Lee DW, Kim MJ, Song KS, Kim HS, Kim HO. Isolation of endothelial progenitor cells from cord blood and induction of differentiation by ex vivo expansion. Yonsei Medical Journal. 2005;46(2):260–7.

[27] O'Neill TJt, Wamhoff BR, Owens GK, Skalak TC. Mobilization of bone marrow-derived cells enhances the angiogenic response to hypoxia without transdifferentiation into endothelial cells. Circulation Research. 2005;97(10):1027–35.

[28] Schmeisser A, Garlichs CD, Zhang H, Eskafi S, Graffy C, Ludwig J, et al. Monocytes coexpress endothelial and macrophagocytic lineage markers and form cord-like structures in Matrigel under angiogenic conditions. Cardiovascular Research. 2001;49(3):671–80.

[29] Du F, Zhou J, Gong R, Huang X, Pansuria M, Virtue A, et al. Endothelial progenitor cells in atherosclerosis. Frontiers in Bioscience. 2012;17:2327–49.

[30] Fadini GP, Losordo D, Dimmeler S. Critical reevaluation of endothelial progenitor cell phenotypes for therapeutic and diagnostic use. Circulation Research. 2012;110(4):624–37.

[31] Hill JM, Zalos G, Halcox JP, Schenke WH, Waclawiw MA, Quyyumi AA, et al. Circulating endothelial progenitor cells, vascular function, and cardiovascular risk. The New England Journal of Medicine. 2003;348(7):593–600.

[32] Van Craenenbroeck EM, Van Craenenbroeck AH, van Ierssel S, Bruyndonckx L, Hoymans VY, Vrints CJ, et al. Quantification of circulating CD34+/KDR+/CD45^{dim} endothelial progenitor cells: analytical considerations. International Journal of Cardiology. 2013;167(5):1688–95.

[33] Van Craenenbroeck EM, Conraads VM, Van Bockstaele DR, Haine SE, Vermeulen K, Van Tendeloo VF, et al. Quantification of circulating endothelial progenitor cells: a methodological comparison of six flow cytometric approaches. Journal of Immunological Methods. 2008;332(1–2):31–40.

[34] Redondo S, Hristov M, Gordillo-Moscoso AA, Ruiz E, Weber C, Tejerina T. High-reproducible flow cytometric endothelial progenitor cell determination in human peripheral blood as CD34+/CD144+/CD3– lymphocyte sub-population. Journal of Immunological Methods. 2008;335(1–2):21–7.

[35] Hristov M, Schmitz S, Nauwelaers F, Weber C. A flow cytometric protocol for enumeration of endothelial progenitor cells and monocyte subsets in human blood. Journal of Immunological Methods. 2012;381(1–2):9–13.

[36] Duda DG, Cohen KS, Scadden DT, Jain RK. A protocol for phenotypic detection and enumeration of circulating endothelial cells and circulating progenitor cells in human blood. Nature Protocols. 2007;2(4):805–10.

[37] Khan SS, Solomon MA, McCoy JP, Jr. Detection of circulating endothelial cells and endothelial progenitor cells by flow cytometry. Cytometry Part B, Clinical Cytometry. 2005;64(1):1–8.

[38] Miller-Kasprzak E, Jagodzinski PP. Endothelial progenitor cells as a new agent contributing to vascular repair. Archivum Immunologiae et Therapiae Experimentalis. 2007;55(4):247–59.

[39] Dong C, Goldschmidt-Clermont PJ. Endothelial progenitor cells: a promising therapeutic alternative for cardiovascular disease. Journal of Interventional Cardiology. 2007;20(2):93–9.

[40] Urbich C, Aicher A, Heeschen C, Dernbach E, Hofmann WK, Zeiher AM, et al. Soluble factors released by endothelial progenitor cells promote migration of endothelial cells and cardiac resident progenitor cells. Journal of Molecular and Cellular Cardiology. 2005;39(5):733–42.

[41] De Falco E, Avitabile D, Totta P, Straino S, Spallotta F, Cencioni C, et al. Altered SDF-1-mediated differentiation of bone marrow-derived endothelial progenitor cells in diabetes mellitus. Journal of Cellular and Molecular Medicine. 2009;13(9B):3405–14.

[42] Li B, Sharpe EE, Maupin AB, Teleron AA, Pyle AL, Carmeliet P, et al. VEGF and PlGF promote adult vasculogenesis by enhancing EPC recruitment and vessel formation at the site of tumor neovascularization. FASEB Journal: Official Publication of the Federation of American Societies for Experimental Biology. 2006;20(9):1495–7.

[43] Shintani S, Murohara T, Ikeda H, Ueno T, Honma T, Katoh A, et al. Mobilization of endothelial progenitor cells in patients with acute myocardial infarction. Circulation. 2001;103(23):2776–9.

[44] Jin DK, Shido K, Kopp HG, Petit I, Shmelkov SV, Young LM, et al. Cytokine-mediated deployment of SDF-1 induces revascularization through recruitment of CXCR4+ hemangiocytes. Nature Medicine. 2006;12(5):557–67.

[45] Langer H, May AE, Daub K, Heinzmann U, Lang P, Schumm M, et al. Adherent platelets recruit and induce differentiation of murine embryonic endothelial progenitor cells to mature endothelial cells in vitro. Circulation Research. 2006;98(2):e2–10.

[46] Rouhl RP, van Oostenbrugge RJ, Damoiseaux J, Tervaert JW, Lodder J. Endothelial progenitor cell research in stroke: a potential shift in pathophysiological and therapeutical concepts. Stroke; A Journal of Cerebral Circulation. 2008;39(7):2158–65.

[47] Chen J, Chen S, Chen Y, Zhang C, Wang J, Zhang W, et al. Circulating endothelial progenitor cells and cellular membrane microparticles in db/db diabetic mouse: possible implications in cerebral ischemic damage. American Journal of Physiology Endocrinology and Metabolism. 2011;301(1):E62–71.

[48] Zhang S, Zhao L, Shen L, Xu D, Huang B, Wang Q, et al. Comparison of various niches for endothelial progenitor cell therapy on ischemic myocardial repair: coexistence of host collateralization and Akt-mediated angiogenesis produces a superior microenvironment. Arteriosclerosis, Thrombosis, and Vascular Biology. 2012;32(4):910–23.

[49] Capobianco S, Chennamaneni V, Mittal M, Zhang N, Zhang C. Endothelial progenitor cells as factors in neovascularization and endothelial repair. World Journal of Cardiology. 2010;2(12):411–20.

[50] Matsumoto T, Mifune Y, Kawamoto A, Kuroda R, Shoji T, Iwasaki H, et al. Fracture induced mobilization and incorporation of bone marrow-derived endothelial progenitor cells for bone healing. Journal of Cellular Physiology. 2008;215(1):234–42.

[51] Yang Z, von Ballmoos MW, Faessler D, Voelzmann J, Ortmann J, Diehm N, et al. Paracrine factors secreted by endothelial progenitor cells prevent oxidative stress-induced apoptosis of mature endothelial cells. Atherosclerosis. 2010;211(1): 103–9.

[52] Jang IH, Heo SC, Kwon YW, Choi EJ, Kim JH. Role of formyl peptide receptor 2 in homing of endothelial progenitor cells and therapeutic angiogenesis. Advances in Biological Regulation. 2015;57:162–72.

[53] Pearson JD. Endothelial progenitor cells—an evolving story. Microvascular Research. 2010;79(3):162–8.

[54] Yoder MC. Endothelial progenitor cell: a blood cell by many other names may serve similar functions. Journal of Molecular Medicine. 2013;91(3):285–95.

[55] Finkenzeller G, Graner S, Kirkpatrick CJ, Fuchs S, Stark GB. Impaired in vivo vasculogenic potential of endothelial progenitor cells in comparison to human umbilical vein endothelial cells in a spheroid-based implantation model. Cell Proliferation. 2009;42(4): 498–505.

[56] Hur J, Yoon CH, Kim HS, Choi JH, Kang HJ, Hwang KK, et al. Characterization of two types of endothelial progenitor cells and their different contributions to neovasculogenesis. Arteriosclerosis, Thrombosis, and Vascular Biology. 2004;24(2):288–93.

[57] Shumiya T, Shibata R, Shimizu Y, Ishii M, Kubota R, Shintani S, et al. Evidence for the therapeutic potential of ex vivo expanded human endothelial progenitor cells using autologous serum. Circulation Journal: Official Journal of the Japanese Circulation Society. 2010;74(5):1006–13.

[58] Krankel N, Luscher TF, Landmesser U. "Endothelial progenitor cells" as a therapeutic strategy in cardiovascular disease. Current Vascular Pharmacology. 2012;10(1):107–24.

[59] Cui B, Huang L, Fang Y, Guo R, Yin Y, Zhao X. Transplantation of endothelial progenitor cells overexpressing endothelial nitric oxide synthase enhances inhibition of neointimal hyperplasia and restores endothelium-dependent vasodilatation. Microvascular Research. 2011;81(1):143–50.

[60] Edelberg JM, Tang L, Hattori K, Lyden D, Rafii S. Young adult bone marrow-derived endothelial precursor cells restore aging-impaired cardiac angiogenic function. Circulation Research. 2002;90(10):E89–93.

[61] Feng Y, Gordts SC, Chen F, Hu Y, Van Craeyveld E, Jacobs F, et al. Topical HDL administration reduces vein graft atherosclerosis in apo E deficient mice. Atherosclerosis. 2011;214(2):271–8.

[62] Feng Y, van Eck M, Van Craeyveld E, Jacobs F, Carlier V, Van Linthout S, et al. Critical role of scavenger receptor-BI-expressing bone marrow-derived endothelial progenitor cells in the attenuation of allograft vasculopathy after human apo A-I transfer. Blood. 2009;113(3):755–64.

[63] Kalka C, Masuda H, Takahashi T, Gordon R, Tepper O, Gravereaux E, et al. Vascular endothelial growth factor(165) gene transfer augments circulating endothelial progenitor cells in human subjects. Circulation Research. 2000;86(12):1198–202.

[64] Friedrich EB, Walenta K, Scharlau J, Nickenig G, Werner N. CD34-/CD133+/VEGFR-2+ endothelial progenitor cell subpopulation with potent vasoregenerative capacities. Circulation Research. 2006;98(3):e20–5.

[65] Kawamoto A, Gwon HC, Iwaguro H, Yamaguchi JI, Uchida S, Masuda H, et al. Therapeutic potential of ex vivo expanded endothelial progenitor cells for myocardial ischemia. Circulation. 2001;103(5):634–7.

[66] Vasa M, Fichtlscherer S, Aicher A, Adler K, Urbich C, Martin H, et al. Number and migratory activity of circulating endothelial progenitor cells inversely correlate with risk factors for coronary artery disease. Circulation Research. 2001;89(1):E1–7.

[67] Agani F, Jiang BH. Oxygen-independent regulation of HIF-1: novel involvement of PI3K/AKT/mTOR pathway in cancer. Current Cancer Drug Targets. 2013;13(3): 245–51.

[68] Brocato J, Chervona Y, Costa M. Molecular responses to hypoxia-inducible factor 1alpha and beyond. Molecular Pharmacology. 2014;85(5):651–7.

[69] Zan T, Li H, Du Z, Gu B, Liu K, Li Q. Enhanced endothelial progenitor cell mobilization and function through direct manipulation of hypoxia inducible factor-1alpha. Cell Biochemistry and Function. 2015;33(3):143–9.

[70] Jiang M, Wang B, Wang C, He B, Fan H, Guo TB, et al. Inhibition of hypoxia-inducible factor-1alpha and endothelial progenitor cell differentiation by adenoviral transfer of small interfering RNA in vitro. Journal of Vascular Research. 2006;43(6):511–21.

[71] Hoenig MR, Bianchi C, Sellke FW. Hypoxia inducible factor-1 alpha, endothelial progenitor cells, monocytes, cardiovascular risk, wound healing, cobalt and hydralazine: a unifying hypothesis. Current Drug Targets. 2008;9(5):422–35.

[72] Kutscher C, Lampert FM, Kunze M, Markfeld-Erol F, Stark GB, Finkenzeller G. Overexpression of hypoxia-inducible factor-1 alpha improves vasculogenesis-related functions of endothelial progenitor cells. Microvascular Research. 2016;105:85–92.

[73] Van Craenenbroeck EM, Bruyndonckx L, Van Berckelaer C, Hoymans VY, Vrints CJ, Conraads VM. The effect of acute exercise on endothelial progenitor cells is attenuated in chronic heart failure. European Journal of Applied Physiology. 2011;111(9):2375–9.

[74] Dimmeler S, Aicher A, Vasa M, Mildner-Rihm C, Adler K, Tiemann M, et al. HMG-CoA reductase inhibitors (statins) increase endothelial progenitor cells via the PI 3-kinase/Akt pathway. The Journal of Clinical Investigation. 2001;108(3):391–7.

[75] Ghani U, Shuaib A, Salam A, Nasir A, Shuaib U, Jeerakathil T, et al. Endothelial progenitor cells during cerebrovascular disease. Stroke; A Journal of Cerebral Circulation. 2005;36(1):151–3.

[76] Chen JZ, Zhang FR, Tao QM, Wang XX, Zhu JH, Zhu JH. Number and activity of endothelial progenitor cells from peripheral blood in patients with hypercholesterolaemia. Clinical Science. 2004;107(3):273–80.

[77] Castejon R, Jimenez-Ortiz C, Valero-Gonzalez S, Rosado S, Mellor S, Yebra-Bango M. Decreased circulating endothelial progenitor cells as an early risk factor of subclinical atherosclerosis in systemic lupus erythematosus. Rheumatology. 2014;53(4):631–8.

[78] Veas C, Jara C, Willis ND, Perez-Contreras K, Gutierrez N, Toledo J, et al. Overexpression of LOXIN protects endothelial progenitor cells from apoptosis induced by oxidized low density lipoprotein. Journal of Cardiovascular Pharmacology. 2016;67(4): 326–35.

[79] Adams V, Lenk K, Linke A, Lenz D, Erbs S, Sandri M, et al. Increase of circulating endothelial progenitor cells in patients with coronary artery disease after exercise-induced ischemia. Arteriosclerosis, Thrombosis, and Vascular Biology. 2004;24(4):684–90.

[80] Hibbert B, Simard T, Ramirez FD, Pourdjabbar A, Raizman JE, Maze R, et al. The effect of statins on circulating endothelial progenitor cells in humans: a systematic review. Journal of Cardiovascular Pharmacology. 2013;62(5):491–6.

[81] Sakatani Y, Miyoshi T, Oe H, Noda Y, Ohno Y, Nakamura K, et al. Pioglitazone prevents the endothelial dysfunction induced by ischemia and reperfusion in healthy subjects. Journal of Cardiovascular Pharmacology. 2014;64(4):326–31.

[82] Raptis AE, Markakis KP, Mazioti MC, Ikonomidis I, Maratou EP, Vlahakos DV, et al. Effect of aliskiren on circulating endothelial progenitor cells and vascular function in patients with type 2 diabetes and essential hypertension. American Journal of Hypertension. 2015;28(1):22–9.

[83] Suzuki R, Fukuda N, Katakawa M, Tsunemi A, Tahira Y, Matsumoto T, et al. Effects of an angiotensin II receptor blocker on the impaired function of endothelial progenitor cells in patients with essential hypertension. American Journal of Hypertension. 2014;27(5):695–701.

[84] George J, Goldstein E, Abashidze S, Deutsch V, Shmilovich H, Finkelstein A, et al. Circulating endothelial progenitor cells in patients with unstable angina: association with systemic inflammation. European Heart Journal. 2004;25(12):1003–8.

[85] Foresta C, Caretta N, Lana A, Cabrelle A, Palu G, Ferlin A. Circulating endothelial progenitor cells in subjects with erectile dysfunction. International Journal of Impotence Research. 2005;17(3):288–90.

[86] Taguchi A, Matsuyama T, Moriwaki H, Hayashi T, Hayashida K, Nagatsuka K, et al. Circulating CD34-positive cells provide an index of cerebrovascular function. Circulation. 2004;109(24):2972–5.

[87] Jiraritthamrong C, Kheolamai P, Y UP, Chayosumrit M, Supokawej A, Manochantr S, et al. In vitro vessel-forming capacity of endothelial progenitor cells in high glucose conditions. Annals of Hematology. 2012;91(3):311–20.

[88] Oikonomou D, Kopf S, von Bauer R, Djuric Z, Cebola R, Sander A, et al. Influence of insulin and glargine on outgrowth and number of circulating endothelial progenitor cells in type 2 diabetes patients: a partially double-blind, randomized, three-arm unicenter study. Cardiovascular Diabetology. 2014;13:137.

[89] Li H, Zhang X, Guan X, Cui X, Wang Y, Chu H, et al. Advanced glycation end products impair the migration, adhesion and secretion potentials of late endothelial progenitor cells. Cardiovascular Diabetology. 2012;11:46.

[90] Balestrieri ML, Servillo L, Esposito A, D'Onofrio N, Giovane A, Casale R, et al. Poor glycemic control in type 2 diabetes patients reduces endothelial progenitor cell number by influencing SIRT1 signalling via platelet-activating factor receptor activation. Diabetologia. 2013;56(1):162–72.

[91] Fabbri-Arrigoni FI, Clarke L, Wang G, Charakida M, Ellins E, Halliday N, et al. Levels of circulating endothelial cells and colony-forming units are influenced by age and dyslipidemia. Pediatric Research. 2012;72(3):299–304.

[92] Zhu XY, Urbieta Caceres VH, Favreau FD, Krier JD, Lerman A, Lerman LO. Enhanced endothelial progenitor cell angiogenic potency, present in early experimental renovascular hypertension, deteriorates with disease duration. Journal of Hypertension. 2011;29(10):1972–9.

[93] Cacciatore F, Bruzzese G, Vitale DF, Liguori A, de Nigris F, Fiorito C, et al. Effects of ACE inhibition on circulating endothelial progenitor cells, vascular damage, and oxidative stress in hypertensive patients. European Journal of Clinical Pharmacology. 2011;67(9):877–83.

[94] Imanishi T, Hano T, Sawamura T, Nishio I. Oxidized low-density lipoprotein induces endothelial progenitor cell senescence, leading to cellular dysfunction. Clinical and Experimental Pharmacology & Physiology. 2004;31(7):407–13.

[95] Imanishi T, Moriwaki C, Hano T, Nishio I. Endothelial progenitor cell senescence is accelerated in both experimental hypertensive rats and patients with essential hypertension. Journal of Hypertension. 2005;23(10):1831–7.

[96] Bozdag-Turan I, Turan RG, Paranskaya L, Arsoy NS, Turan CH, Akin I, et al. Correlation between the functional impairment of bone marrow-derived circulating progenitor cells and the extend of coronary artery disease. Journal of Translational Medicine. 2012;10:143.

[97] Werner N, Wassmann S, Ahlers P, Schiegl T, Kosiol S, Link A, et al. Endothelial progenitor cells correlate with endothelial function in patients with coronary artery disease. Basic Research in Cardiology. 2007;102(6):565–71.

[98] Luppi P, Powers RW, Verma V, Edmunds L, Plymire D, Hubel CA. Maternal circulating CD34 + VEGFR-2+ and CD133 + VEGFR-2+ progenitor cells increase during normal pregnancy but are reduced in women with preeclampsia. Reproductive Sciences. 2010;17(7):643–52.

[99] Matsubara K, Abe E, Matsubara Y, Kameda K, Ito M. Circulating endothelial progenitor cells during normal pregnancy and pre-eclampsia. American Journal of Reproductive Immunology. 2006;56(2):79–85.

[100] Lin C, Rajakumar A, Plymire DA, Verma V, Markovic N, Hubel CA. Maternal endothelial progenitor colony-forming units with macrophage characteristics are reduced in preeclampsia. American journal of hypertension. 2009;22(9):1014–9.

[101] Sugawara J, Mitsui-Saito M, Hayashi C, Hoshiai T, Senoo M, Chisaka H, et al. Decrease and senescence of endothelial progenitor cells in patients with preeclampsia. The Journal of Clinical Endocrinology and Metabolism. 2005;90(9): 5329–32.

[102] Muller-Ehmsen J, Braun D, Schneider T, Pfister R, Worm N, Wielckens K, et al. Decreased number of circulating progenitor cells in obesity: beneficial effects of weight reduction. European Heart Journal. 2008;29(12):1560–8.

[103] MacEneaney OJ, Kushner EJ, Van Guilder GP, Greiner JJ, Stauffer BL, DeSouza CA. Endothelial progenitor cell number and colony-forming capacity in overweight and obese adults. International Journal of Obesity. 2009;33(2):219–25.

[104] Ott I, Keller U, Knoedler M, Gotze KS, Doss K, Fischer P, et al. Endothelial-like cells expanded from CD34+ blood cells improve left ventricular function after experimental myocardial infarction. FASEB Journal: Official Publication of the Federation of American Societies for Experimental Biology. 2005;19(8):992–4.

[105] Mao M, Xu X, Zhang Y, Zhang B, Fu ZH. Endothelial progenitor cells: the promise of cell-based therapies for acute lung injury. Inflammation Research: Official Journal of the European Histamine Research Society. 2013;62(1):3–8.

[106] Xu JY, Lee YK, Wang Y, Tse HF. Therapeutic application of endothelial progenitor cells for treatment of cardiovascular diseases. Current Stem Cell Research & Therapy. 2014;9(5):401–14.

[107] Lasala GP, Silva JA, Kusnick BA, Minguell JJ. Combination stem cell therapy for the treatment of medically refractory coronary ischemia: a Phase I study. Cardiovascular Revascularization Medicine: Including Molecular Interventions. 2011;12(1):29–34.

[108] Li CJ, Gaol RL, Yang YJ, Hu FH, Yang WX, You SJ, et al. Effect of intracoronary infusion of bone marrow mononuclear cells or peripheral endothelial progenitor cells on myocardial ischemia-reperfusion injury in mini-swine. Chinese Medical Sciences Journal 2010;25(3):176–81.

[109] Assmus B, Schachinger V, Teupe C, Britten M, Lehmann R, Dobert N, et al. Transplantation of progenitor cells and regeneration enhancement in acute myocardial infarction (TOPCARE-AMI). Circulation. 2002;106(24):3009–17.

[110] Sharif F, Bartunek J, Vanderheyden M. Adult stem cells in the treatment of acute myocardial infarction. Catheterization and Cardiovascular Interventions: Official Journal of the Society for Cardiac Angiography & Interventions. 2011;77(1):72–83.

[111] Dobert N, Britten M, Assmus B, Berner U, Menzel C, Lehmann R, et al. Transplantation of progenitor cells after reperfused acute myocardial infarction: evaluation of perfusion and myocardial viability with FDG-PET and thallium SPECT. European Journal of Nuclear Medicine and Molecular Imaging. 2004;31(8):1146–51.

[112] Barsotti MC, Magera A, Armani C, Chiellini F, Felice F, Dinucci D, et al. Fibrin acts as biomimetic niche inducing both differentiation and stem cell marker expression of early human endothelial progenitor cells. Cell Proliferation. 2011;44(1):33–48.

[113] Caiado F, Carvalho T, Silva F, Castro C, Clode N, Dye JF, et al. The role of fibrin E on the modulation of endothelial progenitors adhesion, differentiation and angiogenic growth factor production and the promotion of wound healing. Biomaterials. 2011;32(29):7096–105.

[114] Canizo MC, Lozano F, Gonzalez-Porras JR, Barros M, Lopez-Holgado N, Briz E, et al. Peripheral endothelial progenitor cells (CD133 +) for therapeutic vasculogenesis in a patient with critical limb ischemia. One-year follow-up. Cytotherapy. 2007;9(1):99–102.

[115] Karakoyun R, Koksoy C, Yilmaz TU, Altun H, Banli O, Albayrak A, et al. The angiogenic effects of ischemic conditioning in experimental critical limb ischemia. European Journal of Vascular and Endovascular Surgery: The Official Journal of the European Society for Vascular Surgery. 2014;47(2):172–9.

[116] Lara-Hernandez R, Lozano-Vilardell P, Blanes P, Torreguitart-Mirada N, Galmes A, Besalduch J. Safety and efficacy of therapeutic angiogenesis as a novel treatment in patients with critical limb ischemia. Annals of Vascular Surgery. 2010;24(2):287–94.

[117] Tanaka R, Masuda H, Kato S, Imagawa K, Kanabuchi K, Nakashioya C, et al. Autologous G-CSF-mobilized peripheral blood CD34+ cell therapy for diabetic patients with chronic nonhealing ulcer. Cell Transplantation. 2014;23(2):167–79.

[118] Holmen C, Elsheikh E, Stenvinkel P, Qureshi AR, Pettersson E, Jalkanen S, et al. Circulating inflammatory endothelial cells contribute to endothelial progenitor cell dysfunction in patients with vasculitis and kidney involvement. Journal of the American Society of Nephrology: JASN. 2005;16(10):3110–20.

[119] Premer C, Hare JM. Can endothelial progenitor cells treat patients with refractory angina? Circulation Research. 2014;115(11):904–7.

[120] Gutierrez-Grobe Y, Gavilanes-Espinar JG, Masso-Rojas FA, Sanchez-Valle V, Paez-Arenas A, Ponciano-Rodriguez G, et al. Metabolic syndrome and nonalcoholic fatty liver disease. The role of endothelial progenitor cells. Annals of Hepatology. 2013;12(6): 908–14.

[121] Liu F, Liu ZD, Wu N, Wang JH, Zhang HH, Fei R, et al. In vitro interactions between rat bone marrow-derived endothelial progenitor cells and hepatic stellate cells: interaction between EPCs and HSCs. In Vitro Cellular & Developmental Biology Animal. 2013;49(7):537–47.

[122] Laser A, Elfline M, Luke C, Slack D, Shah A, Sood V, et al. Deletion of cysteine-cysteine receptor 7 promotes fibrotic injury in experimental post-thrombotic vein wall remodeling. Arteriosclerosis, Thrombosis, and Vascular Biology. 2014;34(2):377–85.

[123] Alessio AM, Beltrame MP, Nascimento MC, Vicente CP, de Godoy JA, Silva JC, et al. Circulating progenitor and mature endothelial cells in deep vein thrombosis. International Journal of Medical Sciences. 2013;10(12):1746–54.

[124] Ikutomi M, Sahara M, Nakajima T, Minami Y, Morita T, Hirata Y, et al. Diverse contribution of bone marrow-derived late-outgrowth endothelial progenitor cells to vascular repair under pulmonary arterial hypertension and arterial neointimal formation. Journal of Molecular and Cellular Cardiology. 2015;86:121–35.

[125] Xia L, Fu GS, Yang JX, Zhang FR, Wang XX. Endothelial progenitor cells may inhibit apoptosis of pulmonary microvascular endothelial cells: new insights into cell therapy for pulmonary arterial hypertension. Cytotherapy. 2009;11(4):492–502.

[126] Baker CD, Seedorf GJ, Wisniewski BL, Black CP, Ryan SL, Balasubramaniam V, et al. Endothelial colony-forming cell conditioned media promote angiogenesis in vitro and prevent pulmonary hypertension in experimental bronchopulmonary dysplasia. American Journal of Physiology, Lung Cellular and Molecular Physiology. 2013;305(1):L73–81.

[127] Smart N, Riley PR. The stem cell movement. Circulation Research. 2008;102(10):1155–68.

[128] Adams V, Challen GA, Zuba-Surma E, Ulrich H, Vereb G, Tarnok A. Where new approaches can stem from: focus on stem cell identification. Cytometry Part A: The Journal of the International Society for Analytical Cytology. 2009;75(1):1–3.

[129] Egan CG, Caporali F, Garcia-Gonzalez E, Galeazzi M, Sorrentino V. Endothelial progenitor cells and colony-forming units in rheumatoid arthritis: association with clinical characteristics. Rheumatology. 2008;47(10):1484–8.

[130] Szekanecz Z, Koch AE. Vasculogenesis in rheumatoid arthritis. Arthritis Research & Therapy. 2010;12(2):110.

[131] Jung C, Fischer N, Fritzenwanger M, Thude H, Ferrari M, Fabris M, et al. Endothelial progenitor cells in adolescents: impact of overweight, age, smoking, sport and cytokines in younger age. Clinical Research in Cardiology: Official Journal of the German Cardiac Society. 2009;98(3):179–88.

[132] Acosta JC, Haas DM, Saha CK, Dimeglio LA. Ingram DA, Haneline LS. Gestational diabetes mellitus alters maternal and neonatal circulating endothelial progenitor cell subsets. American Journal of Obstetrics and Gynecology. 2011;204(3):254 e8–e15.

[133] Mieno S, Boodhwani M, Robich MP, Clements RT, Sodha NR, Sellke FW. Effects of diabetes mellitus on VEGF-induced proliferation response in bone marrow derived endothelial progenitor cells. Journal of Cardiac Surgery. 2010;25(5):618–25.

[134] Pistrosch F, Herbrig K, Oelschlaegel U, Richter S, Passauer J, Fischer S, et al. PPAR-gamma-agonist rosiglitazone increases number and migratory activity of cultured endothelial progenitor cells. Atherosclerosis. 2005;183(1):163–7.

[135] Esposito K, Ciotola M, Maiorino MI, Giugliano F, Autorino R, De Sio M, et al. Circulating CD34+ KDR+ endothelial progenitor cells correlate with erectile function and endothelial function in overweight men. The Journal of Sexual Medicine. 2009;6(1):107–14.

[136] Han JK, Lee HS, Yang HM, Hur J, Jun SI, Kim JY, et al. Peroxisome proliferator-activated receptor-delta agonist enhances vasculogenesis by regulating endothelial progenitor cells through genomic and nongenomic activations of the phosphatidylinositol 3-kinase/Akt pathway. Circulation. 2008;118(10):1021–33.

[137] Laufs U, Urhausen A, Werner N, Scharhag J, Heitz A, Kissner G, et al. Running exercise of different duration and intensity: effect on endothelial progenitor cells in healthy subjects. European Journal of Cardiovascular Prevention and Rehabilitation: Official Journal of the European Society of Cardiology, Working Groups on Epidemiology & Prevention and Cardiac Rehabilitation and Exercise Physiology. 2005;12(4):407–14.

[138] Laufs U, Werner N, Link A, Endres M, Wassmann S, Jurgens K, et al. Physical training increases endothelial progenitor cells, inhibits neointima formation, and enhances angiogenesis. Circulation. 2004;109(2):220–6.

[139] Aydin Z, Duijs J, Bajema IM, van Zonneveld AJ, Rabelink TJ. Erythropoietin, progenitors, and repair. Kidney International Supplement. 2007(107):S16–20.

[140] Urao N, Okigaki M, Yamada H, Aadachi Y, Matsuno K, Matsui A, et al. Erythropoietin-mobilized endothelial progenitors enhance reendothelialization via Akt-endothelial nitric oxide synthase activation and prevent neointimal hyperplasia. Circulation Research. 2006;98(11):1405–13.

[141] Iwakura A, Luedemann C, Shastry S, Hanley A, Kearney M, Aikawa R, et al. Estrogen-mediated, endothelial nitric oxide synthase-dependent mobilization of bone marrow-derived endothelial progenitor cells contributes to reendothelialization after arterial injury. Circulation. 2003;108(25):3115–21.

[142] Alam MM, Mohammad AA, Shuaib U, Wang C, Ghani U, Schwindt B, et al. Homocysteine reduces endothelial progenitor cells in stroke patients through apoptosis. Journal of Cerebral Blood Flow and Metabolism: Official Journal of the International Society of Cerebral Blood Flow and Metabolism. 2009;29(1):157–65.

[143] Chen DD, Dong YG, Yuan H, Chen AF. Endothelin 1 activation of endothelin A receptor/NADPH oxidase pathway and diminished antioxidants critically contribute to endothelial progenitor cell reduction and dysfunction in salt-sensitive hypertension. Hypertension. 2012;59(5):1037–43.

[144] Herrler T, Leicht SF, Huber S, Hermann PC, Schwarz TM, Kopp R, et al. Prostaglandin E positively modulates endothelial progenitor cell homeostasis: an advanced treatment modality for autologous cell therapy. Journal of Vascular Research. 2009;46(4):333–46.

[145] Verma S, Kuliszewski MA, Li SH, Szmitko PE, Zucco L, Wang CH, et al. C-reactive protein attenuates endothelial progenitor cell survival, differentiation, and function: further evidence of a mechanistic link between C-reactive protein and cardiovascular disease. Circulation. 2004;109(17):2058–67.

Chapter 11

Perioperative Inflammation and Microcirculation in Surgery: Clinical Strategies for Improved Surgical Outcomes

Robert Schier, Philipp Zimmer and Bernhard Riedel

Additional information is available at the end of the chapter

http://dx.doi.org/10.5772/64435

Abstract

Impaired microcirculation secondary to underlying vascular endothelial dysfunction is increasingly recognized to play a central role in the pathophysiology associated with numerous postoperative complications. Noxious stimuli, including direct injury from surgical trauma and hypoxia (e.g., ischemia-reperfusion injury), trigger adrenergic-inflammatory-thrombotic-immune cascades to impair the microcirculation, with consequent perfusion-related postoperative complications. The endothelium, characterized by exquisite sensitivity to inflammation and low proliferative potential, has limited self-repair capacity that is dependent on circulating bone marrow-derived endothelial progenitor cells for regeneration. As such, the extent to which the endothelial physical and functional integrity is preserved mirrors not only underlying cardiovascular health but is also an important factor in susceptibility to postoperative morbidity. This review explores the effect of perioperative inflammation on the microcirculation and some of the current protective strategies available to clinicians. "Prehabilitation," with preoperative exercise to improve the underlying endothelial function and bone marrow responsiveness for endogenous endothelial repair mechanisms, and anti-inflammatory strategies to limit activation of the endothelial-thrombotic-inflammatory cascades may provide clinical strategies to preserve the microcirculation to engender optimal surgical outcomes.

Keywords: microcirculation, endothelial dysfunction, inflammation, perioperative, surgery

1. Introduction

With an estimated 234 million operations performed annually, surgical care is an integral part of health care throughout the world [1]. Furthermore, the World Health Organization (WHO) estimates that the incidence of trauma, predominantly requiring surgery, accounts for 10% of deaths and 16% of disabilities worldwide—considerably more than malaria, tuberculosis, and HIV/AIDS combined [2].

Confounding the underlying comorbidities that patients present with during surgery, patients also suffer a significant biologic perturbation—the "surgical stress response"—a significant stressor to the human body during the perioperative period. A variety of systems are involved in this stress response, including the sympathetic autonomic nervous system, endocrine system, and immune system [3]. Inflammatory mechanisms are intimately tied to the immune system and contribute to direct defense against infection and promote postoperative wound healing. This physiological reaction of the human body can be exaggerated by a systemic inflammatory response syndrome (SIRS) [4]. SIRS results from the release of endogenous factors such as damage-associated molecular patterns (DAMPs) or alarmins [4, 5] after surgical tissue injury [6]. DAMPs activate the complement system, leading to a rapid generation of C3a and C5a [7–9] and initiation of the release of a myriad of inflammatory mediators such as adiponectin, leptin, C-reactive protein, interleukins (IL-8, IL-10, etc.), soluble tumor necrosis factor-receptor 1(sTNF-R1), and 8-isoprostane.

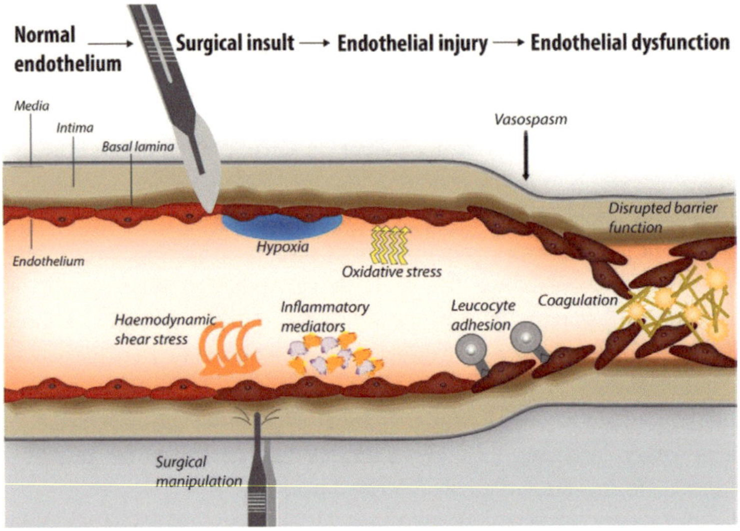

Figure 1. The surgical pro-inflammatory and pro-oxidant milieu may result in both functional and structural alterations in the endothelium, resulting in hemostatic dysregulation and impaired microcirculation with consequent microvascular-related postoperative complications (Illustration courtesy of Dr Marissa Ferguson).

Interestingly, these inflammatory mediators, described as a systemic "inflammome," are increased in obese patients presenting for bariatric surgery [10]. Hence, this suggests that a significant number of patients may present to surgery with an underlying pro-inflammatory state and is also seen in patients with inflammatory comorbidities, such as rheumatoid disease, inflammatory bowel disease, and diabetes mellitus [11, 12]. This inflammatory burden activates cellular processes at affected sites within tissues, with enhanced capillary permeability to soluble mediators, particles, and cellular trafficking. These systems are in a delicate balance, which can be easily disrupted to exacerbate disease or organ dysfunction [13].

Impaired microcirculation, largely driven by vascular endothelial dysfunction, is increasingly implicated as a central pathophysiological feature of postoperative morbidity. Microcirculation is affected by certain noxious stimuli, many of which are common to the perioperative period, including direct injury from surgical manipulation or hemodynamic shear stress, hypoxia (e.g., ischemia-reperfusion injury), and through exposure to inflammatory cytokines and endotoxins. Perioperative inflammation caused in reaction to surgical trauma causes a pro-inflammatory and pro-oxidant milieu that results in both functional and structural alterations in the endothelium. This may lead to microcirculation hemostatic dysregulation with impaired local tissue perfusion and consequent micro- and macrovascular-related postoperative complications (**Figure 1**) [14, 15].

2. Physiology of the endothelium

The endothelial "organ" is estimated to weigh approximately 1 kg in adults and covers the entire vasculature with a single layer of cells, covering a surface area of approximately 100–150 m^2 and comprising 10–60 trillion cells in a single layer.

For a long time, the endothelium was considered to be inert, tasked with passive maintenance of a non-thrombogenic blood-tissue interface. In 1980, however, Furchgott and Zawadzki [16] discovered the endothelium-derived relaxing factor (nitric oxide), and since then our understanding of the importance of the vascular endothelium has undergone a dramatic evolution.

The endothelium is now recognized as a complex tissue composed of key immunoreactive cells that respond to environmental conditions. Sandwiched between the blood compartment and the vascular smooth muscle cells, the single layered endothelium is ideally located to act as a dynamic sensor-effector organ. Most of the endothelial cell mass is found in the endothelial lining of the resistance vessels and capillaries, thereby exposing a relatively large endothelial surface to a small volume of blood (up to 5000 cm^2/ml). This facilitates the exchange of nutrients and metabolic products [17], and thus allows the endothelium to exert significant autocrine, paracrine, and endocrine actions on smooth muscle cells, platelets, and peripheral leukocytes. Endothelial cells, thereby, participate actively and reactively in the regulation of a number of key physiological processes, including vascular tone, vascular permeability, hemostasis (thrombosis, fibrinolysis, and platelet adherence), immune and inflammatory (leukocyte adherence) reactions, angiogenesis, and maintenance of the basement membrane. This dynamic "gate keeping" role of the endothelium, modulated through its metabolic and synthetic functions (such as production of nitric oxide, endothelin, prostaglandins, cytokines, growth factors, and adhesion molecules) and through the expression of endothelial cell receptors and glycoproteins on the abluminal surface, allows the healthy endothelium to maintain a dominant state of vasodilation, anti-thrombosis/pro-fibrinolysis by inhibition of platelet and leukocyte adhesion—a state that is indispensable for body homeostasis [18].

3. Pathophysiology of the endothelium

In contrast, endothelial dysfunction, activation, and injury are characterized by inhibition of vasodilation, promotion of a pro-thrombotic/anti-fibrinolytic state, and promotion of platelet and leukocyte adhesion. Altered release of endothelium-derived factors appears to be pivotal in pathophysiological changes that occur in disease states, such as atherosclerosis, thrombosis, hypertension, pulmonary hypertension, eclampsia, hyperglycemia, diabetes, metastatic disease, immune diseases, inflammatory syndromes, infectious processes, and sepsis. Indeed, there is increasing evidence that perturbations in the vascular endothelium are directly or indirectly involved in the pathophysiology of numerous disease processes, including postoperative morbid events.

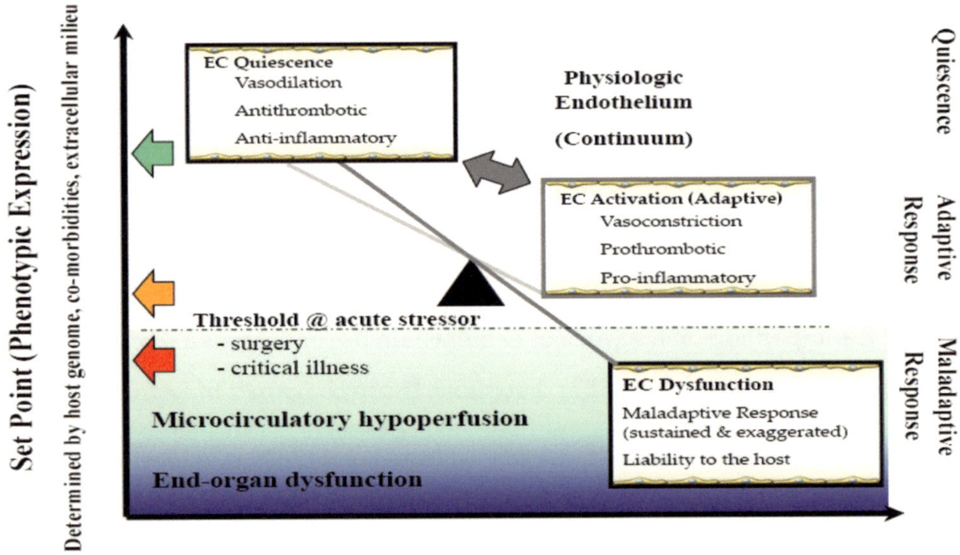

Figure 2. The phenotypic expression of the endothelium can be described as a dynamic "set point" that ranges between a quiescent, activated, or dysfunctional state. Endothelial cell (EC) dysfunction caused by perioperative inflammation in response to an acute stressor (surgery, critical illness) is accompanied by microcirculatory hypoperfusion that can lead to end-organ dysfunction.

The crucial step in the progression of perioperative endothelial dysfunction is the change of the endothelium from a quiescent into an active state. The endothelium, activated by exposure to inflammatory cytokines, becomes prothrombotic, prone to vasoconstriction instead of vasodilation, and more porous with increased fluid extravasation and increased cellular trafficking to the intercellular space. A systemic response to major trauma, associated with a lowered ability to fight infection and susceptibility to sepsis, will further activate the destructive inflammatory response [19].

In those patients presenting with underlying impaired preoperative microcirculatory function now confounded by the pathophysiologic changes to the endothelium that accompanies the surgical stress response will be at higher risk of deterioration of the endothelial reserve below a critical "physiologic threshold" required to sustain microvascular integrity and perfusion (**Figure 2**).

4. Endothelial regeneration

Through reconstitution of the endothelial layer, which generally occurs in the presence of angiogenesis and vasculogenesis, endothelial function can be restored. Neovascularization is mediated through migration and proliferation of endothelial cells within the vasculature. Endothelial colony-forming cells (CFCs) developing endothelial progeny is the key factor in order for mature endothelial cells to proliferate and restore endothelial function [20–22]. For adult vasculogenesis, endothelial progenitor cells (EPCs) play an important role for the *de novo* formation of blood vessels. Historically, the presence of circulating blood cells with the ability to promote vascular repair and regeneration was first described in 1997 [23]. A variety of seemingly endothelial-specific cell surface antigens were displayed on the cells identified as EPCs. Subsequently, numerous experimental studies have assessed the mechanism induced by tissue ischemia, vascular trauma, tumor growth, and inflammation by which EPC are released from the bone marrow, travel to the sites of active neovascularization, and initiate the homing process in the endothelial layer. Furthermore, some studies suggest EPCs as a biomarker for clinical disorders, such as cardiovascular disease [24], cerebrovascular disease [25, 26], sepsis [27], and numerous types of cancer [28, 29]. Interestingly, there is an inverse correlation between the number of bonemarrow released, circulating EPC and the postoperative complication risk. Subsequent experimental data from marrow transplantation demonstrated that these stem cells are recruited to sites of active neovascularization and differentiate into vascular cells *in-situ*. However, the frequency of this occurrence and the identification of the cell type involved need to be fully determined [30].

5. Endothelial progenitor cell populations

A major limitation in this field has been the lack of specific markers and different methods used to identify circulating EPCs. Different methods included flow cytometry, cell culture methods, immunostaining, and consequently render comparison difficult. Three functional populations of EPCs have generally been well defined. A cellular population that expresses the phenotype CD34+ AC133+ KDR+ has gained wide acceptance as a measure of circulating EPC in human subjects [31]. These cells, while being recruited to denuded vessels in ischemic sites, do not become persistent vascular endothelial cells or display de novo in-vivo vasculogenic potential, but rather exhibit potent paracrine properties to regulate new vessel formation through angiogenesis [32, 33]. These cells are referred to as proangiogenic hematopoietic cells [22, 34, 35]. Colony-forming assays, in which plated human CD34+ peripheral blood cells form cellular clusters on fibronectin-coated dishes in-vitro, have identified other populations of EPC. Asahara et al. [23] described that CD34+ peripheral blood cells form clusters, bind acetylated low-density protein (acLDL) and differentiate into spindle-shaped endothelial cells. These cell clusters are referred to as EPC colony-forming units (CFU). A third population of EPCs, identified as yet another type of cell colony emerging from plated peripheral blood mononuclear cells, form tightly adherent cells with a cobblestone appearance and are referred to as endothelial colony-forming cells (ECFC), late outgrowth cells (OEC), or blood outgrowth endothelial cells (BOEC). These cells become part of the systemic circulation of the host and have vessel-forming ability [36] These ECFCs, with *in vivo* human vessel-forming ability, exhibit the greatest features consistent with human postnatal vasculogenic cells [37].

EPC enumeration correlates with cardiovascular risk factors, extent of coronary disease, and risk of future cardiovascular events [24]. EPC enumeration and functional characterization assess the reparative ability and propensity to cardiovascular injury, and thus greatly improves the risk stratification of patients for postoperative morbidity. Given that peripherally circulating EPCs and intrinsic stem cells play an important role in accelerating endothelialization and tissue remodeling following vascular damage from both disease and toxic insults, we anticipate that therapeutic attempts to stimulate mobilization and homing of bone marrow-derived EPC or exogenous administration of cell-based (progenitor) therapies will likely emerge in clinical medicine over the next decade [38–40]. Comorbid disease states and aging associate with decreased regenerative ability by EPCs and may underlie the etiology of postoperative complications and delayed recovery following surgery. For example, diabetes is characterized by poor bone marrow mobilization and decreased proliferation and survival of EPCs [41]. Inhibiting oxidative stress has been shown to modulate EPCs and normalize post-ischemic neovascularization in diabetics. Similarly, EPC mobilization is also reported to improve with insulin therapy in diabetic rats [42]. Whether this effect is mediated by insulin itself or through improved glucose control needs to be clarified.

6. Impaired endothelium-dependent vascular function in the clinical setting

An intact microcirculation is key for the functional success of the cardiovascular system and end-organ perfusion. In the perioperative period, a wide range of microcirculatory alterations associated with surgery itself, including factors such as anesthesia type, hypothermia, hemodilution, inflammatory reaction, and microemboli formation [43,44], impair endothelium-dependent vascular function to decrease blood flow and oxygen supply to the parenchymal cells. An improved understanding of the different types of microcirculatory alterations may also contribute to reducing perioperative complications. Variants of impaired microcirculation include impaired microcirculatory perfusion where obstructed capillaries are observed next to capillaries with flow, often seen in clinical conditions such as sepsis or

http://dx.doi.org/10.5772/64435

reperfusion injury; microcirculatory alterations characterized by increased diffusion distance between oxygen-carrying red blood cells and tissue cells, often seen in hemodilution that accompanies cardiopulmonary bypass; microcirculatory tamponade, often associated with excessive use of vasopressors and/or increased venous pressure. This fluid overload causes tissue edema that consequently leads to a damage of endothelial cells and losses of hemodynamic coherence, glycocalyx barriers, and/or the compromise of adherence and tight junctions [45].

7. Impaired microcirculation during critical illness

Alterations of the cerebral microcirculation may represent a key component for the development of postoperative sepsis-associated encephalopathy. Cerebral hypoperfusion is a common complication of sepsis and its pathophysiology is complex and related to numerous processes and pathways, while the exact mechanisms producing neurological impairment such as delirium in septic patients is not fully understood. Cerebral hypoperfusion is caused by vasoconstriction that may be induced by inflammation and hypocapnia. The underlying endothelial dysfunction in sepsis leads to impairment of microcirculation and cerebral metabolic uncoupling that may further reduce brain perfusion. The natural autoregulatory mechanisms that protect the brain from reduced/inadequate cerebral perfusion can be impaired in septic patients, especially in those with shock or delirium, and this further contributes to cerebral ischemia if blood pressure drops below critical thresholds [46].

Postoperative brain dysfunction (delirium and coma) may relate to impaired microcirculation following surgical trauma and the associated inflammation seen in the postoperative period. Postoperative neurocognitive dysfunction is very prevalent, especially in the elderly surgical patient population. It has been reported to independently associate with prolonged mechanical ventilation, longer and more costly hospitalizations, delayed cognitive dysfunction that persists for months after hospital discharge, and increased mortality [47–53]. Factors implicated in the pathogenesis of acute brain dysfunction, such as inflammation, abnormal cerebral blood flow, and increased blood-brain barrier permeability [54, 55], are known to impact endothelial function. Similarly, critical illnesses, such as sepsis and multiple organ dysfunction syndrome, states that circulating inflammatory cytokines affect endothelial nitric oxide production and expression of adhesion molecules [56, 57]. This results in coagulation system activation, altered perfusion, distorted permeability, and decreased ability for vascular repair [58, 59]. In the brain specifically, structural and functional alterations of blood–brain barrier endothelial cells secondary to inflammatory states have been associated with increased microvascular permeability and impaired microcirculatory blood flow [60–63]. This relationship between endothelial dysfunction and brain dysfunction during critical illness is increasingly reported in critically ill patients. The observed impact of endothelial dysfunction and injury on brain function will also likely reflect that seen in other end organs, including acute lung injury following surgery [64] or during critical illness [65].

8. Therapeutic options to improve perioperative endothelial dysfunction

Therapeutic modulation of underlying subclinical microvascular endothelial dysfunction holds promise for a significant reduction in perioperative morbidity and specifically for complications such as impaired wound healing and end-organ dysfunction related to impaired microcirculation following surgery. Perioperative inflammation can be targeted with non-steroidal anti-inflammatory drugs to limit activation of the endothelial-thrombotic-inflammatory cascades with potential to improve perioperative outcomes [66–68]. Other therapeutic interventions, including preoperative exercise capacity, which aim to improve endothelial-dependent vascular function before surgery in order to cope with the inflammatory burden are currently under investigation in clinical studies [69, 70].

9. Mobilizing of endothelial progenitor cells with preoperative exercise

Numerous factors have an important role in the mobilization of EPCs [71, 72]. These include growth factors (e.g., GM-CSF, GCSF, VEGF, placental growth factor, erythropoietin, and angiopoietin-1), pro-inflammatory cytokines, chemokines (e.g., stromal cell-derived factor-1), hormones (e.g., estrogens, and lipid lowering and antidiabetic drugs), and physical activity [73]. The stimulatory effect of exercise on EPC has been shown in highly trained athletes [74], healthy subjects [71], and importantly also in patients with cardiovascular disease [75]. However, further research is required to understand the potential benefit of exercise to endothelial health in patients with subclinical cardiovascular disease characterized by endothelial dysfunction secondary to comorbidities, including metabolic syndrome or in patients subjected to the acute inflammatory insult of surgery.

Exercise has been shown to improve exercise capacity, specifically the anaerobic threshold (AT) and the maximum oxygen consumption (pVO2), and underlying endothelial reserve. In healthy subjects, Laufs et al. [76] showed that moderate and intense running for 30 min (80–100% velocity of individuals' AT) increased circulating EPC levels, but this was not seen with running occurred at short intervals (10 minutes). In elderly patients with coronary artery disease, a 4-week exercise program achieved significant upregulation of circulating EPCs. More recently, this was achieved after an even shorter (15 days) cardiac rehabilitation program, with an increase in EPCs that correlated with improved exercise capacity [73]. Other markers of improved endothelial function from a cardiac rehabilitation program included: a two-fold increase in EPCs, a three-fold increase in CFU, increased blood nitrite concentration, and reduced EPC apoptosis [75]. The duration and the intensity of exercise that are needed to adequately stimulate EPC mobilization and improve endothelial function require further investigation [77]. Surgical injury induces the mobilization of EPCs, with significantly higher circulating EPC and bone marrow EPC levels observed 24 hours after surgery in an animal model [78]. The ability to mount an EPC response is also seen in critical illness, and the response is significantly greater in patients that survive sepsis [27], and recover from illness, for example, without fibrotic changes after pneumonia [40].

Given that "responders" who mount a "cellular" stress response to injury, with increased EPC mobilization, have improved organ recovery [40] and improved survival [27], it is increasingly clear that a bone marrow-derived cellular component must follow the surgical "stress response" to facilitate repair processes. In a recent pilot study, we were able to demonstrate that patients scheduled for major surgery that exhibited an EPC response to the stressor of preoperative exhaustive exercise with a single cardiopulmonary exercise test up to pVO2 suffered significantly fewer postoperative complications [69]. Whether strategies to improve bone marrow capacity and responsiveness will influence a patient's ability to withstand surgical injury remains to be investigated. Increasing this bone marrow-derived regenerative response through preoperative exercise training may be one potential therapeutic option to optimize patients' health status prior to surgery.

However, discovering an inadequate EPC response during acute illness, such as impaired wound healing, pneumonia, acute lung injury [64], or sepsis [65], is likely too late. Hence, using a surrogate stressor, for example, exercise, to allow for early identification of at-risk patients prior to surgery will enable timely strategies to improve bone marrow responsiveness to be implemented. Importantly, some of the endothelial dysfunction, particularly that acquired in the perioperative period, may be transient or reversible and may not actually involve structural change in the cells of the vascular endothelium, but more likely potentially reversible alterations in function—so these would not require new cells, just repair of a damaged process. Importantly, whether this lack of EPC response is an epiphenomenon, a surrogate marker, or indeed causative of increased postoperative complications, requires further study. The causative nature is supported by animal studies that suggest that exogenous EPC administration can rescue endotoxin-induced acute respiratory distress syndrome (ARDS), with reduced inflammation, improved oxygenation, and improved survival [38, 39].

Jeong et al. [79], investigating whether diabetic neuropathy could be reversed by local transplantation of EPCs, reported that motor and sensory nerve conduction velocities, blood flow, and capillary density were reduced in sciatic nerves of streptozotocin-induced diabetic mice; with recovery after hindlimb injection of bone marrow-derived EPCs that were shown to engraft in close proximity to the vasa nervorum. This study demonstrated that bone marrow-derived EPCs could reverse manifestations of diabetic neuropathy, and that cell-based translational approaches may provide a novel and valid therapeutic alternative in the future.

Exercise [80] and tissue insult from surgery [78] are known to increase the mobilization of EPC. In this manner, cardiopulmonary exercise testing (CPET) can be used as a catalyst to increase the circulating population of EPCs and as a diagnostic tool of a patient's ability to mount an EPC response preoperatively. Additional gas exchange parameters obtained during a diagnostic CPET (anaerobic threshold and peak VO2) can be used to determine patients' individual physiologic capacity and the amount of exercise needed in order to stimulate the population of EPC. Preoperative exercise training could condition patients' individual functional capacity and to improve endothelial reserve by affecting EPC responsiveness. As such, Cesari et al. [73] reported a significant increase in circulating EPCs in those patients that improved their exercise capacity by more than 23%, as assessed by a six-minute walk test, after completion of a rehabilitation program.

10. Exercise and inflammation

Regular exercise has been described to be involved in risk reduction of many chronic pathological alterations such as cancer, cardiovascular, and neurodegenerative diseases. One key mechanism, which is frequently discussed in this context, is that exercise contributes to an anti-inflammatory environment, thereby counteracting a major risk factor of those diseases [81–83]. This hypothesis is supported by a vast body of literature, indicating that acute exercise induces a short-term strong increase in the pro-inflammatory cytokine interleukin-6, which in turn induces a long-term depression of TNF-α and the expression of anti-inflammatory mediators, such as interleukin-10 and soluble receptors of interleukin-1 [84]. Furthermore, recent research suggests that regular exercise suppresses over a life-span the permanent expression of inflammatory cytokines via epigenetic mechanisms. Nakajima et al. [85] showed that the DNA-methylation in the promoter region of the ASC gene, the products of which induce inflammation, is decreased in older subjects. An intermediate exercise intervention resulted in a re-methylation of this region; hence, the methylation pattern of 60- to70-year old was corrected to those of 30- to 40-year-old study participants.

The anti-inflammatory effect of exercise is mediated by cells which secrete protective cytokines, such as interleukin-6, which is expressed by skeletal muscle-tissue during physical activity. However, little is known about the exact mechanism in which exercise triggers the anti-inflammatory component. Evidence rises that regular exercise and higher levels of cardiovascular fitness are related to an increased number of regulatory T-cells. Since these cells have strong anti-inflammatory properties (e.g., by secreting Interleukin-10), they may contribute to the intermediate anti-inflammatory effect of exercise [86].

Exercise is involved in multiple processes establishing an anti-inflammatory environment, which counteracts with perioperative inflammatory stress. Therefore, preoperative exercise, which is feasible over a 1-month time period, may contribute to a reduction of the inflammatory burden that is present in patients undergoing surgery.

11. Other aspects of exercise promoting endothelium-dependent vascular function

Besides the mobilization of EPCs and its anti-inflammatory properties, exercise is known to regulate key factors of vascular functioning. Furthermore, exercise induces the expression of the endothelial nitric oxide synthase (eNOS) and increases the levels of VEGF [87–89]. The first studies revealed that the regulation of these factors is at least partially driven by epigenetic mechanisms. Wu et al. [90] revealed that exercise in rats results in a downregulation of the microRNA155. Interestingly, the messenger RNA of eNOS is known to be inhibited by microRNA155. One essential mediator may be displayed by shear-stress which is also associated with epigenetic modifications of the chromatin (histone modifications) in the eNOS gene region [91, 92]. Fernandes et al. [93] found reduced levels of microRNA126 and 16 in exercising animals. Both microRNAs were previously described to inhibit the expression of

http://dx.doi.org/10.5772/64435

VEGF. Although the previous studies give a premature insight into the underlying mechanism, they display that exercise truly contributes to the improvement of vascular function and regeneration on the molecular level. Further research, especially in humans, is warranted to get more information about the mechanism and dose–response relationship of exercise contributing to endothelial and vascular regeneration.

12. Conclusion/Summary

Impaired microcirculation secondary to underlying vascular endothelial dysfunction is increasingly recognized to play a central role in the pathophysiology associated with numerous postoperative complications. Noxious stimuli, including direct injury from surgical trauma and hypoxia (e.g., ischemia-reperfusion injury), trigger adrenergic-inflammatory-thrombotic-immune cascades to impair the microcirculation, with consequent perfusion-related postoperative complications.

The endothelium, characterized by exquisite sensitivity to inflammation and low proliferative potential, has limited self-repair capacity that is dependent on circulating bone marrow-derived endothelial progenitor cells for regeneration. As such, the extent to which the endothelial physical and functional integrity and bone marrow responsiveness, for the circulating progenitor pool, is preserved mirrors not only underlying cardiovascular health but also as an important factor in susceptibility to postoperative morbidity.

This review explores the effect of perioperative inflammation on the microcirculation and some of the current protective strategies available to clinicians. "Prehabilitation," with preoperative exercise to improve underlying endothelial function and bone marrow responsiveness for endogenous endothelial repair mechanisms, and anti-inflammatory strategies to limit activation of the endothelial-thrombotic-inflammatory cascades may provide clinical strategies to preserve the microcirculation to engender optimal surgical outcomes.

Author details

Robert Schier[1*], Philipp Zimmer[2] and Bernhard Riedel[3]

*Address all correspondence to: robert.schier@gmx.net

1 Department of Anaesthesiology and Intensive Care Medicine, University Hospital of Cologne, Cologne, Germany

2 Department for Molecular and Cellular Sports Medicine, Institute for Cardiovascular Research and Sports Medicine, German Sport University Cologne, Cologne, Germany

3 Perioperative and Pain Medicine, Peter MacCallum Cancer Center, St Andrews Place, East Melbourne, Victoria, Australia

References

[1] Weiser TG, Regenbogen SE, Thompson KD et al. An estimation of the global volume of surgery: a modelling strategy based on available data. Lancet 2008; 372: 139–144

[2] WHO. Global health estimates 2014 summary tables: deaths by cause, age and sex, 2000–2012. 2014, DOI:

[3] Weissman C. The metabolic response to stress: an overview and update. Anesthesiology 1990; 73: 308–327

[4] Zhang Q, Raoof M, Chen Y et al. Circulating mitochondrial DAMPs cause inflammatory responses to injury. Nature 2010; 464: 104–107

[5] Manson J, Thiemermann C, Brohi K. Trauma alarmins as activators of damage-induced inflammation. Br J Surg 2012; 99 Suppl 1: 12–20

[6] Pugin J. How tissue injury alarms the immune system and causes a systemic inflammatory response syndrome. Ann Intensive Care 2012; 2: 27

[7] Burk AM, Martin M, Flierl MA et al. Early complementopathy after multiple injuries in humans. Shock 2012; 37: 348–354

[8] Huber-Lang M, Kovtun A, Ignatius A. The role of complement in trauma and fracture healing. Semin Immunol 2013; 25: 73–78

[9] Neher MD, Weckbach S, Flierl MA et al. Molecular mechanisms of inflammation and tissue injury after major trauma—is complement the "bad guy"? J Biomed Sci 2011; 18: 90

[10] Arismendi E, Rivas E, Agusti A et al. The systemic inflammome of severe obesity before and after bariatric surgery. PLoS One 2014; 9: e107859

[11] Jurjus A, Eid A, Al Kattar S et al. Inflammatory bowel disease, colorectal cancer and type 2 diabetes mellitus: The links. BBA Clin 2016; 5: 16–24

[12] Sjoholm A, Nystrom T. Endothelial inflammation in insulin resistance. Lancet 2005; 365: 610–612

[13] Lwaleed BA, Kazmi RS, Cooper AJ. Inflammation, endothelial dysfunction, and thromboembolism. Semin Thromb Hemost 2015; 41: 547–548

[14] Gokce N, Keaney JF, Hunter LM et al. Risk stratification for postoperative cardiovascular events via noninvasive assessment of endothelial function: a prospective study. Circulation 2002; 105: 1567–1572

[15] Riedel B, Schier R. Endothelial dysfunction in the perioperative setting. Semin Cardiothorac Vasc Anesth 2010; 14: 41–43

[16] Furchgott RF, Zawadzki JV. The obligatory role of endothelial cells in the relaxation of arterial smooth muscle by acetylcholine. Nature 1980; 288: 373–376

[17] van Hinsbergh VW. The endothelium: vascular control of haemostasis. Eur J Obstet Gynecol Reprod Biol 2001; 95: 198–201

[18] Levi M, ten Cate H, van der Poll T. Endothelium: interface between coagulation and inflammation. Crit Care Med 2002; 30: S220-224

[19] Lord JM, Midwinter MJ, Chen YF et al. The systemic immune response to trauma: an overview of pathophysiology and treatment. Lancet 2014; 384: 1455–1465

[20] Ingram DA, Mead LE, Moore DB et al. Vessel wall-derived endothelial cells rapidly proliferate because they contain a complete hierarchy of endothelial progenitor cells. Blood 2005; 105: 2783–2786

[21] Ingram DA, Mead LE, Tanaka H et al. Identification of a novel hierarchy of endothelial progenitor cells using human peripheral and umbilical cord blood. Blood 2004; 104: 2752–2760

[22] Yoder MC, Mead LE, Prater D et al. Redefining endothelial progenitor cells via clonal analysis and hematopoietic stem/progenitor cell principals. Blood 2007; 109: 1801–1809

[23] Asahara T, Murohara T, Sullivan A et al. Isolation of putative progenitor endothelial cells for angiogenesis. Science 1997; 275: 964–967

[24] Hill JM, Zalos G, Halcox JP et al. Circulating endothelial progenitor cells, vascular function, and cardiovascular risk. N Engl J Med 2003; 348: 593–600

[25] Ghani U, Shuaib A, Salam A et al. Endothelial progenitor cells during cerebrovascular disease. Stroke 2005; 36: 151–153

[26] Rafat N, Beck G, Pena-Tapia PG et al. Increased levels of circulating endothelial progenitor cells in patients with Moyamoya disease. Stroke 2009; 40: 432–438

[27] Rafat N, Hanusch C, Brinkkoetter PT et al. Increased circulating endothelial progenitor cells in septic patients: correlation with survival. Crit Care Med 2007; 35: 1677–1684

[28] Nowak K, Rafat N, Belle S et al. Circulating endothelial progenitor cells are increased in human lung cancer and correlate with stage of disease. Eur J Cardiothorac Surg 2010; 37: 758–763

[29] Rafat N, Beck G, Schulte J et al. Circulating endothelial progenitor cells in malignant gliomas. J Neurosurg 2010; 112: 43–49

[30] Voswinckel R, Ziegelhoeffer T, Heil M et al. Circulating vascular progenitor cells do not contribute to compensatory lung growth. Circ Res 2003; 93: 372–379

[31] Peichev M, Naiyer AJ, Pereira D et al. Expression of VEGFR-2 and AC133 by circulating human CD34(+) cells identifies a population of functional endothelial precursors. Blood 2000; 95: 952–958

[32] Estes ML, Mund JA, Ingram DA et al. Identification of endothelial cells and progenitor cell subsets in human peripheral blood. Curr Protoc Cytom 2010; Chapter 9: Unit 9.33, pages 1–11

[33] Medina RJ, O'Neill CL, Sweeney M et al. Molecular analysis of endothelial progenitor cell (EPC) subtypes reveals two distinct cell populations with different identities. BMC Med Genomics 2010; 3: 18

[34] Richardson MR, Yoder MC. Endothelial progenitor cells: quo vadis? J Mol Cell Cardiol 2011; 50: 266–272

[35] Timmermans F, Plum J, Yoder MC et al. Endothelial progenitor cells: identity defined? J Cell Mol Med 2009; 13: 87–102

[36] Melero-Martin JM, Khan ZA, Picard A et al. In vivo vasculogenic potential of human blood-derived endothelial progenitor cells. Blood 2007; 109: 4761–4768

[37] Critser PJ, Yoder MC. Endothelial colony-forming cell role in neoangiogenesis and tissue repair. Curr Opin Organ Transplant 2010; 15: 68–72

[38] Cao JP, He XY, Xu HT et al. Autologous transplantation of peripheral blood-derived circulating endothelial progenitor cells attenuates endotoxin-induced acute lung injury in rabbits by direct endothelial repair and indirect immunomodulation. Anesthesiology 2012; 116: 1278–1287

[39] Lam CF, Roan JN, Lee CH et al. Transplantation of endothelial progenitor cells improves pulmonary endothelial function and gas exchange in rabbits with endotoxin-induced acute lung injury. Anesth Analg 2011; 112: 620–627

[40] Yamada M, Kubo H, Ishizawa K et al. Increased circulating endothelial progenitor cells in patients with bacterial pneumonia: evidence that bone marrow derived cells contribute to lung repair. Thorax 2005; 60: 410–413

[41] Avogaro A, Albiero M, Menegazzo L et al. Endothelial dysfunction in diabetes: the role of reparatory mechanisms. Diabetes Care 2011; 34 Suppl 2: S285–290

[42] Fadini GP, Sartore S, Schiavon M et al. Diabetes impairs progenitor cell mobilisation after hindlimb ischaemia-reperfusion injury in rats. Diabetologia 2006; 49: 3075–3084

[43] Bauer A, Kofler S, Thiel M et al. Monitoring of the sublingual microcirculation in cardiac surgery using orthogonal polarization spectral imaging: preliminary results. Anesthesiology 2007; 107: 939–945

[44] De Backer D, Dubois MJ, Schmartz D et al. Microcirculatory alterations in cardiac surgery: effects of cardiopulmonary bypass and anesthesia. Ann Thorac Surg 2009; 88: 1396–1403

[45] Kara A, Akin S, Ince C. The response of the microcirculation to cardiac surgery. Curr Opin Anaesthesiol. 2016 Feb;29(1):85-93

[46] Taccone FS, Scolletta S, Franchi F et al. Brain perfusion in sepsis. Curr Vasc Pharmacol 2013; 11: 170–186

[47] Ely EW, Gautam S, Margolin R et al. The impact of delirium in the intensive care unit on hospital length of stay. Intensive Care Med 2001; 27: 1892–1900

[48] Ely EW, Inouye SK, Bernard GR et al. Delirium in mechanically ventilated patients: validity and reliability of the confusion assessment method for the intensive care unit (CAM-ICU). JAMA 2001; 286: 2703–2710

[49] Ely EW, Shintani A, Truman B et al. Delirium as a predictor of mortality in mechanically ventilated patients in the intensive care unit. JAMA 2004; 291: 1753–1762

[50] Girard TD, Jackson JC, Pandharipande PP et al. Delirium as a predictor of long-term cognitive impairment in survivors of critical illness. Crit Care Med 2010; 38: 1513–1520

[51] Milbrandt EB, Deppen S, Harrison PL et al. Costs associated with delirium in mechanically ventilated patients. Crit Care Med 2004; 32: 955–962

[52] Pisani MA, Kong SY, Kasl SV et al. Days of delirium are associated with 1-year mortality in an older intensive care unit population. Am J Respir Crit Care Med 2009; 180: 1092–1097

[53] Shehabi Y, Riker RR, Bokesch PM et al. Delirium duration and mortality in lightly sedated, mechanically ventilated intensive care patients. Crit Care Med 2010; 38: 2311–2318

[54] Girard TD, Pandharipande PP, Ely EW. Delirium in the intensive care unit. Crit Care 2008; 12 Suppl 3: S3

[55] Sharshar T, Carlier R, Bernard F et al. Brain lesions in septic shock: a magnetic resonance imaging study. Intensive Care Med 2007; 33: 798–806

[56] Aird WC. The role of the endothelium in severe sepsis and multiple organ dysfunction syndrome. Blood 2003; 101: 3765–3777

[57] Shapiro NI, Schuetz P, Yano K et al. The association of endothelial cell signaling, severity of illness, and organ dysfunction in sepsis. Crit Care 2010; 14: R182

[58] Ait-Oufella H, Maury E, Lehoux S et al. The endothelium: physiological functions and role in microcirculatory failure during severe sepsis. Intensive Care Med 2010; 36: 1286–1298

[59] Sakr Y, Dubois MJ, De Backer D et al. Persistent microcirculatory alterations are associated with organ failure and death in patients with septic shock. Crit Care Med 2004; 32: 1825–1831

[60] Abbott NJ, Ronnback L, Hansson E. Astrocyte-endothelial interactions at the blood–brain barrier. Nat Rev Neurosci 2006; 7: 41–53

[61] Gavins F, Yilmaz G, Granger DN. The evolving paradigm for blood cell-endothelial cell interactions in the cerebral microcirculation. Microcirculation 2007; 14: 667–681

[62] He F, Peng J, Deng XL et al. RhoA and NF-kappaB are involved in lipopolysaccharide-induced brain microvascular cell line hyperpermeability. Neuroscience 2011; 188: 35–47

[63] Taccone FS, Su F, Pierrakos C et al. Cerebral microcirculation is impaired during sepsis: an experimental study. Crit Care 2010; 14: R140

[64] Burnham EL, Taylor WR, Quyyumi AA et al. Increased circulating endothelial progenitor cells are associated with survival in acute lung injury. Am J Respir Crit Care Med 2005; 172: 854–860

[65] Becchi C, Pillozzi S, Fabbri LP et al. The increase of endothelial progenitor cells in the peripheral blood: a new parameter for detecting onset and severity of sepsis. Int J Immunopathol Pharmacol 2008; 21: 697–705

[66] Heidemann SM, Ofenstein JP, Sarnaik AP. Ibuprofen attenuates cardiopulmonary dysfunction by modifying vascular tone in endotoxemia. Prostaglandins Leukot Essent Fatty Acids 1999; 60: 181–185

[67] Ou HC, Lee WJ, Wu CM et al. Aspirin prevents resistin-induced endothelial dysfunction by modulating AMPK, ROS, and Akt/eNOS signaling. J Vasc Surg 2012; 55: 1104–1115

[68] Tsai KL, Huang PH, Kao CL et al. Aspirin attenuates vinorelbine-induced endothelial inflammation via modulating SIRT1/AMPK axis. Biochem Pharmacol 2014; 88: 189–200

[69] Schier R, El-Zein R, Cortes A et al. Endothelial progenitor cell mobilization by preoperative exercise: a bone marrow response associated with postoperative outcome. Br J Anaesth 2014; 113: 652–660

[70] Schier R, Hinkelbein J, Marcus H et al. A novel technique for the assessment of preoperative cardiovascular risk: reactive hyperemic response to short-term exercise. Biomed Res Int 2013; 2013: 837130

[71] Aicher A, Zeiher AM, Dimmeler S. Mobilizing endothelial progenitor cells. Hypertension 2005; 45: 321–325

[72] Asahara T, Takahashi T, Masuda H et al. VEGF contributes to postnatal neovascularization by mobilizing bone marrow-derived endothelial progenitor cells. EMBO J 1999; 18: 3964–3972

[73] Cesari F, Sofi F, Caporale R et al. Relationship between exercise capacity, endothelial progenitor cells and cytochemokines in patients undergoing cardiac rehabilitation. Thromb Haemost 2009; 101: 521–526

[74] Redondo S, Hristov M, Gordillo-Moscoso AA et al. High-reproducible flow cytometric endothelial progenitor cell determination in human peripheral blood as CD34+/CD144+/CD3-lymphocyte sub-population. J Immunol Methods 2008; 335: 21–27

[75] Sandri M, Adams V, Gielen S et al. Effects of exercise and ischemia on mobilization and functional activation of blood-derived progenitor cells in patients with ischemic syndromes: results of 3 randomized studies. Circulation 2005; 111: 3391–3399

[76] Laufs U, Urhausen A, Werner N et al. Running exercise of different duration and intensity: effect on endothelial progenitor cells in healthy subjects. Eur J Cardiovasc Prev Rehabil 2005; 12: 407–414

[77] Moyna NM, Thompson PD. The effect of physical activity on endothelial function in man. Acta Physiol Scand 2004; 180: 113–123

[78] Condon ET, Wang JH, Redmond HP. Surgical injury induces the mobilization of endothelial progenitor cells. Surgery 2004; 135: 657–661

[79] Jeong JO, Kim MO, Kim H et al. Dual angiogenic and neurotrophic effects of bone marrow-derived endothelial progenitor cells on diabetic neuropathy. Circulation 2009; 119: 699–708

[80] Rehman J, Li J, Parvathaneni L et al. Exercise acutely increases circulating endothelial progenitor cells and monocyte-/macrophage-derived angiogenic cells. J Am Coll Cardiol 2004; 43: 2314–2318

[81] Paneni F, Beckman JA, Creager MA et al. Diabetes and vascular disease: pathophysiology, clinical consequences, and medical therapy: part I. Eur Heart J 2013; 34: 2436–2443

[82] Sfanos KS, Hempel HA, De Marzo AM. The role of inflammation in prostate cancer. Adv Exp Med Biol 2014; 816: 153–181

[83] Singhal G, Jaehne EJ, Corrigan F et al. Inflammasomes in neuroinflammation and changes in brain function: a focused review. Front Neurosci 2014; 8: 315

[84] Pedersen BK, Febbraio MA. Muscle as an endocrine organ: focus on muscle-derived interleukin-6. Physiol Rev 2008; 88: 1379–1406

[85] Nakajima K, Takeoka M, Mori M et al. Exercise effects on methylation of ASC gene. Int J Sports Med 2010; 31: 671–675

[86] Weinhold M, Shimabukuro-Vornhagen A, Franke A et al. Physical exercise modulates the homeostasis of human regulatory T cells. J Allergy Clin Immunol 2015, DOI: 10.1016/j.jaci.2015.10.035

[87] Montero D. The association of cardiorespiratory fitness with endothelial or smooth muscle vasodilator function. Eur J Prev Cardiol 2015; 22: 1200–1211

[88] Nualnim N, Barnes JN, Tarumi T et al. Comparison of central artery elasticity in swimmers, runners, and the sedentary. Am J Cardiol 2011; 107: 783–787

[89] Vital TM, Stein AM, de Melo Coelho FG et al. Physical exercise and vascular endothelial growth factor (VEGF) in elderly: a systematic review. Arch Gerontol Geriatr 2014; 59: 234–239

[90] Wu XD, Zeng K, Liu WL et al. Effect of aerobic exercise on miRNA-TLR4 signaling in atherosclerosis. Int J Sports Med 2014; 35: 344–350

[91] Illi B, Nanni S, Scopece A et al. Shear stress-mediated chromatin remodeling provides molecular basis for flow-dependent regulation of gene expression. Circ Res 2003; 93: 155–161

[92] Marin T, Gongol B, Chen Z et al. Mechanosensitive microRNAs-role in endothelial responses to shear stress and redox state. Free Radic Biol Med 2013; 64: 61–68

[93] Fernandes T, Magalhaes FC, Roque FR et al. Exercise training prevents the microvascular rarefaction in hypertension balancing angiogenic and apoptotic factors: role of microRNAs-16, -21, and -126. Hypertension 2012; 59: 513–520